Contents

Laboratory Management

Principles and Processes

Second Edition

enise M. Harmening, PhD, MT(ASCP), CLS(NCA)

Professor
University of Maryland School of Medicine
Department of Medical & Research Technology
Baltimore, Maryland

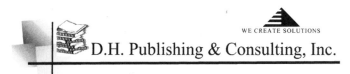

WE CREATE SOLUTIONS

D.H. Publishing & Consulting, Inc.

St. Petersburg, Florida 33711

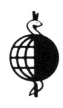

Distributed by F.A. Davis Company/Publishers

This book was previously published by: Pearson Education, Inc., formerly known as Prentice-Hall, Inc.

Library of Congress Cataloging-in-Publication Data

Laboratory management : principles and processes / [edited by] Denise M. Harmening.
    p. ; cm.
Includes bibliographical references and index.
    ISBN-13: 978-0-8036-1599-1
    ISBN-10: 0-8036-1599-X
  1. Medical laboratories—Management. I. Harmening, Denise.
    [DNLM: 1. Laboratories--organization & administration. QY 23 L223 2007]
    RB36.3.F55L332 2007
    610'.284—dc22

                      2006022186

Publisher: *D.H. Publishing & Consulting, Inc.*
Director of Production and Manufacturing: *Jesse A. Javens*
Production Editor: *Denise Harmening*
Cover Designer: *Jesse Javens*
Reviewer: *Virginia C. Hughes*
Editorial Assistant: *Janelle Kidd-Spence*
Composition: *Pine Tree Composition, Inc.*
Printing and Binding: *Book Masters*
Distribution Publisher: *F.A. Davis Company, 1915 Arch Street Philadelphia, PA., www.fadavis.com*

WE CREATE SOLUTIONS

D.H. Publishing & Consulting, Inc.

ISBN 10:0-8036-1599X
ISBN 13:978-0-8036-1599-1

Dedication

This book is dedicated to my family especially, my husband, who has always supported all of my works and who has encouraged me to fulfill my potential............
And
To all laboratory personnel- past, present, and future- who have touched and will continue to touch the lives of so many students and patients..........

I also dedicate this book to you in the hope of inspiring an unquenchable thirst for knowledge.

Preface

Currently, there is a great demand for laboratory managers, with a national vacancy rate of 15%. The rapidly changing laboratory environment is constantly responding to diverging trends in healthcare. This mandates the requirement for effective management. Laboratory managers will need to create new solutions to today's problems. This book is designed to give a problem-based approach to teaching the principles of laboratory management. The focus is to present underlying managerial concepts and then assist the learner in the successful application of theoretical models to real-life situations. Each chapter begins with an illustrative case to present a management problem followed by thought-provoking questions to stimulate the learners critical thinking skills. In addition, each chapter contains an outline and educational objectives that can be used in teaching. Internet and website references permit the learner to acquire advanced and current information in each of the major topic areas. Problem-based learning activities are listed at the end of each chapter to serve as a guide for instruction and reinforcement of the content presented. Eighteen chapters are divided into four major areas of management: Basic Principles and Organizational Structure, Human Resource, Finance, and Operations. Unique to this book is a chapter on Education and Training, a chapter on Ethical Issues in Laboratory Management, a chapter on Career Planning and a glossary of key terms. The Author and contributors of Laboratory Management: Principles and Processes 2nd Edition present detailed management and educational information along with real-life problem-based learning activities designed to engage learners by assuming managerial roles. Learners are encouraged to use these problem-based activities not only to review knowledge presented in this text but also to gain further knowledge related to the management and educational aspects of laboratory science. I would like to acknowledge and thank my husband, Jesse A. Javens, for his contribution, dedication and support of this book. I would also like to thank Virginia C. Hughes, MS, MT(ASCP)SBB for reviewing the chapters and sharing her expertise and time for this second edition.

Denise M. Harmening, PhD, MT(ASCP), CLS(NCA)

Contributors

Lani Barovick, MS
Assistant VP for Administrative
  Computing
eUMB and Human Resources
Baltimore, Maryland

Elaine M. Brett, MS, MT(ASCP)
Performance Development Consultant
EMB Associates
Bowie, Maryland

Sandra S. Brown, MBA, MT(ASCP)
Laboratory Manager
Maryland Heights, Missouri

Marie A. Cato, MBA, MT(ASCP)
Vice President of Operations, Wisconsin
Aurora Consolidated Laboratories, Inc.
West Allis, Wisconsin

Jeanne M. Donnelly, MBA, RHIA
Assistant Professor
Department of Health Information
  Management
Saint Louis University
St. Louis, Missouri

Sharon Ehrmeyer, PhD, MT(ASCP)
Director, Clinical Laboratory Science/
  Medical Technology Program
Professor, Department of Pathology and
  Laboratory Medicine
University of Wisconsin Medical School
Madison, Wisconsin

Vicki S. Freeman, PhD, MT(ASCP)SC
Chair and Professor
Department of Clinical Laboratory Science
School of Allied Health Services
University of Texas Medical Branch
Galveston, Texas

Paul Griffey, MBA, MT (ASCP)
Manager
LifeBridge Health
Department of Pathology
Baltimore, Maryland

Janet Hall, MS, CC(NRCC)
Associate Administrator, Laboratories
  of Pathology
Outreach Referral and Business
  Services
University of Maryland Medical Center
Baltimore, Maryland

Denise Harmening, PhD, MT (ASCP),
  CLS (NCA)
Professor, Department of Medical
  & Research Technology
University of Maryland School of
  Medicine
Baltimore, Maryland

Jan Heier DBA, CPA
Associate Professor of Accounting
Auburn University Montgomery
Montgomery, Alabama

Ellen Hope Kearns, MS, SH(ASCP)H
Professor and Graduate Coordinator
Division of Health Sciences, School
  of Health
California State University Dominguez
  Hills
Huntington Beach, California

Michael Kurtz, MS, MBA
Laboratory Administration/Marketing
  Manager
Clinical Laboratories
Saint Louis University Hospital
St. Louis, Missouri

Ronald H. Laessig, PhD
Professor, Preventive Medicine
Professor, Pathology and Laboratory
    Medicine
Director, Wisconsin State Laboratory of
    Hygiene
University of Wisconsin Medical School
Madison, Wisconsin

Randall S. Lambrecht, PhD, MT(ASCP),
    CLS(NCA)
Dean and Professor, College of Health
    Sciences
University of Wisconsin-Milwaukee
Milwaukee, Wisconsin

Brian N. Lenz, MT(ASCP)
Business Development Coordinator
Regional Pathology Services
University of Nebraska Medical Center
Omaha, Nebraska

Irina Lutinger, MPH, H(ASCP), DLM
Senior Administrator-Director of
    Laboratories
New York University Medical Center
New York, New York

Kelly McLeay, RN, MSN
MSICU/NSU Nurse Manager
Morton Plant Hospital
Clearwater, Florida

Thomas H. Peters, Jr., MT(ASCP)
Director, Vanderbilt Pathology Labora-
    tory Services
Vanderbilt Medical Center
Nashville, Tennessee

Dale C. Scutro, BS, MT(AMT)
Laboratory Manager
Morton Plant Hospital
Clearwater, Florida

Adil E. Shamoo, PhD
Professor, Department of Biochemistry
    and Molecular Biology
University of Maryland School of
    Medicine
Baltimore, Maryland

Fang Sun, PhD
Assistant Professor, Division of Health
    Services
College of Health and Human Services
California State University Dominguez
    Hills
Carson, California

Ann Tiehen, MT(ASCP)SBB
Project Coordinator
Department of Pathology & Laboratory
    Medicine
Evanston Hospital
Evanston, Illinois

Christine V. Walters, MAS, JD, SPHR
Independent Consultant
Glyndon, Maryland

In order for laboratory managers to be effective on the job, they must not only be technically competent in their specific area(s) of laboratory medicine but also familiar with the nontechnical side of management. This "other side" includes all of the topics addressed in this text. For ease of learning, these topics are combined into five sections as noted in the table of contents and the introduction of each section.

Section I introduces the learner to the global concept of organizational structure followed by specific discussions of leadership, management functions, and managerial problem solving and decision making. As one might imagine, some of the issues discussed in this section are appropriately brought out in more than one chapter where they best apply.

Section I Contents:

CHAPTER 1

Organizational Structure: A Look at Concepts and Models

ELAINE M. BRETT, MS, MT(ASCP)

Chapter Outline

Objectives

Following successful completion of this chapter, the learner will be able to:

1. Describe some of the historical influences on organizational structures.
2. Define mechanistic and organic models of organizations.
3. Use Open Systems thinking to evaluate organizational needs.
4. Propose new structures based on customer/patient needs and environmental forces.
5. Identify and describe the impact of five organizational trends.

Key Terms

Congruence Model

Functional Structure

Matrix Organizations

Mechanistic Structure

Network Structures

Open Systems

Organic Structure

Self-contained Unit Structure

Case Study: Organizational Structure

Use your own laboratory or one with which you are familiar in the following situation. You have been asked to participate in a strategic planning exercise representing the laboratory for a multisite health system. Your hospital has had a traditional approach to managing the organization. The health system desires to take a "fresh look" at all aspects of the organization.

Issues and Questions to Consider

1. *Describe the current structure of the health system, the hospital, and the laboratory.*
2. *Looking at the laboratory as an open system, list some things external to the laboratory that will influence its operation and structure.*
3. *What are some factors internal to the laboratory that you will need to consider in making any changes to the system?*
4. *Consider the structural models described in this chapter. Visualize your laboratory in each of these structures. Prepare a rough sketch of your laboratory using each of the models*
   a. *Functional*
   b. *Self-contained Units*
   c. *Matrix*
   d. *Network*

Which one works best for your system? Why?

INTRODUCTION

An organization is a collection of people working together under a defined structure for the purpose of achieving predetermined outcomes through the use of financial, human, and material resources. There are a number of approaches to the structure and management of organizations. Structure is defined as the hierarchical structure which defines how the work is divided. Selection of the management organizational structure will depend on factors such as size, content, complexity, and distribution in the laboratory.

As laboratories move into the new century, they must redefine and explore the possibilities of our organizations. We live in a world of communities and organizations. These are **systems** made up of individuals who share a common purpose and perform tasks in service of that purpose. Success of any organization is a function of the capabilities of the individuals rather than the way in which they are organized. Talented personnel will perform well in most organizational structures and much better in a good organization. The structures of these organizational systems are both a creation of our behavior and creators of our behavior. Organizations provide vision and focus, they consist of technical and social components, they provide boundaries and creative freedom, and they are open to the changing environment yet contain their own culture within.

Organizations serve the following functions:

- Provide society with products and services.
- Offer employment and economic exchange for members.
- Give a framework for a social system (i.e., organizations are social habitats for people).

Albert Einstein said: "We cannot solve the problems we have created with the same thinking that created them." Organizations, like individuals, must learn from past successes and failures and look for creative ways to find solutions for the future. Organizations perform best where information flows rapidly. Information must flow both internally and externally to permit accurate decisions to be made. The clinical laboratory is no different from any other system in this regard.

The clinical laboratory is typically an organization within an organization. It functions as part of the larger health system and provides specific services that are vital to the overall mission of providing patient care. The laboratory may also function across health systems, providing specialized services and "centers of excellence." Understanding basic concepts of organizational structure and function can give insight into how we act and react in our own systems. Optimizing the technical and social aspects of the organization can enhance and maximize performance and outcomes. In almost any laboratory you will find an organization chart that can help you understand the levels of authority and lines of communication. By convention, the organizational chart with boxes and lines describes a structural plan. This chapter provides information about the background of **organizational structures.** It describes a broader concept of the organization as a complex system and its design as an "architecture" that includes work and social components in addition to formal structure. It examines organizations through several different lenses: historical, system models, and design/structure. In addition, it describes 21st century organizational trends.

Fundamentally, a look at organizations should help answer the question "How do we divide up the work?" To adequately function in the complex healthcare **environment,** it is important for the clinical laboratory scientist to understand the structure and politics of their organization. Such an appreciation can foster better communication, better understanding of system decisions, and help in career advancement opportunities.

HISTORICAL PERSPECTIVE

The structures of organizations in the West are really "recent" inventions. The most familiar structures developed as the 19th century shifted from a basically agrarian society to an industrial society. The effect, as we shall see, was to provide a dedicated workforce that required a top-down flow of information and instructions. The concepts were based on a bureaucratic approach derived from military organizations. The **cultural** changes that unfolded as a result of our moving into the Information Age in the last quarter of the 20th century require that our organizations take on new and different forms. Unfortunately, many of the modern day organizations—including those in healthcare—are still using a 19th century model!

In the early part of the 1900s, the stage was set for modern organizations. As the Industrial Age took hold, the need for managing large numbers of people in complex activities required an efficient way to organize people. Max Weber, a German sociologist, introduced the concept of **bureaucracy** or *rational-legal* system. The structure and processes required a strong hierarchy of authority, extensive division of labor for optimum functional performance, impersonal rules and rigid procedures that account for nearly every contingency, and decision making based on rules and tactics developed to guarantee consistent and effective pursuit of organizational goals. The model presents the image and characteristics of a "well-oiled" machine working particularly well in businesses involving routine tasks that can be specified in writing and that do not change quickly or frequently.

Near the turn of the 20th century, Frederick Taylor introduced the discipline of scientific management as a means to organize work. In the introduction to his book, *The Principles of Scientific Management*, he states, "In the past the man has been first; in the future the system must be first." Taylor dealt with the problem of how to get more productivity out of workers and used time and motion studies to break jobs into smaller repetitive tasks and find the best way to do a job. He introduced several principles including the following:

- Specialization—the creation of specialist jobs and "thinking departments"
- "Piecework" pay-systems designed to increase motivation and reduce "slacking-off" by workers

Taylor advocated a strong division of labor between management (thinking) and worker (doing). It was the manager's job to understand the task and plan a method of executing it, and then coerce the worker to do it, by motivating the worker with pay.

The essence of Weber and Taylor and other classic theorists was to organize working groups in a rational manner, a noble effort for their times. These were days of assembly lines and unskilled immigrant labor. These approaches had many desirable features in terms of motivation, efficiency, and, use of expertise. However, the pure application of the theories was challenged in the studies of the effects of social factors on morale and productivity in the decades that followed. The beginnings of a "human relations movement" came out of studies from the Hawthorne plant of the Western Electric Company in the late 1920s and early 1930s. In short, these studies, which influenced the organization of the workforce through the 1960s, suggested that informal social structures had much to do with the way an organization runs. Feelings and attitudes about the work, the environment, and the supervisor all contributed to performance. "Just doing their job" left workers feeling alienated and dispirited. Formal organization provides the direction and the stability of the infrastructure. The informal organization has well-developed social structures, histories, and culture. Informal groups have a powerful influence on productivity, sometimes more so than economic incentives. Human relations approach advocated paying greater attention to workers' needs, training in interpersonal skills for supervisors, and generally "humanizing" the workplace.

The inclusion of the human element in organizations continued. In the 1950s and 1960s the development and application of behavioral and social sciences in combination with advancements in industrial and information technology created new questions about the work environment. Global competition and demands for greater efficiency and productivity prompted efforts to redesign existing processes.

One influencing approach was sociotechnical systems theory, which was based on the premise that an organization is a combination of social and technical parts and is open to its environment. Both parts must work together to accomplish tasks and produce both physical products or services and social/psychological outcomes. The social and technical parts are jointly optimized in contrast with traditional methods that first design the technical component and then "fit" the people to it. Implementation of sociotechnical systems is highly participative, involving all relevant stakeholders and promoting employee involvement at all levels in the work design. Process changes evolved with formation of self-managing work groups, training of group members in multiple skills, and delegation of the work. Sharing of information, knowledge, and learning is characteristic of this approach. In the context of clinical laboratory, this means organizing a department by considering the instrumentation and technology *and* by focusing on people issues, communication, and social interactions.

In 1961, after observing trends in many organizations, Burns and Stalker described a range of organization structures that they referred to as mechanistic to organic systems. A ***mechanistic structure*** may be appropriate in an environment of slow change and relative stability. The organization is highly structured with direction and communication from the top-down and relies on authority-obedience relationships. In the extreme, there is centralized decision making, strict division of labor, and insistence on loyalty and conformity to policy and procedures. At the opposite end is the ***organic structure,*** which is preferred in an environment of high change. This system features decentralized decision making and a fluid design, which facilitates flexibility and adaptation and encourages a wide sharing of responsibility.

In the 1980s and 1990s, different types of process improvements influenced organizational structures in business and healthcare. French and Bell summarized the variety of interventions that have affected structural changes in organizations over the past several decades. Table 1–1 provides basic definitions of some of these approaches as well as some of the consequences to the organization. Many of these approaches foster a team concept to the work and a regard for both the technical and social aspects of the organization. The changes represent a more results-focused application of processes and a collaborative sharing of information.

TABLE 1-1.   A Summary of Structural Interventions and Their Consequences on the Organization

Intervention	Objective	Consequence
Self-managed Teams	Provide teams with a grouping of tasks that make up a major unit of the total work to be performed.	Flattening the organization, improved productivity; reconceptualizing roles of managers as coordinators and coaches.
Work Redesign Theory	Motivation and performance can be enhanced by redesigning jobs.	Redistribution of tasks; greater individual accountability.
MBO—Management by Objectives	Assumes the need for systematic (quantifiable) goal setting linking the goals of superiors to subordinates.	May range from autocratic, unilateral mechanisms to enforce compliance to collaborative process with increased focus on organizational objectives.
Quality Circles	A form of group problem solving with primary focus on enhancing product quality.	Formation of cross-functional and multifunctional teams; greater employee participation; more creative integration.
Quality of Work Life	Restructuring of several dimensions of the organization to solve a problem and introduce sustained change.	Increase in employee participation in decision-making work teams.
Total Quality Management	A combination of approaches including quality circles, statistical quality control, self-managed teams. Focus is on customer needs and continuous improvement process.	Increase in employee participation and teamwork. Higher productivity. Supports participative management.
Reengineering	Focuses on redesigning business processes.	Top-down program. Combining, eliminating, restructuring activities to affect efficiency and productivity.

It appears that the structure of organizations is evolving. The traditional top-down mechanistic model that exists in many organizations will give way to an organic or network model where employees on the front line drive critical decisions to serve customer/client needs. The organization of the future will take on open system characteristics discussed in the next section.

AN OPEN SYSTEMS PERSPECTIVE

Models help to categorize the large amount of information about a system. We see organizations as *open systems* and can use this thinking to evaluate the needs of the organization. Using a simple abstract model, such as a biologic organism, organizational systems can be thought of as interdependent, interconnected elements that constitute an identifiable whole. Biologic systems are generally thought of as open systems that function as **input-throughput-output mechanisms.** As shown in Figure 1–1, systems exhibit activities that take input from the environment, do "something" to the input through transformation or conversion, and export a changed product back into the environment. In a single cell organism, the system is totally dependent on the flow of energy and matter. Beginning with intake of food, water, and air to the elimination of energy, waste, and, by-products, the components of the system are organized to handle the flow of energy and they possess the capacity to change and adapt. In *Leadership and the New Science*, Dr. Margaret Wheatley expands on the metaphor: " Our concept of organizations is moving away from the mechanistic creations that flourished in the age of bureaucracy. We now speak in earnest of more fluid, organic structures, of boundaryless and seamless organizations. We are beginning to recognize organizations as whole systems, construing them as 'learning organizations' or 'organic' and noticing that people exhibit self organizing capacity."

If we look at our organizations as open systems, we can start to see the interactions and influences of one part of the system with others. It can help us understand why some organizations perform well and why others may experience conflict. The clinical laboratory is an excellent example of the open system model. The laboratory receives input including specimens, test requests, and supplies from many sources. The laboratory staff, instruments, and processes "transform" the inputs to provide test results and information for patients and clinicians.

Open systems share the following characteristics:

1. There is an implied purpose or goal that is the reason for the system's existence. The primary mission or task of a system determines its distinct nature. The clinical laboratory, for example, may be dedicated to the output or production of

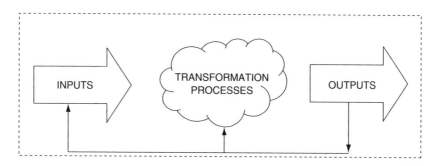

FIGURE 1–1   Simple open system configuration.

timely and meaningful delivery of test results. This purpose will be a "guiding light" that helps all members accept direction and focus.

2. The external environment drives significant change. The requirements of the environment will direct and define the purpose. The environment consists of external elements and forces that affect an organization's ability to establish and reach its objectives. If the environment no longer requires the output of the system, the system will no longer have purpose and may cease to exist. Consider the medical need for laboratory testing and the influence of new technologies. There is a constant change in the demand for the kind of testing and the delivery of testing. An example is the influence of point-of-care testing. The external environment (patients, clinicians) demand testing closer to the patient where immediate results could be obtained and decisions regarding treatment made. The available technology made this testing possible, streamlining the diagnostic process. These external influences have driven significant change on the laboratory organization and delivery of test results.

3. Systems have clearly defined boundaries. Physical structure, technology, or the type of work give the system uniqueness and label its purpose and function. The individual parts or members within the system interact and work together toward a common purpose. An open system, however, is permeable to its environment and exchanges information and resources with the environment. The members of the Clinical Laboratory are recognized by the boundaries of the department or system and will act synergistically within the boundaries to provide quality test results. The laboratory boundary, however, must be open to the needs, processes, and contributions of the health system and the community that is served.

4. Like biological systems, organizations seek to maintain a state of stability or equilibrium. Part of the plan of a successful organization is to maintain harmony with the potentially disruptive forces of the environment. The more complex and turbulent those forces are, the bigger the challenges and demands on the system. The paradox is that to achieve stability and equilibrium, a system must constantly change. It is a challenge and a frustration to leaders and managers who must find the most agreeable ways to maintain order in the workplace and at the same time make continuous adjustments to meet the demands of the external environment. In modern organizations leaders must acknowledge that there may be multiple paths and multiple adjustments to reach a particular outcome or goal. This becomes quite evident by observing many different laboratory organizations. All laboratories have similar purpose—generating quality results. Yet each laboratory is unique in the way it accomplishes the tasks to meet the needs of its particular community.

5. As a system grows and becomes more complex, it forms differentiated, specialized components or subsystems including work teams, sections or departments. The subsystems seek to be unique and different and eventually evolve into a hierarchy. In the hospital laboratory specialization takes place on several levels. Even though the laboratory has its unique purpose in receiving specimens and delivering data, it functions as a subsystem in the larger hospital organization. The laboratory, in turn, is differentiated into sections, such as blood bank, virology, or molecular diagnostics, that function as self-contained sub-subsystems and meet special needs and technical requirements.

6. Feedback is important to the alignment and performance of the system. Positive feedback will inform whether the purpose and goals are aligned with the environmental needs and whether the targets are appropriate. Adjustments in the system can be made to serve the purpose. Negative feedback challenges whether the system is on course with the purpose and goals and prompts corrective action. For the laboratory, interdepartmental meetings and communications are important feedback mechanisms that can help monitor performance, provide information, and prompt necessary changes.

Despite their behavior as open systems, many laboratory organizations remain in a relatively closed system framework. Table 1–2 compares certain organizational elements and behaviors in Open and Closed Systems. Closed system, being less considerate of external forces, is internally focused. The closed system uses mechanistic structures as previously described. Top-down authority and reliance on policy and procedures are typical. As previously stated, in a relatively stable, slow changing environment, the closed, mechanistic approach may be appropriate. It is a challenge for the laboratory manager to recognize inconsistencies and to be able to implement changes that improve the organization.

One way of approaching the changes is to look more closely at what must happen within an open system to support a state of equilibrium. The *congruence model* described by David Nadler shows a little more detail of the elements of an

TABLE 1–2. A Comparison of Open and Closed Organizational Systems

	Relatively Closed System	Relatively Open System
Leadership Style	Independent Superior-Subordinate basis	Collaborative Collegial basis
Decision Making	Hierarchically determined	At the level where the problem and the information reside
Authority and Responsibility	Located together Single accountability	May be separate with multiple accountability
Conflict	Eliminate or suppress	Manage
Performance Appraisal	Hierarchical or external	Self-review
Distribution of Work	Allocate jobs to people	Negotiate work among groups
Thinking Mode	Euclidean Sequential and logical	Multiple frames of reference
Power Base	Hierarchy or status	Control over uncertainty
Managing Arena	Within the system	At the system boundary

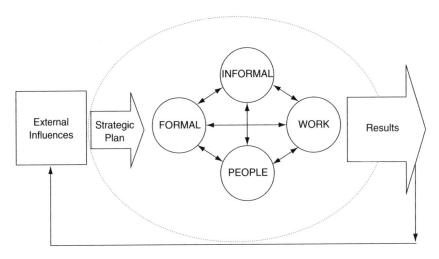

FIGURE 1–2. A congruence model showing the organization as an open system. *Source:* Adapted from David A. Nadler, *Champions of Change*, p. 41.

TABLE 1–3. Application of Elements of the Clinical Laboratory to the Congruence Model

Inputs	Operating Organization	Outputs
Environmental Influences • Patient needs • Healthcare regulations • Health system requirements • Sample delivery • Competitors • Unions	*Formal Organization* • Structure • Policies • Procedures • Regulatory compliance	*System Information* • Test results • Diagnostic information • Consultation
Resources • Financial • Information • People • Supplies • Technology	*People* • Individual skills and knowledge • Needs and preferences • Expectations	*Department Contribution* • Financial performance • Patient response
Organization's History • Vision and mission • Values and norms • Location	*Work* • Test performance • Process flow • Automation/Instrumentation • Point of care	*Individual* • Academic contribution • Teaching/learning • Personal growth and recognition
	Informal Organization • Informal working arrangements • Behavior of leaders • Patterns of relationships • Culture and climate • Communication patterns	

organization as an open system and some of the dynamics involved. The model can be used to analyze environmental relationships of an organization and assess the internal interdependence and alignment of its parts. In the model, the elements of the transformation process or, more appropriately, the operating organization are the major components that transform the inputs to the outputs through the implementation of a strategy. In Figure 1–2 the following components are represented and their interrelationships are shown as arrows:

- Work—the tasks performed to provide the products or services
- People—including skills, knowledge, and workforce expectations
- Formal Organization—formal structures, policies, and procedures for performing the work
- Informal Organization—culture and informal rules and understanding about how the system works

Table 1–3 provides examples of how some elements of the clinical laboratory might be represented in the congruence model.

Constituents of the system must be considered and must be congruent with each other to obtain maximum efficiency in transforming strategies to performance. The lack of fit between any of the components of the operating organization—between formal and informal structures, people and work requirements—will compromise the system and can produce huge problems including operational inefficiencies, tension among personnel, morale problems, miscommunication, and overall dysfunction. Table 1–4 poses questions that may test how well your organization demonstrates "goodness of fit" between the four components of the operating organization. This assessment may help us understand how well the laboratory system is functioning and identify inconsistencies.

ORGANIZATION DESIGN: A STRUCTURAL PERSPECTIVE

Focus on regulatory policies and quality initiatives along with advances in technology have resulted in most laboratories being technically good and demonstrating acceptable clinical competency. Changes in organizational design can further affect efficiencies, productivity, cost-containment, and personnel needs. Whereas system models help categorize the many aspects of the system, structural models show function and linkage of how groups in the organization relate to each other.

Five factors influence the design and structure of the organization:

- Organizational goals and strategic direction.
- Technologic capabilities, including information technology.
- Size (the laboratory subsystem and the larger health system).
- Environment (especially client/patient needs).
- Leadership style, member behaviors, and organization culture.

Four structural models illustrate the range from mechanistic to organic networks. These models include functional, self-contained units, matrix, and net-

TABLE 1–4. Assessment of "Goodness of Fit" Among the Four Components of the Operating Organization Based on the Congruence Model

Fit	Issue	Questions
People—Formal Organization	Individual needs are met by the organization. Individuals are clear on organizational expectations and individual system goals are aligned.	Are goals communicated clearly? Are individuals aligned with the mission of the laboratory? the health system? Are people working for or against the system? Are reward systems adequate?
People—Work	Individual needs are met by the work. Individuals are prepared with skills and knowledge for the work.	Is the work fulfilling? Is there enough creative freedom to do the job? Are people adequately trained? Are the right people in the job?
People—Informal Organization	Individual needs are met by the informal organization. The informal organization makes use of individual resources.	Do leadership behaviors promote the values and mission? Is the culture and climate conducive to achieving desired performance? Can individuals express themselves in a safe environment?
Work—Formal Organization	Organizational arrangements support the task. The organization motivates behavior that is consistent with expected performance.	Does the organization structure support the departmental task? Is the work being done consistent with the mission and values of the organization? Are work expectations being met? Are the right resources in place to successfully meet the goals? Are job descriptions appropriate?
Work—Informal Organization	The informal organization helps or hinders the performance of the work.	Does the culture support the execution of the tasks?
Formal—Informal Organization	The elements of the informal organization are consistent with the formal organization.	Are interdepartmental and intradepartmental communications supported? Are the goals and rewards of the informal organization consistent with the formal organization? Is alignment evident?

work structures. Although these models are not exclusive, they illustrate some basic advantages and disadvantages of recognizable approaches. Understanding the design helps us understand how the work is divided and how work efforts are coordinated. In reality a clinical laboratory may be a hybrid of several of the structural models.

The *functional structure* is hierarchical and, in the extreme, rigidly bureaucratic. In this structure specialized units report in an upward chain of command, and there is clear understanding of responsibility and authority. As with the closed system model, these organizations can function best in a stable, controlled environment where the organization is small to medium in size and departments are engaged in repetitive, efficient, routine tasks. The disadvantages of the functional structure are that communication among groups can be compromised with departments acting as silos and focused on only their areas of responsibility. There is a possibility that coordination between departments may become competitive and unresponsive. Functional laboratory organizations may have both a medical/technical and an administrative reporting scheme structure at the top of the organization. Specialized units such as Chemistry, Hematology, Microbiology, and others may be represented as sections or departments with a hierachy of supervision and management as shown in Figure 1–3a.

In the restructuring of clinical laboratories, efforts at consolidation and creating more cost-effective structures have resulted in a flattening of the hierarchical structure and elimination of some supervisory and management layers. Although there may be fewer steps in the decision-making process, the top-down control remains (Figure 1–3b).

The *self-contained unit structure* is organized around a common basis. This may be a discipline, a location, a customer group, or a technology. Each unit contains all relevant skills and processes to successfully operate. The grouping of disciplines in the laboratory (e.g., Chemistry, Hematology, Microbiology) in large health system environments with their own functional expertise and supervisory structure are examples of self-contained units. Also, satellite laboratories or service specialty areas responsible for their own outcomes may be self-contained "pods" providing their own special skills and services. Figure 1–4 represents one approach to a self-contained unit or team approach where members of each unit are grouped by function around centralized support and management services. Team approaches work well if resources are coordinated toward a common goal. Good communication plans and sharing of information maximize efficiency. A disadvantage to this structure is that there can be duplication of resources and expertise.

Matrix organizations take advantage of skills and function. Matrix designs allow departments or areas to simultaneously concentrate on specialized functions and on production. In the clinical laboratory, restructuring from a functional system with specialty disciplines such as Chemistry, Hematology, or Microbiology toward a production focus as a core or rapid response laboratory may result in the matrixing of technical and production operations responsibilities as shown in Figure 1–5. Vertical lines represent responsibility for functional and operational

A.

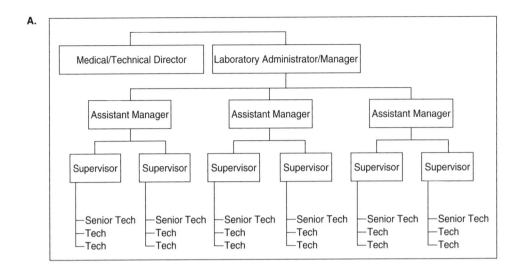

B.

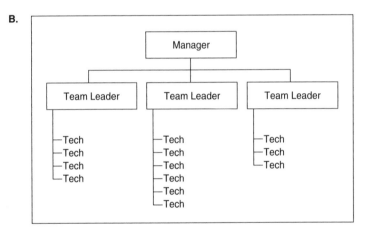

FIGURE 1–3 Functional laboratory organizational chart. a. Traditional multilayer design. b. "Flattened" design.

issues; horizontal lines provide subject or discipline expertise; circles designate teams that are formed for optimal skills and performance. A matrix design works best when the demands of the environment are changing and uncertain and where there is a high interdependency on technical expertise and specialization. This type of structure promotes skill diversification (cross-training) and efficiency in sharing human resources. The disadvantage of matrix structures is that roles and reporting structures can be confusing and ambiguous. An individual may report to more than one boss and may be asked to assume different roles depending on

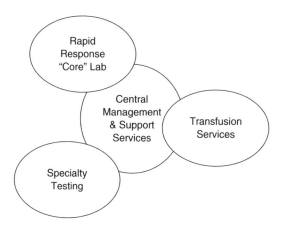

FIGURE 1–4 Example of a self-contained unit structure. Circles represent overlapping teams, each with specialized functions and tasks.

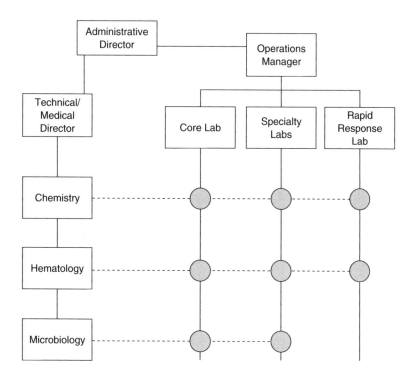

FIGURE 1–5 Matrix structure. (Solid lines indicate formal direct reporting; dashed lines indicate informal reporting. Circles represent functional departments or teams.)

the team they are on. Employees may feel "pulled in many directions" until they completely understand the structure and access to resources.

Network structures are evolving as information technology allows instantaneous access and distribution of data and information. For many years organization structures emulated machine structures. References to "well-oiled" parts and "lean-machines" implied control of knowledge and resources. Networked organizations reflect information technology models with customer focus and information sharing. Network structures consist of specialized units, either internal or external to the organization, that are linked together by informal or formal agreements. Networks may take on a variety of forms because they run from the customer/patient back, not from the top down. They combine innovation and responsiveness of small entrepreneurial structures with the economies of scale of large organizations.

One concept is the human network organization patterned after a **browser-server model** as portrayed by H. Dent in Figure 1–6. On the front line, employees serve client needs and make critical decisions. Employees on the back lines, who specialize in a particular skill or knowledge base, support the front line. Unlike traditional organizations, network organizations have a center, not a top. The role of management is to coordinate, facilitate, and serve. In a laboratory setting, the front line may represent those activities that are closest to the patient such as point-of-care testing and client services. The next layer, front-line support, represents less urgent batched testing. Back-line support includes specialized technical areas that offer more complex and esoteric tests. The back line also serves as a resource for front line in technical or clinical matters. A central management provides necessary resources and serves as support of functions such as information systems, faclities, and personnel.

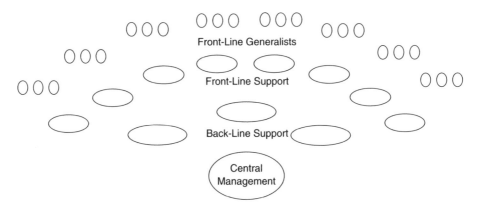

FIGURE 1–6 **Human network organization. Adapted from H. Dent,** *The Roaring 2000s,* **p. 150.**

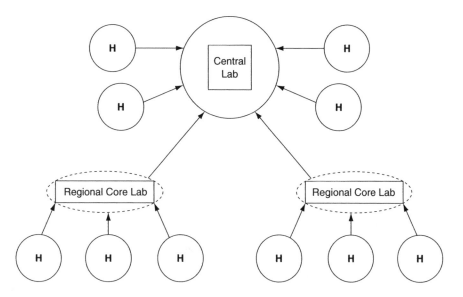

FIGURE 1–7   **A health system network. Adapted from S. Lu, et al., p. 509.** *Laboratory Medicine,* **September/October, 1996.**

Another network model used in the clinical laboratory incorporates the need to consolidate services, reduce duplications, and expand revenue-generating services while delivering high-quality cost-effective results. Depending on the scope of the health system, the network may incorporate, point-of-care, internal (inpatient) operations, and external (outreach) functions. The network may also have alliances and partnerships with other systems or centers of excellence. Figure 1–7 shows a model of three levels of service from point-of-care to core laboratory in a large geographic region. In this network model hospitals or outreach laboratories (labeled H) handle immediate testing that requires quick turnaround. Batched tests typically with next-day turnaround are done in regional core laboratories. A central laboratory provides low-volume and esoteric testing and serves as a medical and technical resource. This networked system depends on strong collaborative leadership, an efficient information system, appropriate clinical instrumentation, and flexible staffing.

Network structures have emerged to respond to the dynamically changing environment that is growing more and more complex and interdependent. Our access to information is overwhelming and individual customers/patients demand personalized and immediate attention. The network structure is highly flexible and streamlines responses. However, the model requires radical change in how we view working relationships and leadership/management roles. Without that change, it is difficult to manage the equilateral interactions across organizations and to maintain commitment of members to the network.

21st Century Organizational Trends

In general, some trends in organizations will be prompted by the requirements for efficiency, speed, cost-effectiveness, and customer/patient focus.

1. Technology advancements continue to evolve providing faster, more comprehensive platforms that will become more and more accessible. Information handling, telecommunications, and emerging point-of-care and noninvasive medical devices will have significant effects on the structure of laboratory systems. The balance of economies of scale through consolidated platforms along with the demand for patient-focused (customer) testing will create a healthy tension that will challenge the traditional clinical laboratory system and will necessitate new models for service delivery.

2. Diversity in both the workforce and the consumer population emerges as a key issue to organizational structure, culture, and management. Changing demographics resulting a workforce that is more heterogeneous sexually, ethnically, culturally, generationally, and individually are a source of both innovation and conflict. How an organization copes with different styles of interaction, communication, and appearance will challenge its structure.

3. Flexibility and organizational agility are necessary to respond to demands of patients and healthcare providers. Rigid structures that are bound by rules and regulations will give way to those that can quickly respond with innovative solutions. Structures that are flexible allow greater autonomy and encourage decision making at the point-of-care. Systems will emphasize lifetime employability by creating learning environments rather than lifetime employment through career tracks.

4. Flattening of organizations will result in fewer management levels and empowerment of employees to make decisions. The access to information through more robust technology means less need for the communication and control functions managers have traditionally held. In some ways the role of management is challenged with the "automation of management" by accessibility of information systems capable of storing and "sharing" organizational goals, plans, policies, and procedures. Aspects of the management role that can be programmed free up managers to be facilitators and coaches instead of "corporate cops." In addition, the expectation of employees to be self-directed and accountable reduces requirements for managers as caretakers. Adequate learning environments that promote leadership development and individual empowerment will need to be created.

5. Trends toward strategic alliances, partnerships, mergers, and industry information sharing contribute to a networked approach to organizational structures. Internal signs that organizations are trending toward networks include an increase in direct communications across unit and department boundaries, formation of cross-functional teams, and decentralization of services to meet customer/patient demands. The increased use of the Internet and health system *intra*nets will complement the trend toward point-of-care and self-testing and broaden the network even more. Patients will take on the perspective of consumers of laboratory and other medical information and will expect faster, more efficient delivery of services.

SUMMARY

Laboratory professionals should be challenged to look for new and creative designs to the meet the needs of the environment, particularly customers and patients. There is no single structure and no "right way" to divide up the work. Each organization must evaluate their unique situation and anticipate the future trends. The leadership of the system must find and recognize the future and not be blinded by the day-to-day business at hand or paralyzed by past practices. We must ask the questions that help us understand the interdependencies of the components of the organization. We must look at the forces in our environment that will drive change and create new opportunities. We must look to align processes and the people in our organizations to carry out strategic plans that will guide us to the organization's goals and vision.

SUGGESTED PROBLEM-BASED LEARNING ACTIVITIES

Chapter 1: Organizational Structure: A Look at Concepts and Models

Instructions: Use Internet resources, books, articles, colleagues, etc., to present solutions to the problems listed below. There is no one correct solution to any problem.

Note to Instructor: Students in class may be divided into groups and given the problem-based learning activity to discuss and solve. Once the group has reached consensus as to a solution, the group will present it to the other students in the class. This activity will provide all students with information regarding solutions to the problem.

Problem #1
Design a traditional organizational chart for an institution and then restructure the chart for a client-focused design. Discuss formal and informal structures related to this organizational chart.

Problem #2
A new administration has taken charge in your institution and you (the laboratory manager) have been directed to form self-directed work groups to focus on each component of the mission of your department.

Problem #3
Your hospital administration has asked you to develop an organizational structure to facilitate productivity and cost-effectiveness.

BIBLIOGRAPHY

Bradford, DL and Burk, WW: *Reinventing Organizational Development*, Pfeiffer, San Francisco, CA., 2005.

Dent Harry S Jr: *The Roaring 2000s*, Touchstone—Simon and Schuster, Inc., New York, NY., 1998.

Farwell DC: Hospital laboratory consolidation. *Clin Lab Manage Rev*, 9(5):411–20, 1995.

French WL, Bell CH Jr: *Organization Development*, Prentice Hall, Inc., Upper Saddle River, NJ., 1999.

Friedman BA: Integrating laboratory processes into clinical processes, web-based laboratory reporting, and the emergence of the virtual clinical laboratory. *Clin Lab Manage Rev*, 26 (5):333–38, 1998.

Holman, D et al: *The Essentials of the New Workplace: A Guide to the Human Impact of Modern Working Practices,* John Wiley & Sons, Indianapolis, IN., 2004.

Howells, J: *The Management of Innovation,* Sage Publications USA, Thousand Oaks, CA., 2005.

Lu, Susie et al: Outreach, consolidation, and networking: Columbia's approach to successful integration of laboratory services in California. *Clin Lab Manage Rev*, 10(5):507–17, 1996.

Nadler, DA, Nadler, MB: *Champions of Change,* Jossey-Bass, Inc., San Francisco, CA., 1998.

Rothwell, WJ, et al: *Practicing Organization Development: A Guide for Consultants*, Jossey-Bass/Pfeiffeer, San Fransisco, CA., 1995.

Taylor, FW: *The Principles of Scientific Management*, Kessinger Publishing, Whitefish, MT., 2004.

Wheatley, MJ: *Leadership and the New Science.* Barrett-Koehler Publishers, San Francisco, CA., 1999.

Internet Resources

Business Open Learning Archive
www.sol.brunel.ac.uk/Jarvis/bola.

Department of Organizational Studies, Boston College
www.analytictech.com.

Web site for the Tavistock Institute
www.tavinstitute.org.

Web site for Systems Thinking Press a resource for publications on systems thinking and strategic management
www.systemsthinkingpress.com.

AQP, The Association for Quality and Participation, is an international not-for-profit membership association dedicated to improving workplaces through quality and participation practices
www.aqp.org.

2

Principles of Leadership: Past, Present, and Future

ELLEN HOPE KEARNS, MS, SH(ASCP)H
FANG SUN, PhD

Chapter Outline

Objectives

Following successful completion of this chapter, the learner will be able to:

1. Discuss three work-related situations and describe appropriate effective versus ineffective leadership styles and behaviors.
2. Briefly explain leadership theories X, Y, and Z.
3. Compare and contrast leadership versus management.
4. Briefly describe three key functions of a formal leader.
5. Assess one's own leadership qualities according to attributes presented.
6. Describe four competencies for effective leadership.
7. Explain the Blake-Mouton Managerial Grid.
8. Assess one's own leadership style according to leadership styles presented.

Key Terms

Behavioral Approach
Influence Approach
Keirsey Four Types Sorter
Leadership
Myers-Briggs Type Indicator

Reciprocal Approach
Situational Contingency Approach
Theory X-Theory Y
Theory Z
Trait Approach

Case Study: Leadership Styles

Congratulations! You have just been promoted to Laboratory Manager in a medium-sized community hospital after six years of working in the Chemistry Section. You are well respected by your peers and knowledgeable of laboratory practices. However, some of the staff have questioned why you got the job since you have had very little formal management or supervisory training.

The administrator asks you to lead a task force to increase outreach business for the hospital. She tells you that you must increase market share in the next six months.

Issues and Questions to Consider

1. *What management characteristics will you need to exhibit?*
2. *What leadership attributes will be needed to achieve success?*
3. *Name at least three things you will do first to get this project going.*
4. *Describe how you can use the leadership styles in Table 2-5 to maximize your effectiveness.*
5. *What are your strengths?*
6. *What traits or styles will you need to improve?*
7. *What do you anticipate are some leadership challenges that you will need to overcome?*

INTRODUCTION

The chronology and history of leadership research have revealed a variety of central themes including relationships between leadership styles and behaviors, leadership skills, leader and follower characteristics, personality traits of leaders, situational leadership, organizational leadership theories, leaders versus managers, visionary leadership, transformational leadership, and the role of leaders and leadership. The Southwest Educational Development Laboratory Report highlights some of the major works of leadership research published in the 1900s.

In this chapter, examples are cited of popular leadership theories, paradigms, and principles written by contemporary scholars who have inspired us and influenced our understanding of leadership. This chapter begins with an historical perspective on researchers' approach to leadership and includes definitions of leadership and a section on leadership development. Whether you are reading this chapter because you are taking a required course, have recently accepted a new leadership role in the laboratory, or are already a leader, it is our hope that you will understand your leadership role better after your reading.

WHAT WE MEAN BY LEADERSHIP

Leadership is not domination, but the art of persuading people to work toward a common goal.

Daniel Goleman on Emotional Intelligence(1)

Leadership is defined in many different ways; however, many definitions of leadership contain common elements. For example, Susan Komives and her colleagues suggest that leadership is viewed and valued differently by various cultures and disciplines and that a multidisciplinary approach to leadership fosters a shared understanding of similarities and differences in leadership principles and practices across disciplines and cultures.(2) In health care services, Longest and his colleagues note that leadership is "a process of one individual influencing another individual or group to achieve particular objectives".(3) Southwest Airlines' view of leadership is "a dynamic relationship based on mutual influence and common purpose between leaders and collaborators in which both are moved to higher levels of motivation and moral development as they affect real, intended change".(4) It is interesting to note that Southwest Airlines uses the word "collaborator" instead of "follower", a more commonly used term in leadership discussions. In their view, "collaborator" better describes the individuals at Southwest Airlines because leadership is what Southwest leaders and their collaborators do together. John Snyder, an outstanding leader in clinical laboratory sciences and higher education administration, defines leadership as "the ability to persuade others to seek defined objectives enthusiastically. It is the human factor which binds a group together and motivates it toward goals. Management activities such as planning, organizing, and decision-making are dormant cocoons until the leader triggers the power of motivation in people and guides them toward goals".(5) Notice that these leadership definitions include groups, individuals, organizations, management tasks, goals and objectives, attitudes and behaviors. And, influence is a common element. Influence will be discussed under "Power and Influence".

LEADERSHIP VERSUS MANAGEMENT

Leadership and management are often thought of as the same thing. However, like other authors, we contend that there is an important distinction between the two. The primary difference between the two concepts is addressed in Michael Maccoby's article "Understanding the Difference Between Management and Leadership".(6) Maccoby suggests that **managers** are primarily administrators who are able to influence decisions and actions, whereas **leaders** influence the opinions and attitudes of others to accomplish a mutually agreed on task while advancing the group's integrity and moral purpose. Simply put, the leader is the central person who guides the group toward achieving a goal. In other words, leadership takes place anytime that one attempts to influence the behavior of a group, whether it is to accomplish one's own goals or those of the organization.

John Kotter, in *Leading Change*, makes the distinction of management versus leadership in the following way. He describes management as a set of processes (such as planning, budgeting, organizing, and problem solving) that can keep a complicated system of people and technology running smoothly.(7) Leadership, on the other hand, creates organizations or adapts them to significant changes in circumstance. Leadership defines the future and establishes direction, aligns the people and processes with a vision, and inspires the organization to make it happen. Zalesnick views managers and leaders as different types of people. In his view "managers and leaders differ in attitudes toward goals, conceptions of work, behavior toward risk taking, relations with others, and their sense of self".(8) Further, Zalesnick suggests that different personality traits exist between leaders and managers. Leadership traits will be discussed under the heading of "Attributes of Effective Leadership".

If this were a perfect world, all managers would be effective leaders that people would want to follow. However, based on feedback from our colleagues, a number of managers are ineffective and often resemble "the boss" portrayed in the poem entitled "The Leader", written by an unknown author, which appears below:

The boss drives group members, the leader coaches them.
The boss depends upon authority; the leader on good will.
The boss inspires fear; the leader inspires enthusiasm.
The boss says "I"; the leader says "we."
The boss assigns the task, the leader sets the pace.
The boss says, "Get there on time"; the leader gets there ahead of time.
The boss fixes the blame for the breakdown; the leader fixes the breakdown.

The boss knows how it is done; the leader shows how.
The boss makes work drudgery; the leader makes it a game.
The boss says, "Go"; the leader says, "Let's go."

According to Kevin Cashman, "Leadership is authentic self-expression that creates value." He continues "It involves awakening our inner identity, purpose and vision so that our lives are dedicated to a conscious, intentional manner of living".(9)

POWER AND INFLUENCE

An effective leader must be able to get followers to follow. In other words, a leader must have the capability to influence others to follow his/her advice, suggestion, or directive in pursuing the common goals of the groups or organizations to which they all belong. Therefore, before we introduce various leadership approaches, we need to briefly discuss the topics of power and influence, which are relevant and important to leadership. *Power* is defined as the capacity to influence others' behavior. When we say Person A has power over Person B, we mean A can get B to do what A wants, rather than what B himself or herself wants. Power is a different concept than authority, which is obtained by a manager when she or he takes a position and has the legitimacy to expect compliance from subordinates. Power refers to A's ability to influence B, not A's right to do so.

Power is no doubt essential to a manager to become a true leader. There are several theories on where power comes from. According to Emerson's *dependency theory,* individual/group A will have power over an individual/group if B is dependent on A.(10) Most of the time, we will find this dependence to be resources-related. A will have power over B, if A controls the resources that are desirable to B and B will not be able to gain access to such resources other than through A. The desired resources could be money, materials and space for work, tools and equipment, knowledge and expertise, political networks, and the like.

Another theory on the sources of power was developed by psychologists John French and Bertram Raven.(11) According to French and Raven, based on the difference in sources, power can be categorized into the following groups: legitimate power, reward power, coercive power, expert power, and referent power.

Legitimate power is derived from a person's position or job in an organization. Being put in the manager's position, a person is authorized by the organization with the legitimate right to require and demand compliance from his or her subordinates. In today's culture, such compliance by subordinates is well expected. It is understood in today's culture that people have a tendency to comply with the requests and demands of their bosses at work. Traditionally, medical laboratories have functioned under this type of "bossiness". While there is no clear explanation for this, this tendency is believed to have something to do with our life experiences with parents, teachers, and law enforcement officials.

Reward power exists in those who have the capacity to influence others by providing positive rewards. The rewards that are perceived to be valuable may include: raises, promotions, favorable job performance evaluations, assignment of preferred tasks, better working conditions, recognition, and compliments, to name a few. *Coercive power* is the capacity to apply punishments to those who refuse to comply with requests or demands. The punishments in organizations include, but are not limited to, docking pay or other benefits, assignment of unfavorable tasks, blocked promotion, disciplinary actions, criticisms, and being isolated. Both reward and coercive powers are based on the expectation of those supposedly influenced that they may either loose the chance to get desired rewards or simply get punished if they refuse to comply with the demands or requests.

Expert power derives from powerholders' superior knowledge, skills and abilities. People tend to be influenced by experts who know how to perform and have experience in performing their jobs well. The more crucial and unusual this expertise, the greater the expert power will be. It is not surprising that expert power is especially common in scientific and technical areas such as the medical laboratory. Such power, once obtained, is not easy to loose because of the difficulty in replacing the superior skills, abilities and knowledge.

Referent power exists when the powerholder is liked, respected, or admired by others. As human beings, we are more likely to be influenced by the people who we like and are attracted to. We may easily welcome their opinions, often seek their approval, sometimes even use them as role models, and we tend to ignore their failures. Referent power represents a more profound base of power than those based on incentives or threats. Both referent and expert power are most likely to generate true commitment and enthusiasm on the followers' side with regard to the manager's requests or demands.

In general, the power possessed by a manager is a combination of legitimate power, reward power, coercive power, referent power, and expert power. By taking the manager's position, an individual is given the authority to make demands and requests of the subordinates. Normally with such authority comes the ability in various levels to give rewards or apply punishment to the subordinates. It is also likely that the manager is a true expert in his/her technical area and/or a charismatic person who is greatly admired by his/her colleagues. In actuality, often times this is the major reason for a person being promoted. Therefore, managers can use a variety of strategies to build and accumulate power.

Firstly, newly promoted managers should be willing and feel comfortable to give orders or make demands, realizing the general tendency of employees to comply with such orders and demands. By confidently and appropriately exercising the authority to give orders, managers can enhance their legitimate power. Secondly, managers should constantly absorb new knowledge and develop their skills in the technical areas related to their work. This is particularly important in the medical laboratory setting. If they are already technical experts, managers should be willing to demonstrate their expertise by helping employees to solve technical problems. If they are not yet technical experts themselves, they should be able to delegate a technical specialist and be ready to listen to, and learn from, that individual. Repetitive mistakes in making technical decisions will greatly harm a managers' reputation and ultimately discount the effectiveness of their leadership. Although technical instrument failures, laboratory personnel errors, and erroneous test results may be unavoidable in a medical laboratory arena, laboratory managers must take swift corrective action to avoid repetitive mistakes in order to safeguard their patients, clients, and overall reputation of the laboratory.

Thirdly, managers should consciously cultivate friendly interpersonal relations with subordinates, peers, bosses, and outsiders to gain the referent power within organizations. Although it is often difficult and sometimes impossible to be liked by everybody at work, managers should try their best to win as much respect as possible from their colleagues. Arguably, many of the traits that make a person likable may not be learnable. However, many behaviors that make a person respectable are indeed learnable, like being loyal and committed to others, treating everyone fairly, being righteous and responsible, and self-sacrificing when needed (refer to the section of "ATTRIBUTES FOR EFFECTIVE LEADERSHIP" of this chapter for more detailed discussion of such behaviors). If you as a manager have these behaviors, you are on your way to win the respect of your colleagues.

Finally, managers should use every opportunity on the job to gain control of resources that are desirable to their employees. Among such resources are not only financial resources, desirable tools and equipment, preferred work space, and chances for promotion and career advancement, but also political connections and professional networks. With more resources under direct control, managers increase their ability to reward employees. On the other hand, managers should also negotiate wisely both before and after taking their positions so that their own employees will not be prevented from obtaining rewards and will not be subject to reprisals or sanctions. Although good managers may not necessarily resort to coercive mechanism to increase their ability to influence employees, it is nice to have such mechanism available if it is ever needed. (Relevance?)

APPROACHES TO LEADERSHIP

During the 20th century, there has been a significant transformation in the approach to leadership. In the first half of the century, the **trait approach** to leadership produced varying lists of personal traits that purportedly guaranteed successful leadership to persons who possessed varying outstanding characteristics such as heights, charisma, intelligence, and the like. The trait approach focused on addressing the question "what a leader is" or "who becomes a leader". The major problem of this approach is its assumption that there was a definite set of characteristics that made a leader and that leadership can not be learned.

In the 1950s and 1960s, trait theories were disputed by writers such as Ralph Stogdill, a distinguished leadership researcher, who were more interested in the **behavioral approach** to leadership and focused attention on what a leader "does," rather than what a leader "is." The behavioral approach took the position that leadership can be learned through education, training, and life and work experience. Within this approach, different patterns of leaders' behavior were grouped together and labeled as leadership styles. However, the behavioral approach did not address the issue of how a manager should select the most effective leadership style in a specific situation.

Since the 1960s, *situational contingency approach* had emerged, focusing on the importance of the context of the situation in explaining leader effectiveness. The central point of the contingency approach is that the leadership style needed would change with the situation. Various models of the contingency approach had been proposed to help to choose the appropriate leadership style for a particular circumstance.(12), (13)

The trait, behavioral, and contingency approaches have traditionally been the foundation of most of leadership theories. This chapter is also firmly based on these approaches in introducing various leadership concepts and principles. However, it is noteworthy that there are other approaches to leadership. From the mid 1920s to the late 1970s, advocates of the influence approach asserted that leadership is an influence or social exchange process, followed by the present day *reciprocal approach* that leadership is a relational and shared process that includes a strong emphasis on followership. In the book *Exploring Leadership*, Komives and colleagues summarized the chronology, assumptions, criticisms, and theories associated with each of the aforementioned approaches.(2) Other perspectives of leadership have emerged, including those on transformational leadership, transactional leadership and charismatic leadership.(3), (14), (15), (16)

LEADERSHIP AND TEMPERAMENT

As we pointed out previously, the efforts that intended to isolate specific personal traits as determinants of leadership abilities in the early years of leadership research led to the conclusion that no single trait separates leaders from non-leaders. On the contrary, various studies since the 1970s suggested that people of various characters and personalities all have the potential to become effective leaders. Among the studies is the *Keirsey Temperament Theory.*

David Keirsey proposed a modified model of the *Myers-Briggs Type Indicator* questionnaire for identifying actions and attitudes associated with 16 personality types.(17) Keirsey's questionnaires, called the Keirsey Temperament Sorter II, are self-scoring questionnaires designed to identify 16 combinations of four temperament types. Following the Myers-Briggs model, Keirsey elected to label each of the temperament types with a combination of letters, seen in parentheses to describe elements of personality traits represented in the four basic types shown in Table 2–1. Table 2–2 lists 16 personality types within the four temperament types

TABLE 2–1. Letters and Descriptions of Keirsey's Four Temperament Types

Artisan	(SP)	S stands for Observant and P stands for Probing
Guardian	(SJ)	S stands for Observant and J stands for Scheduling
Idealist	(NF)	N stands for Introspective and F stands for Friendly
Rational	(NT)	N stands for Introspective and T stands for Tough-minded

TABLE 2–2. Keirsey's Sixteen Types of Personality Grouped by Four Temperament Types

A	Artisans	(Promoter, Crafter, Performer, Composer)
G	Guardians	(Supervisor, Inspector, Provider, Protector)
I	Idealists	(Teacher, Counselor, Champion, Healer)
R	Rationals	(Field marshal, Mastermind, Inventor, Architect)

proposed by Keirsey, who suggests that temperament is an integral part of a person's character and personality that drives one's behavior. Moreover, he provides valuable insight into the self-image, values, interests of, and social roles played by the artisan (SP), guardian (SJ), idealist (NF), and rational (NT) types.

In his book, *Please Understand Me II*, Keirsey pointed out that, although several great world leaders including Mohandas Gandhi, Winston Churchill, George Washington, and Abraham Lincoln are so different from each other in personalities, they are all well recognized for their effective leadership. Keirsey suggested that certain kinds of temperament are needed for certain circumstances to make a leader an effective one. Keirsey and Myers-Briggs questionnaires have served as valuable research tools and sustained public interest over the years as evidenced by the scores of people who take them each year. The questionnaires and interpretation of the results are both published in Keirsey's book. A modified version of the questionnaire is posted on his website (http://www.keirsey.com). Take the Keirsey Temperament Sorter tests online to ascertain your personality temperament types. Once you complete the questionnaire, you will be provided with an interpretation of the results based on your responses.

ATTRIBUTES FOR EFFECTIVE LEADERSHIP

Whereas we recognize the fact that people of different personalities all have the potentials to become effective leaders, we also suggest that there are certain attributes commonly shared by effective leaders. Take a moment to visualize the leaders in your organization who you admire and trust. What are the reasons you would work harder for them rather than someone else? Jot down the attributes that you believe they possess. After you are finished, compare and contrast your list with ours. Our list begins with **character.** We may think of character as learning *how to be* rather than *how to act*. It is the essence of being a leader that opens up possibilities. Qualities of character include authenticity, purpose, creating value, trust, congruence, and compassion. Character is the foundation of Win/Win, a philosophy of human interaction, moral strength, on which everything else builds according to Stephen Covey, an internationally respected leadership authority and teacher.(18) Win/Win is based on the paradigm that there's enough for everyone, that one person's success is not accomplished at the exclusion of the success of others. **Integrity,** the value we place on ourselves and on others, is a key attribute for effective leadership. Integrity, sincerity, and honesty engender trust and respect. In other words, we admire leaders who "talk the talk and walk the walk"! Leaders need to have a **vision**. The leaders need to be visionaries who are able to see the "big picture", and be able to effectively communicate the strategic direction of their vision to the organization. Having self-confidence and a keen understanding of others is essential for being self-empowered and empowering others to be part of a solution or the change process. **Passion** for the job enables great leaders to get through the painstaking tasks of creating change, an inevitable outcome of the leadership process. Passion inspires and creates followership. Effective leaders must be believable. **Credibility** is based on excellent credentials, substantive knowledge, and sound practical experience. Leaders must be willing to assume greater responsibility for changing group outcomes. **Courage** is essential for creating a new vision, taking risks, and challenging the status quo. Personal **insight** and perception into the realities that exist in and outside of the organization are important attributes for effective leadership. **Humility** is a hallmark characteristic of a strong leader, good listener, and a perpetual learner who is willing to admit that others also have good ideas and accept that one can be wrong. Next on the list is a **sense of humor.** If you're going to be a leader, a good sense of humor will help you and others. When appropriately used, humor is a valuable tool, especially for ameliorating stress. **Emotional intelligence,** a concept proposed by Daniel Goleman in his book by the same name, consists of basic emotional competencies that describe the abilities needed to manage ourselves and our relationships effectively.(1) These include self-awareness, self-management, social awareness and social skills. Finally, with a **positive self-esteem,** a leader works selflessly to support people working toward the common good of the organization. A successful leader has positive self-esteem and self-respect, evidenced by the leader's positive behaviors such as taking risks confidently and communicating with clarity. Rate yourself according to the leadership qualities presented in Table 2–3 and prepare to work on areas in need of

TABLE 2–3. Key Attributes for Effective Leadership: Self-Assessment

Attribute	I Really Need Help!	I'm Working On It!	I Have It!
1. Character			
2. Integrity			
3. Vision			
4. Passion			
5. Credibility			
6. Empowerment			
7. Courage			
8. Insight			
9. Humility			
10. Sense of humor			
11. Emotional intelligence			
12. Positive self-esteem			

improvement. You may wish to use this exercise as an index to monitor your personal growth and professional development as a leader. Leadership development programs are available. Refer to examples of successful programs later in this chapter.

COMPETENCIES FOR EFFECTIVE LEADERSHIP

Key competencies for effective leadership include: creating and inspiring a shared vision communicating, diagnosing, problem solving, and adapting. Vision points direction and gives purpose to the organization's work. Effective communication of the vision is an art and leaders spend more time communicating than performing other activities. The communication process is dependent on varying message forms including written and spoken words, as well as nonverbal behavior such as facial expressions, body language, and listening. Researchers indicate that people spend approximately 45% of their communication time listening. Nevertheless, the average listener understands and retains about 50% of what is said immediately after a presentation. This level diminishes to approximately 20% within 48 hours. These data suggest that listening is one of the most crucial skills in the communication process. Other informal survey data suggest that communication is the number 1 problem in the workplace and in interpersonal relationships. The results of a national survey of laboratory directors by the American Society for Clinical Pathology ranked "effective communication skills" on top of the list of preferred skills for potential employees. Being able to understand the situation or a problem you are trying to influence is another important part of the leadership process. The leader must be able to analyze the current situation/problem and develop an effective strategy for intervention. Having the ability to adapt to change is key to successful leadership. The leader must adapt to behaviors and other available resources in such a way as to close the gap between the current situation and what he or she wants to influence.

LEADERSHIP STYLES

Becoming a leader is synonymous with becoming yourself. It's precisely that simple, and it's also that difficult.

Warren Bennis, On Becoming a Leader (19)

Although the concept of leadership remains debatable and elusive, there is consensus among researchers that leadership is, and effective leaders are, crucial to the success of an organization. Like parenting, leadership is not an exact science. Leadership must and can be learned. The learning process starts from first understanding various styles of leadership and identifying "what effective leaders do". These styles are different from competencies or responsibilities of leaders. Styles are concerned with the observed manner of the leader's behavior and actions.

Until today, much of the research done in the area of leadership styles focuses on some combination of high/low production and high/low concern for people.

The Blake-Mouton Model

Robert Blake and Jane Mouton proposed one classic research model on leadership style in 1964 called the managerial grid.(20) They visualized leadership styles in terms of a balance between concerns for getting the job done and the working relationships that must be integrated to achieve effective leadership. In the Blake-Mouton managerial grid, five different types of leadership, based on concern for production (task) and concern for people (relationship), are positioned in four quadrants (Figure 2–1). Concern for production is illustrated on the horizontal axis and concern for people on the vertical axis. The strength of a concern is rated on a scale from 1 to 9, with a 9/1 (*Task*) indicating the maximum commitment to working objectives, with little to no concern given to people's feelings. A 1/9 (*Country Club*) suggests a preoccupation with relationships and satisfying the needs of others at the expense of the task that needs to be done. A 1/1 (*Impoverished*) would be characteristic of a low-profile manager, who exerts minimal effort to get the job done and has minimal contact with others. The 5/5 (*Middle Road*) managers tend to maintain a satisfactory balance between the need to get the work done and the morale of the people doing the work. Like McGregor's Y, the belief of the 9/9 manager is that people have an inherent desire to perform well at work provided they are given the opportunity and encouraged to do so. All styles except the 9/9 (*Team*) suggest an expectation of conflict between keeping people happy and getting the job done.

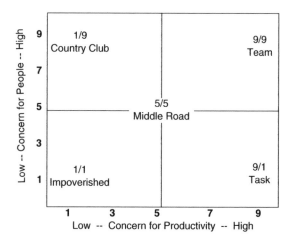

FIGURE 2–1 Blake and Mouton's Managerial Grid. Adapted from Hersey and Blanchard, The Managerial Grid leadership styles, pg. 100. In Hersey, P., Blanchard, KH, "Management of Organizational Behavior: Utilizing Human Resources." Prentice Hall, Englewood Cliffs, NJ, 5th Edition, 1988.

The Lorenzi-Riley Model

Derived from the task-oriented and people-oriented model developed by Hersey and Blanchard(13), Nancy Lorenzi and Robert Riley proposed the following styles of leadership behaviors: the on-the-job retirees, the whip crackers, the schmoozers, and the team builders.(21) On-the-job retirees are low on task skills, low on interpersonal relationships, and are usually procrastinators. The whip crackers are usually very task oriented, low on interpersonal skills, and see the task to be done as their primary responsibility, no matter what the cost. The whip crackers motto is "damn the torpedoes, full speed ahead! Schmoozers, taken from the Yiddish word for one who chats and idly gossips, rank low on task and high in interpersonal relationships. They can be enthusiastic about a project, but have a problem getting their group to get the job done. The last category, team builders, ranks high in both task and interpersonal skills. They empower their staff and they know what questions to ask and when to offer support.

Theories X, Y, and Z

Another model on leadership styles is the *Theory X-Theory Y* model proposed by Douglas McGregor in 1960. This model is somewhat different and more classic than the two other models introduced above. McGregor suggests that managers operate from two sets of expectations about employees' attitudes and abilities that ultimately influence their work performance.(22) McGregor's X-philosophy implies that employees are basically lazy, that they detest work, and that they need direction and control to protect them from the anathema of work. The X-oriented manager is likely to have to compensate for the worker's shortcomings. X-oriented managers tend to be dictatorial and autocratic. By contrast, McGregor's Y-philosophy suggested an optimistic set of expectations that workers view work as natural as play, that they are highly motivated, self-disciplined, and exercise creativity in problem solving. The Y-oriented manager's role then is one of capitalizing on the strengths of the workers. Y-oriented managers have a participative leadership style.

In more recent years, a modified *Theory Z* model has been introduced. Proponents of the Z-model suggest that the self-disciplined and highly motivated characteristic of employees in the Theory-Y model is cultural. This concept evolved from efforts to incorporate some of the Japanese moves into our American management practices as a possibility for increasing productivity and job satisfaction. The Z-philosophy is that changing societal goals must be included in the workplace and that productivity and rewards are not the only objectives of workers, but other issues such as quality of their work lives have a significant impact on their performance. Goldsmith refers to the Japanese Theory Z approach as a "magic potion" that, when applied to ailing U.S. industries and government, can solve problems of turnover, productivity, and alienation.(23) The Japanese magic formula contains elements such as lifetime employment; a company's concern for their employees' total well being; consensus decision making; and a consistent system of promotions, among other elements. Quality circles and total

TABLE 2–4. Leadership Style, Behavior, and Situation

Style	Authoritative	Democratic	Laissez-Faire
Behavior	"Telling." Leader identifies a problem, considers solutions, chooses one, and then tells others what they are to do	"Consulting." Leader gives people a chance to influence a decision from the start; members asked for ideas and leader then selects most promising solution	"Joining." Leader is "just another member" and agrees in advance to carry out decision group makes
When Style is Effective	Time is limited; people lack skills; group doesn't know each other	Time is available; group is motivated; people have some degree of skills	Group is highly motivated; sense of team exists; routine is familiar to group members
When Style is Ineffective	Strong sense of team; people have some degree of skills/ knowledge; group wants spontaneity in work	Group is unmotivated; people have no skills; high level of conflict present	Low sense of team; people have low degree of skills; group expects to be told what to do

quality management "TQM" are an outgrowth of the Japanese approach to management taught to them by the American W. Edwards Deming and others.(24)

Leadership Styles and Situations

Most people have a leadership style that they prefer and feel comfortable with. What you must realize is that different leadership behaviors may be required for different situations in order to get the job done. Leadership is not static, but rather a dynamic, fluidic, complex process involving a combination of three factors: the group, the environment, and the task. The most effective leadership style for a laboratory manager depends on the strength of the leader's abilities, the work environment, the group dynamics and morale, and the motivations of each of the workers. Hence, successful and effective leaders have the ability to adapt their style to fit the requirements of the situation. Table 2–4 lists conventional leadership styles, associated behaviors, and in what situation each style is effective and ineffective.

LEADERSHIP DEVELOPMENT PROGRAMS

This section consists of just a few examples of successful leadership development programs for those who wish to further explore leadership potential and/or enhance a current leadership role. Further information on each of these development programs, with the exception of the National Coalition for Allied Health

Leadership (see the section for specific source), may be obtained using the corresponding Internet resources located at the end of this chapter.

National Coalition for Allied Health Leadership

In 1998, the Association for Schools of Allied Health Professions (ASAHP), in partnership with the National Network of Health Career Programs in Two Year Colleges (NN2), and the Health Professions Network (HPN), sponsored a national program designed to develop leaders in the allied health professions. As a part of the leadership role of the American Society for Clinical Pathology (ASCP), the Society invited members to participate in this unique program, "Coalition for Allied Health Leadership." Participants attended two conferences in Washington, DC during which they learned decision-making and problem-solving skills (see Chapter 4 for more details on these concepts) and discussed leadership roles and responsibilities. They were also expected to make group presentations and complete workgroup projects, some of which were published in the summer of 2000.(25), (26) At the time of this writing, this special leadership development program is still attracting participants from across the United States.

A Laboratory for Leaders

The Toastmasters Club functions as a laboratory for developing leadership skills. The national organization structure of Toastmasters provides support to club members at the area, division, and district levels. Toastmasters offers an innovative success/leadership program in a series of educational workshops-style modules. The club also publishes a high performance leadership manual that is a hands-on, skill building program in which an individual conducts a project and serves as its leader. The Internet reference provided at the end of this chapter includes information on activities and locations of Toastmasters Clubs.

Leadership Learning Laboratory

The University of California, Davis offers a course entitled "The Leadership Learning Laboratory." This introductory course is designed to explore one's organizational culture and leadership needs, discuss challenges of leading and opportunities for leadership, and identify specific leadership competencies through self knowledge and awareness.

Change Leadership Certificate Program

Georgetown University's Professional Development Program offers a certificate program for project leaders, mid-level managers, directors, and executives leading organizational changes. The program includes personal assessment of leadership skills, strategies, and tools for implementing change, and development of leadership capabilities.

LEADERSHIP STYLES FOR THE FUTURE

A leader is someone you choose to follow to a place you wouldn't go by yourself.

Joel A. Barker in Leadershift

The challenge for the future is to be able to inspire leadership at all levels and to be comfortable with ambiguity and chaos. As organizations get more complex, structures flatten, and decision making gets closer to the place of the customer interface, leadership characteristics become an expectation throughout. Corporate leaders like Max DuPree of Herman Miller, Inc. and Dee Hock of VISA International see their organizations as communities often exhibiting a high degree of chaos.(27, 28) They create a space for more leaders with inspiring goals and trust that employees guided by vision and goals will do the right thing. Effective leaders use the tools of community building to create an environment in which many leaders can emerge.

Peter Block redefines "leadership" for the future in terms of "stewardship."(29)

Stewardship is…the choice to preside over the orderly distribution of power. This means giving people at the bottom and the boundaries of the organization choice over how to serve a customer, a citizen, a community. It is the willingness to be accountable for the well-being of the larger organization by operating in service, rather than in control of those around us. Simply stated, it is accountability without control or compliance.

The concept of stewardship fits well with emerging organizational structures, team concepts, and shared accountabilities. It is one thing to describe the concepts and theories; it is another to understand *how leaders shall act* and *how leaders shall be*. Peter Drucker, the acknowledged "father of modern management," has studied leaders and leadership for more than 50 years. In *The Leader of the Future*, he concludes that effective leaders know four simple things:

1. A leader is someone who has followers.
2. The effective leader gets followers to do the right things. He/she might not be popular but he/she gets results.
3. Leaders are visible; they set examples.
4. Leadership is not about rank or title; it is about responsibility.(30)

"Get results" is a resounding answer to the question "What do leaders do?" Using extensive research tools, Daniel Goleman has described six distinct leadership styles that appear to have a direct impact on the performance of an organization.(31) The effectiveness in these styles is not in the exclusive use of any one, but in the mental and emotional agility to choose the right style for the right situation. Table 2–5 delineates the styles and some of their dimensions. If a leader can use these styles to challenge, support, and inspire members of the organization, they will spark optimum performance and get the desired results. The most effective leaders are those who can be flexible with their style and fluid in action. Mastery of at least four of the six styles—especially the authoritative, affiliative, democratic, and coaching—creates the best organizational climate and best business performance.

TABLE 2–5. Leadership Styles for the Future

Styles:	Coercive	Authoritative	Affiliative	Democratic	Pacesetting	Coaching
The leader's modus operandi	Demands immediate compliance	Mobilizes people toward a vision	Creates harmony and builds emotional bonds	Forges consensus through participation	Sets high standards for performance	Develops people for the future
What they say	"Do what I tell you"	"Come with me"	"People come first"	"What do you think?"	"Do as I do, now"	"Try this"
Underlying emotional intelligence competencies	Drive to achieve, initiate, self control	Self-confidence, empathy, change catalyst	Empathy, building relationships, communication	Collaboration, team leadership, communication	Conscientious, drive to achieve, initiative	Developing others, empathy, self-awareness
When to use the style	In a crisis, to kick-start a turnaround	When changes require a new vision, or when a clear direction is needed	To heal rifts in a team or to motivate people during stressful circumstances	To build buy-in or consensus or to get input from valuable individuals	To get quick results from a highly motivated and competent team	To help individuals improve performance or develop long-term strengths
Long-term impact	Negative	Most strongly positive	Positive	Positive	Negative/Positive	Positive

Adapted from Goleman D: Leadership That Gets Results, pg. 82–83.

The leaders of the future will need to demonstrate mental and emotional agility, guiding organizations through new and complex situations. It begins with appropriate use of self—self-awareness and self-leadership. Leaders need to take inventory of personal attributes and values and to understand the vision and purpose that motivates them to lead. As organizations move from a mentality of "chain-of-command" management to an attitude of "web-of-influence" leaders, we highlight three fundamental dimensions for leaders:

- *Embrace Vision and Change.* Create an "invisible force" that gives organizational clarity and purpose and future direction. Embrace change and your role as a change agent. Get agreement of goals and values, which will allow people the freedom to develop and make choices for which they will be accountable.
- *Share Information.* We no longer think of Knowledge as Power, but rather applying the knowledge as a means of nourishment for the organization.
- *Develop Collaborative Relationships.* Creating a web of influence through relationship building provides strength and energy to the organization. The quality and diversity of collaborative relationships will help identify resources and foster a learning environment.

SUMMARY

In this chapter we presented definitions, theories, concepts, principles, and styles of leadership in the context of the medical laboratory setting. The themes throughout this chapter support our notion that leadership means change for the common good of the laboratory community. Leadership involves the abilities to create and communicate a vision that acts as an invisible guide, to build a rich diversity of relationships that energize teams, and to share information to nurture change. We hope that the information and exercises in this chapter will serve as a useful guide while working with others to accomplish change as we face the challenges of living and working in the 21st century.

SUGGESTED PROBLEM-BASED LEARNING ACTIVITIES

Chapter 2: Principles of Leadership: Past, Present, and Future

Instructions: Use Internet resources, books, articles, colleagues, etc. to present solutions to the problems listed below. There is no correct solution to any problem.

Note to Instructor: Students in class may be divided into groups and given the problem-based learning activity to discuss and solve. Once the group has reached consensus as to a solution, the group may present it to the other students in the class. This activity will provide all students with information regarding solutions to the problem.

Problem #1
Use a personality trait assessment tool (e.g. The Keirsey Four Types Sorter or Myers-Briggs Type Indicator) to type students in your class and stratify them into working groups. Observe the working behaviors of group members during problem-based learning exercises.

Problem #2
Identify a leadership style and use it to explain how it could be used in dealing with a problem employee.

Problem #3
You have implemented a participative management process within your department. When input is requested, you receive minimal if any responses from your supervisors. Discuss what leadership skills may be used to best facilitate and accomplish this process.

REFERENCES

1. Goleman, D. (1997). *Emotional intelligence*. New York: Bantam Books.
2. Komives, S. R., Lucas, N., & McMahon, T. R. (1998). *Exploring leadership* (p.5). San Francisco: Jossey-Bass Publishers.
3. Longest, B. B., Rakich, J. S., & Darr, K. (2000). *Managing health services organizations and systems* (p. 737). Baltimore: Health Professions Press.
4. Freiberg, K., & Freiberg, J. (1997). *NUTS! Southwest Airlines' crazy recipe for business and personal success* (p. 298). New York: Broadway Books.
5. Snyder, J. R. & Senhauser, D. A. (1989). *Administration and supervision in laboratory medicine* (p. 93). Philadelphia: J.B. Lippincott Company.
6. Maccoby, M. (2000). Understanding the difference between management and leadership. *Research Technology Management, 43* (1), 57–59.
7. Kotter, J. (1996). *Leading change*. Boston: Harvard Business School Press.
8. Zalesnick, A. (1977). Managers and leaders: Are they different? *Harvard Business Review, 55* (3), 67–78.
9. Cashman, K. (1998). *Leadership from the inside out*. Provo: Executive Excellence Publishing.
10. Emerson, R. M. (1962). Power-dependence relations. *American Sociological Review, 27*, 31–41.
11. French, J., & Raven, B. (1959). The base of social power. In D. Cartwright (Ed.), *Studies in Social Power* (pp. 150–167). Ann Arbor: University of Michigan Press.
12. Fiedler, F. E. (1967). *A theory of leadership effectiveness*. New York: McGraw-Hill.
13. Hersey, P., & Blanchard, K. H. (1988). *Management of organizational behavior: utilizing human resources*. Englewood Cliffs, NJ: Prentice Hall.
14. Burns, J. M. (1977). *Leadership*. New York: Harper and Row.
15. Trishy, N. M., & Devanna, M. A. (1986). *The transformational leader*. New York: John Wiley.

16. House, R. J. (1977). A 1976 theory of charismatic leadership. In J. G. Hunt & L. L. Larson (eds.) in Leadership: The Cutting Edge.
17. Keirsey, D. (1998). *Please Understand Me II. Delmar*, CA: Prometheus Nemesis Books.
18. Covey, S. R. (1990). *The 7 habits of highly effective people*. New York: Simon and Schuster.
19. Bennis, W. G. (1989). *On becoming a leader*. Reading, MA: Addison-Wesley.
20. Blake, R. R., & Mouton, J. S. (1981). *The versatile manager: a grid profile*. Homewood, IL: Irwin.
21. Lorenzi, N. M. & Riley, R. T. (1994). *Organizational aspects of health informatics: managing technological change*. New York: Springer-Verlag.
22. McGregor, D. (1966). *Leadership and motivation*. Cambridge, MA: MIT Press.
23. Goldsmith, S. B. (2005). *Principles of health care management: compliance, consumerism, and accountability in the 21st century* (p. 161). Boston: Jones and Bartlett Publishers.
24. Drucker, P. P. (1971). What we can learn from Japanese management. *Harvard Business Review, 59* (3), 110–122.
25. Gonzales, L., Hope Kearns, E., Lafferty, S., & Lampigno, J. (2000). The middle school mentoring program in allied health: a proposed model. *Journal of Allied Health, 29* (2), 114–119.
26. Wilson, S.L. (2000). Allied health leadership development program. *Journal of Allied Health, 98* (2), 98.
27. DuPree, M. (1992). *Leadership jazz*. New York: Dell Publishing.
28. Hock, D. (1999). Birth of the chaordic age. San Francisco: Berrett-Koehler.
29. Block, P. (1996). *Stewardship*. San Francisco: Berrett-Koehler.
30. Hesselbein, F., Goldsmith, M., & Beckhard, R. (1996). The leader of the future. San Francisco: Jossey-Bass.
31. Goleman, D. (2000). Leadership that gets results. *Harvard Business Review, 78* (2), 78–90.

BIBLIOGRAPHY

Bennis, W. G. (2000). *Managing the dream*. Cambridge, MA: Perseus Publishing.
Dunn, R. (2002). *Haimann's healthcare management*. Chicago, IL: Health Administration Press.
Hunt, J. and Larson, L. (Eds.) (1977). *Leadership: The cutting edge* (pp. 189–207). Carbondale, IL: Southern Illinois University Press.
Varnadoe, L. A. (1996). *Medical laboratory management and supervision operations, review, and study guide*. Philadelphia: FA Davis.
Wallace, M. A. & Klosinski, D. D. (1998). *Clinical laboratory science education and management*. Philadelphia: W.B. Saunders.
Wheatley, M. J. (1999). *Leadership and the New Science*. San Francisco: Barrett-Koehler Publishers.

INTERNET RESOURCES

Southwest Educational Development Laboratory
www.sedl.org/change/leadership/history.html
Toastmasters Club: A Laboratory for Leaders
http://www.ecommercemarket.com/toastmasters/message3.html
UC Davis Leadership Learning Laboratory
http://sdps.ucdavis.edu/browse/hr/hrs021.htm
The Website for the Keirsey Character Sorter Questionnaire
http://www.keirsey.com
Website for Emotional Intelligence information
www.eiconsortium.com
Georgetown University Change Leadership Program
www.changeleadership.com
Website for *Joel Barker's Leadershift: Five Lessons for Leaders in the 21st Century*
www.employeeuniversity.com

3

Management Functions

RANDALL S. LAMBRECHT, PhD, MT(ASCP), CLS(NCA)
MARIE CATO, MBA, MT(ASCP)

Chapter Outline

Objectives

Following successful completion of this chapter, the learner will be able to:

1. Identify the major roles and functions associated with effective laboratory management.
2. Discuss the qualities and style an effective manager should possess.
3. Describe how laboratory management has evolved over the past 20 years.
4. List important basic components of the planning process and be able to explain their role on short-term and long-term goals.
5. Provide a list of steps or functions essential for organizing a plan of implementation.

6. Identify effective means of communication and describe the benefits of taking a collaborative approach to problem solving.
7. Apply key management principles in response to a problem-based case study situation.
8. Outline assessment tools that provide a measurement of successful management and operational performance outcomes.

Key Terms

Collaboration
Communication
Controlling
Coordination
Directing
Implementing

Management
Organizing
Outcomes Assessment
Personnel Development
Planning
Supervisory

INTRODUCTION

The effectiveness of any organization is determined by the way work is organized and by the way people work with or against each other. The way in which people co-operate with each other, with management, and with the community, indeed the extent of their commitment to their organization, depend on the style of management. *Management* can be and has been defined in many different ways over the years. The most contemporary rendition of this term in the business world involves the concept of achieving organizational goals in an effective and efficient manner by working with and through people. Management, and in particular health care management, has undergone significant changes over the last 10 to 20 years. Historically, laboratory management had a primary function of organizing and directing the staff to ensure the production of quality laboratory results. In today's healthcare environment, the production of quality laboratory results is only one of many expected outcomes that must be achieved for a medical laboratory to attain success. The ability to handle change is one of the most important skills a manager who is a leader can have. As organizations develop, management and leadership traits such as transformational, charismatic and visionary rise in importance as workforces become more diverse, technology becomes more complex, and competition heightens. Other facets leading to success include marketability, cost management, benchmarking, reengineering, personnel management, *personnel development*, staff empowerment, collaboration, standardization, and providing exceptional service. The competition among healthcare providers today rivals that among the major business corporations. However difficult the competition becomes, successfully managed organizations invest in their people; and they do so wisely.

The philosophy of management has also undergone a type of metamorphosis and continues to evolve. In the past, management tended to function from a more autocratic and "power of position" focus often perceived as being controlling inflexible and lacking inclusivity. There were, however, important advantages related to this approach, such as firmer and quicker decisions, predictability, and for the manager, a zone of comfort. Today's management style has evolved to power derived from leadership rather than power derived from position. Leadership is a quality that evolves with time and experience and requires a high degree of confidence in addition to competence to facilitate a more global view and a broad-based approach to issues. Leadership also requires the ability to form and communicate a vision as well as build teams of individuals who work together toward common goals. There is an old axiom that says, a leader cannot lead if there are no followers. Today's leadership is much more democratic and participatory. It increases the roles of facilitator, coach, and communicator for the manager and has the advantages of greater employee involvement, broader based decisions, and greater creativity. In earlier years, employees were often hesitant to question management authority. In today's environment the employee does not hesitate to ask questions or seek answers. Today's manager must be able to respond to challenge and be prepared to explain decisions rather than simply being dismissive.

The management of a laboratory is complex and varies depending on its size, geographic location, patient/client population, goals of the institution, and the board that oversees it. Aligning the clinical laboratory's vision, goals, programs, resources, facilities, and expectations with mission, strategic plans, and objectives is critical to it's efficiency and performance. Evaluation and assessment should focus on both the planning and achievements that encompass the laboratory's function. Effective management is a process that begins with establishment of goals and ends with assessment of the achievement of those goals. Within this process are functions that enable these goals to be realized. These basic functions include planning, organizing, and implementing and controlling (Figure 3–1). Embedded within each of these functions are more specific and very important responsibilities and activities. The primary task for each of these management functions is listed in Table 3–1. For example within the management function of organizing are the critical roles of prioritizing and implementing. Similarly, the function labeled implementing contains controlling, monitoring, assessing, and making adjustments when needed. In reality, the boundaries separating each function are somewhat obscure because there is much overlap and crossover as a result of mutual reliance between functions. Important to the entire process is the recognition that coordination, collaboration, communication, personnel management and development, innovativeness, and vision are critical to the realization of successful outcomes.

As a result of the combination of changes in management style and the tools available to measure success, the functions of today's healthcare manager are much more diverse, complex, and interdependent. It is imperative that a manager is skilled in all of these functions to attain both job and personal satisfaction. Obtaining management and leadership skills is often a factor of experience. Even though certain individuals may naturally possess some of the building blocks required to manage, expertise and experience must still be developed. A manage-

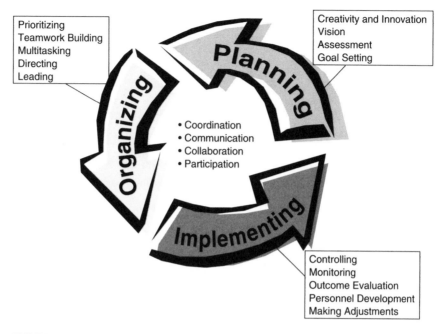

FIGURE 3–1 The basic functions of management.

ment position requires conceptual (thinking) skills, people skills, and technical skills. As you progress from lower levels of management toward upper levels of management, the mix of these required skills changes. In the lower levels of management (e.g., **supervisory**), the technical skills are more frequently used along with the people skills. In the upper levels of management (e.g., director), conceptual or cognitive skills are more frequently used along with people skills. The increase in conceptual and people skill levels is often a function of experience and not something that can simply be taught. Figure 3–2 shows how time spent on various management functions changes in relation to the management level.

To summarize, the three primary components of the management function process are interdependent and critical to making the laboratory a productive and competitive organization. We have chosen to consider the function of

TABLE 3–1. Primary Components of the Management Function Process

Planning	Clarifies the process of attaining organizational goals
Organizing	Identifies the steps needed to implement a successful plan
Implementing and Controlling	Puts plan into operation and measures implementation progress

First Level (Supervisors)

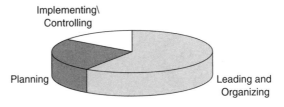

Middle Level (Managers)

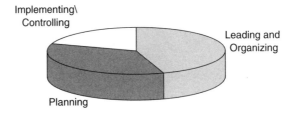

Top Level (Vice Presidents/CEOs)

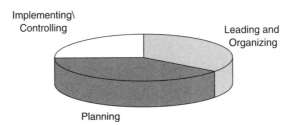

FIGURE 3–2   Relative functions within management levels.

controlling as embedded within implementing because of the high degree of interdependence and because they are often concurrent. Throughout the management function cycle of planning, organizing and controlling phases are embedded the 3 Cs (coordination, communication, and collaboration), which invite participation of all stakeholders.

The basic functions of management represent a consistent strategy that can be used when addressing any of the responsibilities that managers face. Management **functions** should not be confused with the **tasks** and responsibilities associated with management duties. The former (functions) describes a process and strategy for dealing with issues of change, whereas the latter (responsibilities) deals with the routine tasks for which laboratory managers are held responsible and accountable.

This chapter is designed to introduce the learner to the basic management functions (planning, organizing, and implementing and controlling) using a case study approach. Each subsection begins with a case study followed by questions to consider. A discussion of the management function(s) covered provides the learner with background and descriptive information to ponder and use to determine suitable answers to the case questions. It is important to note that more than one answer may be appropriate for a given question. Learners are encouraged to share their thoughts on these cases with their instructors and other students. This approach will allow everyone to consider all of the possible answers.

MANAGEMENT FUNCTIONS
Planning
Case Study

You are the laboratory manager of a medium-sized 120-bed hospital and are called to a hospital leadership meeting by the CEO of the facility. You are told that the hospital is having problems meeting some debt responsibility and there is a possibility that budgetary cutbacks will be needed to alleviate the situation. Each departmental manager is being given 1 week to plan how to accomplish a cost reduction of 10% within his/her department should it become necessary. You are also told that this situation is highly confidential because it is not yet known whether the cost reduction will be needed.

Issues and Questions to Consider
1. *Identify the steps in developing short-term goals to address the potential reduction in resources described above.*
2. *What type of information will you need to gather to assess your current state and develop a plan?*
3. *What criteria will you use to determine the best plan of action?*
4. *What type of long-range planning should be considered?*

Planning is the management function that clarifies the process of attaining the desired goals of an organization. It includes activities such as data gathering, assessment, calculation of risks, and determination of a strategy. Planning requires an emphasis on creativity, innovation, vision, and thinking "beyond traditional methods." In other words, a manager should not be constrained by preconceived notions or doing things as they have been done in the past. A simple lesson when trying to effect change is that if you do things the way they have always been done, you will get the same results as in the past. Planning is concerned with the future impact of today's decisions and is the fundamental function of management from which the other functions stem. The need for planning is easy to postpone in the short-run and too often apparent after the fact. The organizing, staffing, leading and controlling functions stem from the planning function. The determination of whether or not goals are being accomplished and standards met is based on the planning function. The planning function provides the goals and standards that drive the controlling function. Planning is important at all levels of management. However, its characteristics vary by level of management. Planning represents the cognitive (thinking) function of management. Management often finds it difficult to allocate sufficient quality time to this phase despite its importance to the entire process. There is a dangerous tendency to immediately jump into action rather than thinking through the options and implications. Planning requires attention to detail, creativity, globalization, flexibility, logic, predictability, decisive decision making, vision, as well as a deep understanding of the organization's purpose. It might be better to refer to strategic planning as *strategic management,* as it is often regarded as the first step in the functional role of management. The major components of the planning function are listed in Table 3–2.

Planning is a process that is essential to:

1. Make advanced rational decisions about the future.
2. Anticipate and react positively to changes.
3. Analyze information and make improvements.
4. Reduce ambiguity and anxiety among staff.
5. Accomplish goals and objectives in a timely and efficient manner.
6. Remain competitive and cost effective.
7. Be proactive rather than reactive.

Planning begins with fully understanding the institution's "purpose for being." Planning has as its components:

Vision: Provides nonspecific, directional, and motivational guidance for the entire organization. Top managers are eager to provide a vision for the business. The vision is usually the most emotional of the levels in the hierarchy of purposes.

Mission: An organization's reason for being. It is concerned with the scope of the business and what makes the enterprise distinct from similar operations. Missions reflect the culture and values of the institution or laboratory enterprise.

Objectives: Objectives address key issues within the organizational mission such as market standing, innovation, productivity, physical and financial resources, profitability, management and worker performance and efficiency. They are expected to be general, observable, challenging, and untimed.

Goals: Goals are specific statements of anticipated results that further define the organization's objectives. They are expected to be **SMART:** *S*pecific, *Mea*surable, *A*ttainable, *R*ewarding, and *T*imed.

TABLE 3–2. Major Components of the Planning Function

- Mission statements and core principles
- Innovation and vision
- Assessment
- Goal setting
- Tactics

Tactics: Tactics are another level of planning and are the most specific plans that describe how, who, what, when, and where activities will take place to accomplish a goal.

Every healthcare provider and/or medical laboratory service should have a **mission statement** that is clear and consistent. The mission statement articulates the purpose, attitude, and core competencies of the institution in as concise a declaration as possible. The mission statement should highlight what the healthcare organization and the laboratory do best or excel at most. Policies, practices, and behaviors should all evolve around the mission statement, and management decisions should be consistent with supporting the mission statement. Although it is common and healthy for changes and adaptations to occur in any organization, the mission statement should remain steadfast because it exemplifies the core principle of why an organization exists, and the assumptions on which the organization was built. The mission statement, together with the assumptions that shape an organization's behavior, should dictate any decisions an organization makes. If an organization has been struggling to survive for a long time, it may need to review its mission statement and assumptions to see if they no longer fit with reality or have become outmoded, but for the most part, the mission statement describes the heart of an organization's existence and is therefore nonnegotiable. Peter Drucker, the author of *Managing in a Time of Great Change* coined the phrase *Theory of the Business* to describe the clear, consistent, and focused assumptions that usually define the principles by which a business or organizational unit operates. The healthcare system in the Unites States currently exists in a dynamic and rapidly changing environment; thus, healthcare providers who are slow to accept change or are unreceptive to adapting to meet the needs of the future will soon find themselves uncompetitive and struggling to survive. Careful planning and anticipation for the future are essential for an organization to remain in business.

The planning stage should be participatory. This will increase the scope of ideas and will also help with "buy-in" from those who are involved. In addition, it will help identify and dilute any preconceived notions or biases you as an individual may bring to the process. Planning is a critical step of the process and, unfortunately, is often rushed or short-changed. The act of planning will allow you to set a direction. A simple but instructive analogy would be taking a vacation by automobile. You must identify your final destination and then determine a route and direction that will take you there. Planning requires that you have a comprehensive understanding of your starting point. If you misinterpret that point, you may well miss your final destination or target. The plan represents the road map of your automobile vacation.

Planning can take place over different time periods. Short-term goals will usually have fewer benchmarks, but that does not decrease their importance, as you will also have less time for adjustment. The short-term plan often defines less lofty goals, but is much quicker to accomplish than the long-term plan, which is more complex and whose goals are generally more difficult to achieve. Advantages of short-term goals are that they are usually good for morale during the longer planning process, and they provide "quick wins" in terms of witnessing accomplishments in a short period. Irrespective of the period, there are a number of approaches to good effective planning. The first step usually involves an assessment or survey of the organization's strengths, weaknesses, opportunities, and threats. Regardless whether long term or short term, the plan must include goals that are clear and concise, as well as attainable. Plans that are not realistic are nothing more than organized dreams.

A careful study of the assessment survey is necessary to identify areas that need improvement and to help the organization meet its goals, which are usually the endpoint of most management efforts. The assessment tool should look at issues such as environment, safety, space, equipment and personnel needs, employee morale, productivity output, technology, demographic trends, cost issues and qualitative outcomes, as well as external items such as healthcare trends and government-legal and political climate. The assessment phase should attempt to develop baseline data. For the assessment to be comprehensive and of greatest use, it should involve input from as many groups and individuals as possible, keeping in mind, however, that decision making is both the privilege and the burden of managers.

Establishing **goals** helps the institution define its mission, control its destiny, motivate its employees, and ensure that everyone understands the purpose of the enterprise. Setting goals helps move an institution forward. Goals should be challenging but achievable, visionary but realistic, and supported by available resources with measurable outcomes. A laboratory needs to decide where and what it wants to be in the future. Does it want to have a particular focus or expertise? Can it do all things equally well, or does it have a particular niche whereby it is regarded as an invaluable resource. Long-term goals are broad ambitions that are often met through a series of smaller, more focused **objectives.** Objectives are often developed as directives for accomplishing the established goals.

In addition to identifying opportunities in the planning function, management must identify possible threats, uncertainties, or negative consequences inherent in a plan. These need to be anticipated, as each one can become such an enormous unexpected factor that they may render an institution paralyzed, leaving any future planning futile if not counterproductive. Planning for surprise events involves peering into the future and forecasting potential problems in an attempt to avoid them. Many uncertainties have already occurred and, with experience, can be anticipated and avoided if history is not forgotten. A good plan will also help the manager and staff sharpen their focus, thereby accomplishing goals more quickly and efficiently. Another benefit of planning that should not be underestimated is the value of discussion and preparing those involved for change. Change itself is often less dramatic or stressful than the unknown, and individuals are less resistant to change if the process is clearly outlined. Planning will reduce that fear of the unknown. If open discussions cannot be held in the planning stage, it should be incorporated as soon as possible, and your plan should allow for refinement or revision based on acquired input.

Organizing

Case Study

After you have presented your proposal to hospital administration and it has been accepted, you are informed that the impending cost reductions will need to be implemented. You are told to meet with your supervisory staff to organize the implementation of your plan. The CEO will be holding hospital employee briefings beginning the next afternoon to provide the employees with an overview of the situation confronting the hospital. Over the next 2 to 3 days you will be meeting with your supervisory staff and then with the laboratory employees to provide additional detail specifically as it pertains to the laboratory and its staff. Your goals are to have your employees fully understand the situation and its implications, allow them to communicate their thoughts and concerns, and to finally accomplish buy-in from the staff regarding the proposal you must implement.

Issues and Questions to Consider

1. What steps or functions are key to organizing the plan for implementation?
2. Who needs to be included in this process and why?
3. What are the various means of communication that could be used in this situation? Which one(s) is chosen and why?
4. What areas of collaboration or coordination, if any, will be needed with the supervisory staff, pathology staff, bench staff, medical staff, other hospital staff?
5. What situations could require mentoring and/or motivating of staff?

Organizing is the process of determining the steps needed to implement a successful plan. It includes identifying the various steps that need to take place in addition to determining the appropriate personnel for accomplishing those steps. This step also includes allocating or reallocating resources including equipment, funds, and/or staffing. Staffing is one of the most important managerial activities that ensure qualified people for all positions in the laboratory. Recruiting, hiring, training, evaluating and compensating are the specific activities included in the function. Directing is another organizing activity that influences people's behavior through motivation, communication, group dynamics, leadership and discipline. The purpose of directing is to channel the behavior of all personnel to accomplish the organization's mission and objectives while simultaneously helping them accomplish their own career objectives. There are at least four key elements of laboratory organization that include: the assays and tasks to be performed, the individual task performers, teams of laboratory personnel working together, and the physical environment of the workplace. Organization plays an important role in determining the effectiveness of the clinical laboratory by defining the relationship among those key elements. Organizing brings structure to your plan by detailing what has to be done, who has to do it, and how it is going to be done.

Organizing for a specific activity usually entails being cognizant of the organizational structure with which the laboratory operates. There are a number of organizational charts and modeled hierarchal structures that describe many types of organizational management systems in health care. These include multilevel pyramids (Figure 3–3) or vertical charts with clear delineation about who's on top and who's not. They profile the lines of authority and communication, as well as illustrate patterns of coordination. Conflict in an organization is inevitable, but may be reduced through clarity of organizational relationships. Although organizational diagrams can sometimes help depict how different units or disciplines relate to each other and to administration, it may be difficult to glean activities between units that are integrated and interdisciplinary. Few areas of a laboratory are independent with the exception of highly specialized laboratories that require segregation and separate treatment for security, safety, or other purposes (drug testing laboratory for example).

A dual form of organization as a result of the traditional dichotomous relationship between medical staff and administrators often characterizes healthcare institutions. The ultimate authority and responsibility for the management of the overall institution rest with its governing board. Because of licensure, medical governance boards, and accreditation policies, there are usually two lines of authority, each with their own hierarchical structure, whereby the board appoints a chief executive officer and a chief of the medical staff. In an attempt to consolidate authority, some institutions will designate a high-level administrative position to whom both the CEO and Chief of the Medical Staff report. The same dual reporting structure (administrative and medical) may hold true within the medical laboratory depending on its size.

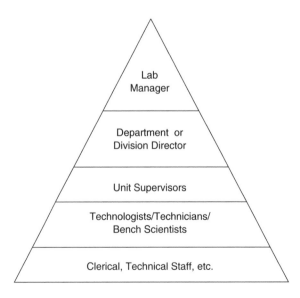

FIGURE 3–3   Typical laboratory pyramidal hierarchy.

Organizational structures have become more flexible recently as institutions and managers have recognized the need to effect change and have witnessed the benefits in having a flexible structure that can respond more readily to external and internal pressures and changing environments. Several successful strategies include forming interdisciplinary task forces, establishing temporary cross-disciplinary teams, encouraging cross-training and multitasking, and using a matrix organization approach. Matrix organizational design involves creating a flexible and adaptable organizational structure by combining workers from several different functional units to form a collaborative group to work on a specific project. The structure is thought of in terms of a lattice or grid because it combines the talents and expertise of individuals across disciplines and improves the communication and understanding among different units.

As a management function, organizing is a skill that contains a number of activities and responsibilities. Effectively organizing and leading a workforce requires prioritizing, coordinating, communicating, collaborating, team building, and directing. The primary tasks for the organizing function are listed in Table 3–3.

When organizing for a specific task at the workplace, there are some underlying premises:

1. Everyone is working toward a common goal.
2. The goal has been articulated in detailed plans in terms of scope and priorities.
3. Responsibilities are clearly outlined and delegated.
4. There is a command structure and an understanding of authority.

Inherent in the organizing function is the prioritizing function. Prioritizing involves ordering the functions or tasks to be accomplished. Priority may be established based on urgency, availability of resources, or foundation (i.e., step a must precede step b). Prioritizing will allow you to more appropriately allocate the resources identified earlier in the organizing function. Clearly, setting priorities for the laboratory is a primary responsibility of the laboratory manager.

The Importance of the 3 Cs: It is perhaps the organizing function for which the 3 Cs—coordination, collaboration, and communication—are most important. All three are dependent on participation and have profound influence on the "people side" of the equation.

TABLE 3–3.   **Major Components of the Organizing Function**

- Prioritizing
- Coordination
- Communication
- Collaboration
- Team building
- Staffing & Directing

Coordination is the blending of functions so that they are intertwined and build on each other. Coordination ensures that you are minimizing the risks of duplication or redundancy. It will also minimize the risk of allowing something to be overlooked or "falling through the cracks." Coordination requires that various portions of the plan move at specified speeds so they remain synchronized. Coordination requires significant attention to detail and continual monitoring to allow for any needed adjustments.

The second C, *collaboration,* is the act of working together to achieve a common end. Collaboration may be required both internal and external to the department. Collaboration is difficult to attain without cooperation. Collaboration requires definite managerial expertise regarding people skills. Although collaboration is designed to align people, if not carefully planned and implemented, it actually may have the opposite effect.

The third C, *communication,* may well be the most critical element to the success of a manager. Studies have shown that information needs to be communicated a minimum of seven times to ensure that people have actually heard the correct message. There is a saying within management that you can never communicate too much. When appropriate and timely communication is not present, the rumor mill or grapevine will fill the gap. In some ways the grapevine is one of the most effective ways of communication in that it is faster than formal communication and often is clear, accurate, and factual; however, it can be damaging if it is not factual. Experienced managers will find ways to use the grapevine to their advantage. Today's computer technology is, to some extent, making the grapevine obsolete. With electronic mail (e-mail) availability, the manager is able to disseminate accurate information to all personnel in a timely manner. As with any written communication, however, there should be a mechanism for employees to ask for and receive clarification. This type of communication does not eliminate the need for face-to-face discussion; however, it should serve as a foundation for such discussion. Another form of communication that is available to the manager is called the chance encounter. Chance encounters are those times when a manager is walking through the workplace and is approached spontaneously regarding an issue or question. Chance encounters are informal and may involve only a single employee but still provide an additional opportunity for communication. Most employees see chance encounters as positive because they are less formal, tend to be one-on-one with management, are spontaneous, and indicate that the manager is willing to take the time to listen to the employee's concerns.

Organizing is often accomplished through work teams that are brought together based on common responsibility, needed skills or expertise, or some combination. It is critical for the manager to solicit involvement from employees at this point if it could not be accomplished previously. The staff and supervisory level know and understand the details of the workplace more thoroughly than upper level management. In addition, the plan and its implementation will in all likelihood affect the staff more directly than management. Inclusion of staff in this function will result in a better-defined organizational plan in addition to increasing the "buy-in" of employees. Good communication among all employees and the sense of belonging and involvement will lead to positive morale, which in turn will result in greater productivity.

Directing, or **leading,** as it is often called, accounts for a large percentage of the organizing function. Depending on the level of management, directing makes up 40% to 50% of a manager's efforts. Directing is vital to organizing and implementing a plan. Managers who are good at directing are capable of matching organizational goals to the abilities and interests of their employees and work groups. A leader can make things happen through inspiring goal-directed behavior and by his/her directing, which is leadership put into action. Directing can reward, punish, strengthen, motivate, and influence individuals, all in support of the task at hand. There are many different types of management/leadership styles, from autocratic to participative, from bureaucratic to laissez-faire. The type of style has a tremendous impact on the amount of effort employees exert toward the organizing process. When working with professionals, a participative leadership style is usually effective at inspiring organization effort. The manager consults with employees concerning goals, work assignments, and directives during the decision-making process. This approach is an attempt to capitalize on the talents and contributions that others have to offer, and it is difficult for participants not to accept the final outcome when they've been a part of it. A leadership style in which the manager is viewed as a facilitator is usually effective when building participation and consensus. Nonetheless the manager is still responsible for giving directives to accomplish the task. This is a major responsibility of the manager and is instrumental to moving the organizing function forward. Issuing directives involves attentions to timing, language, and precision so as to avoid misunderstanding. Directing doesn't stop with the organization function, but rather is carried through the implementation phase where it becomes part of the controlling function. It should be emphasized that the three primary management functions overlap and their boundaries are not distinct. It is unlikely that conflict and disagreement can be totally avoided, but if the planning and organizing of a project have been effectively managed, negative and unpleasant events can be reduced.

Every organization should have an organizational structure. By action and/or inaction, managers provide structure to the organization. Ideally, in developing an organizational structure and distributing authority, managers' decisions reflect the mission, objectives, goals and tactics that grew out of the planning function. Specifically, they have responsibility for making decisions concerning: hiring, division of labor, delegation of authority, departmentalization, scope of responsibility, and coordination.

Organizing depends on good planning, devoted employees, and competent leadership. Staff development and mentorship are qualities that can nurture good employees and make them invaluable to the organization. A manager who is a leader will recognize leadership qualities or other special talents in others and will encourage that individual to take advantage of those skills. Likewise, encouraging a network of individuals who have something in common and are willing to promote each other and the organization in a mutually beneficial manner is a win-win situation for everyone. Through a network, recommendations and ideas may be shared, which will benefit the process. Allowing the staff to seek development and networking opportunities is an investment in their professional growth, as well as contributions they will make to the organization. Investments in staff development will positively influence morale, stimulate enthusiasm, and avoid job stagnation and staff turnover, thereby providing for the retention of good employees and decreasing the need for employee recruitment.

Implementing and Controlling

Case Study

You and your team are ready to begin implementation of your cost reduction plan (see case study in the organizing section for details). The plan will be implemented in phases because of its complexity and the required time lines for some of the ideas.

Issues and Questions to Consider

1. *Define the managing role in the actual implementation.*
2. *What types of challenges could you encounter during implementation, and how would you address them?*

Your plan has been underway for two weeks. You have been asked by hospital administration to attend a leadership meeting and report on the status of your cost reduction plan.

Issues and Questions to Consider

1. *What type of monitors would be helpful to ensure that the implementation is progressing according to plan?*
2. *What methodologies or processes might you use to accomplish any adjustments to the implementation?*
3. *What do you consider to be the key factors indicating your plan's degree of success?*

Implementing and *controlling* could be separate management functions but are discussed together under one function because in practicality they should occur simultaneously. The major core components of the implementing and controlling functions are listed in Table 3–4. Weaved throughout effective control systems are also the following characteristics: control at all levels, acceptability to

TABLE 3–4.   **Major Components of the Implementing and Controlling Functions**

- Monitoring
- Outcomes evaluation
- Personnel management and staff development
- Making adjustments

those responsible for assurance, flexibility, accuracy, timeliness, cost-effectiveness, balance between objectivity and subjectivity. Implementing is the action that starts to put the plan into operation. As implementation takes place, monitoring must be in place to observe plan's performance; otherwise no conclusion will be able to be drawn regarding achieving the desired outcome and goal. Controlling is actually an extension of the directing activity that occurred during the organizing phase, but with the manager playing a much greater role during implementation, as decision making must be swift and deliberate. The control function completes the management function cycle through its outcomes and assessments.

The word *controlling* is often seen as negative, especially in today's work environment. In this context, it is not meant to refer to an exclusive dictatorial or autocratic management, but rather to indicate the process of measuring implementation progress, with the control resting with the manager. Controlling is a performance measurement of implementation whereby adjustments and corrective actions can be made to ensure that organizational goals are achieved. Controlling can take the form of a feedforward (checking ahead of action) to anticipate deviation in implementation and outcomes and prevent it. It can also take the form of concurrent or feedback mechanisms whereby deviations are addressed as they happen or after they occur. The manager is in control of the operation and closely supervises its performance.

The control process should be designed during the organizing to allow for adequate measurement and assessment. It should have as one phase a set of acceptable standards, a second phase of measurement performance, and a third phase for correcting problems or making adjustments. Standards may be quantitative or qualitative and are actually the outcomes that are to be measured. Examples of standards might be related to speed of performance, economics and cost, greater productivity, higher quality, or enhanced reporting. Standards may include benchmarking of an organization's activities to that of another organization, or it may compare output and productivity to some other respectable target. There are standards that are intangible (not measurable) but provide valuable information. Intangible standards include such things as job satisfaction and employee engagement. A well-organized plan should solicit feedback on all aspects of implementation. Listening to feedback and being open to making adjustments are essential to successful implementation. A common critical mistake is to be so locked into the plan that you jeopardize its entire success because you don't make minor adjustments. Needed adjustments and/or the assessment of outcomes will likely reinitiate the planning function and refuel the continuous management process.

In summary, controlling should be both anticipatory and retrospective. The process anticipates problems and takes preventive action. With corrective action, the process also follows up on problems whereby each person in the business views control as his or her responsibility. Controlling is related to each of the other functions of management and builds on planning, organizing and leading. Our final ***outcome assessment*** will be when we reach our objectives and qualitatively (purposeful and enjoyable?) and quantitatively (cost and time?) evaluate the experience of having attained our goals.

SUMMARY

Although the functions of a healthcare manager can be grouped into three primary categories—planning, organizing, and implementing/controlling—they do not exist separately but rather are interconnected in a type of concentric circle. If one of the functions is weak or nonexistent, the success of the project may be compromised. Without continuity, the manager may be seen as weak and ineffective and may not be considered a leader by staff, peers, or executive leadership.

One of the most critical attributes of a successful manager is the ability to balance multiple responsibilities. In the most basic interpretation, this refers to the ability to multi-task, prioritize, organize, and keep agendas moving forward. This balancing act becomes more complicated when there are two or more sides to an issue that require the manager to weigh and consider all potential outcomes (Table 3–5).

This can be a delicate balancing act with the manager as the fulcrum straddling the center. Although it would be ideal to keep everything evenly balanced, this goal is not realistic. If the manager is to be successful and keep advancing the agendas of his/her department, she/he will need to maintain flexibility as urgent situations and priorities warrant. Over the longer term however, balance in the organization must be reestablished and in a reasonable time frame.

In addition to the ongoing struggle to maintain a balance of functionality, a myriad of external pressures are also brought to bear on laboratory management. In this example, external refers to those issues not directly related to testing or producing the product. These issues will pull or stretch the manager in one direction or another at various times. The following diagram illustrates some of these "gravitational external forces" (Figure 3–4).

Health care management functionality is complex and diverse. It requires formal learned skills, experiential skills, and a high level of dedication and commitment; it presents those involved with significant challenges on a daily basis. In

TABLE 3–5. Management Balancing Act

People centered	versus	Task centered
Personnel resources	versus	Capital resources
Laboratory issues	versus	Hospital or corporate issues
Financial goals	versus	Service goals
Opportunities	versus	Threats
Speed	versus	Detailed process
Perceptions	versus	Facts

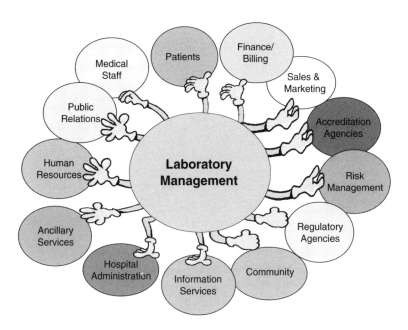

FIGURE 3–4 Laboratory external forces.

return, however, the successful manager will experience a significant degree of achievement and satisfaction.

SUGGESTED PROBLEM-BASED LEARNING ACTIVITIES
Chapter 3: Management Functions

Instructions: Use Internet resources, books, articles, colleagues, etc., to present solutions to the problems listed below. There is no one correct solution to any problem.

Note to Instructor: Students in class may be divided into groups and given the problem-based learning activity to discuss and solve. Once the group has reached consensus as to a solution, the group may present it to the other students in the class. This activity will provide all students with information regarding solutions to the problem.

Problem #1
You have just been hired as the manager of a laboratory. How do you introduce yourself? What is your initial plan of action for being in charge? What are the first steps you intend to take in the running of your laboratory?

Problem #2
Suppose you terminated an employee who has now filed a discrimination complaint. How do you handle this situation?

Problem #3
You are requested to set up an offsite laboratory at a community outreach facility. How would you proceed in the implementation of such a laboratory?

BIBLIOGRAPHY

Daft RL: *Management*, 5th ed. The Dryden Press, Orlando, FL, 2000.

Allen RW: A behavior known as performance. The Dreyden Press, Orlando, FL., 2000.

Bishop JW, Scott KD, Burroughs SM: Support commitment, and employee outcomes in a team environment. *Journal of Management* 2000; 26:1113–1132

Drucker PF: The theory of the business. In *Managing in a Time of Great Change*, Truman Talley Books/Plume, Penquin Putnam, Inc. New York, 1998, pp. 21–38.

DuBrin AJ: *Essentials of Management*, 3rd ed. College Division South-Western Publishing Co., Cincinnati, OH., 1994.

Garcia LS, Balselki BS, Burke MD Schwab DL (eds). Clinical laboratory management 2004. ASM Inc.

Hudson J: Principles of clinical laboratory management : A study guide and worbook, 2003. Prentice Hall.

Jones GR, Gerorge JM, Hill CW: *Contemporary Management*, 2nd ed. Irwin McGraw Hill. Boston, MA., 1998.

Liebler JG, McConnell CR: Part II. The management functions: from theory to application. In *Management Principles for Health Professionals*. Aspen Publications Inc., Gaithersburg, MD., 1999, pp. 85–278.

Robbins SP: *Organizational Behavior*, 9th ed. Prentice Hall, Inc., Upper Saddle River, NJ., 2000.

Snyder JR, Wilkinson DS: Management functions in the clinical laboratory. In Snyder JR, Wilkinson DS (eds): *Management in Laboratory Medicine*, 3rd ed. Lippincott-Raven Publishers, New York, NY., 1998.

Turnbull DC: Communicating successfully in the workplace. *Lab Med* 2005; 36:4 205–08

Workman RD, Lewis MJ, Hill BT: Enhancing the financial performance of a health system laboratory network using an information system. *Am J Clin Pathol* 2000;114(1):9–15.

Internet Resources

Management Functions and Principles
http://books.google.com/books?q=management+ functions+and+principles&oi=print

McNamara, C: Free Basic Guide to Management and Supervision
http://search.msn.com/results.aspx?srch=105&FORM=AS5&q=Free+Basic+Guide+to+Management+and+Supervision
Understanding the Manager's Job
http://search.msn.com/results.aspx?srch=105&FORM=AS5&q=Understanding+the+Manager%e2%80%99s+Job

Managerial Problem Solving and Decision Making

VICKI S. FREEMAN, PhD, MT(ASCP)SC

Chapter Outline

Objectives

Following successful completion of this chapter, the learner should be able to:

1. Define problem solving and decision making.
2. Differentiate decision making from problem solving.
3. Describe the five steps that managers should take to make the best decisions.
4. Explain the eight traps that affect decision making and lead managers to make poor decisions.
5. Describe the PDCA (plan, do, check, act) cycle of group decision making.
6. Contrast PDCA cycle to Six Sigma Methodology for problem solving.
7. Define tools that are used in the decision-making process.
8. Apply the problem-solving process to a relevant laboratory management issue.

Key Terms

Brainstorming
Cost/Benefit Analysis
Decision Making
Decision Tree
Fishbone Diagram

Pareto Chart
Plus/Minus/Interesting
Problem Solving
Scatter Diagram

Case Study: Managerial Problem Solving and Decision Making

You are the manager of a clinical laboratory at a mid-sized (200 bed) community hospital. Physicians and nurses are concerned about the turnaround time for laboratory tests ordered on early morning rounds. It appears that the samples are collected by the phlebotomy team on the 6:00 AM rounds. Physicians begin their patient rounds at 7:30 AM. The physicians prefer to review the results of the laboratory tests ordered at the time they see the patient. They explain to you that they cannot make decisions with regard to further patient treatment or discharge without these results. Time is of the essence, as the hospital is cutting the budget, and it is important to decrease patient length of stay. You are expected to look into this matter and make recommendations regarding the most efficient and effective way to address this problem.

Issues and Questions to Consider
1. *What is the best method of addressing this problem?*
2. *What management techniques/styles might be used?*
3. *Who should be included in a team assigned to address this issue?*
4. *What decision traps might be encountered, and how can they be avoided?*
5. *What decision-making tools would facilitate the analysis of the problem?*

INTRODUCTION

The day-to-day operation of the laboratory requires strong leadership and management. The laboratory manager must serve as an advocate for the laboratory, providing quality patient care while ensuring an effective and efficient customer-centered operation. As physicians, nurses, and other allied health professionals have come to rely on the laboratory to provide them with timely, accurate information to diagnosis and treat the patient, it is important that the laboratory be responsive to any problems that arise and impede the flow of test results. The laboratory manager must intervene and find ways to solve the problem by researching the problem, identifying the causes, and solving it by making a decision from a cadre of alternatives. A proactive manager will welcome this opportunity as a chance to improve the laboratory process and service rather than viewing it as an intrusion.

Problem solving and decision making are interrelated. *Problem solving* is the process of identifying and defining the problem, and determining what happened to cause it and what steps or possible solutions will be necessary to solve it. Problem solving focuses on solving an immediate tangible problem. It consists of multiple steps and includes the decision-making step. *Decision making,* on the other hand, is the process of choosing among several alternatives. It may or may not be the result of an immediate problem, but is usually goal directed. An effective manager uses a systematic process in decision making to choose among the various options using clearly defined criteria. In decision making, the end is first defined and then the means to achieve that end are identified.

This chapter is designed to introduce the learner to the problem-solving process. A discussion of the five associated steps is followed by a detailed description of the problem-solving component known as decision making. Traps associated with decision making, tips for using these components in groups, and strategies and tools used in the decision-making process are also discussed.

STEPS IN THE PROBLEM SOLVING PROCESS

Problems can be structured or unstructured. Structured problems tend to be routine, recurring, and involve an almost automatic process. They have a high degree of certainty with regard to outcome. With structured problems, managers have established rules or guidelines to follow as they have made decisions about the same type of problem many times. Quite often, preplanned actions have been developed to apply to the situation when it arises. An example of a routine problem is the reordering of laboratory supplies on a regular basis or the scheduling of personnel. In contrast, unstructured problems are nonroutine, nonrecurring, have an uncertain outcome, and require new and often unique solutions. These are unusual situations that have not been often addressed. There are no rules to follow, as the decision is new. These decisions are made based on information gathered and a manager's intuition and judgment. Examples of nonroutine problems include the decision to investigate in a new technology or instrumentation in the laboratory or the reorganization of a laboratory section.

There are five steps in the problem-solving process: (1) problem identification, (2) problem analysis, (3) criteria establishment, (4) alternative development and decision making, (5) problem solution feedback.

Problem Identification

Once a manager has identified whether a problem is routine or unique, the problem must be defined. One approach to problem solving is grounded in John Dewey's[1] analysis of the steps in the reflective thinking process. This process emphasizes the detailed analysis of the problem before discussion of solutions and then a systematic evaluation of alternatives. In this model, problem solving consists of five steps. The first step is identifying and defining of the problem. According to Hersey and Blanchard,[2] a problem exists when there is a discrepancy between what one would like to happen and what is actually happening. This discrepancy may be in the eyes of the manager, a subordinate, or a customer. In the laboratory setting, a common complaint heard from individuals outside the laboratory is the time it takes for a laboratory result to be generated and returned to the patient's chart (called turnaround time). In the laboratory, technologists may believe that they are completing the laboratory tests in record time, but from a nurse or physician standpoint, when patient care is the primary concern, the time may seem much too long. The manager must define what ideally should be happening (how long should it take to get a test result back?) and where the discrepancy lies (is it really taking too long? Is the problem pre, post, or during the analytical phase?). At this point, symptoms and evidence that a problem exists are looked at, but not the causes or why a problem exists. Also, information about the problem is collected, potential resources for data collection identified, and unfamiliar terms and concepts defined. It is important that the problem be clarified before proceeding to the next step.

Problem Analysis

The second step in the problem-solving process is the analysis of the problem. After evidence has been collected, the existence of the problem identified, and the problem defined, the manager's attention turns to analyzing the evidence more thoroughly and looking for relevant data that may explain why the problem exists. This step in the procedure is a matter of evaluating the data that has been collected in step 1 and the sources from which that data come. In the turnaround time example, the manager will collect data on the time of the request for the test, the time the specimen is obtained and received in the laboratory, how the specimen is processed, when the test is performed, and when the result is reported back to the patient's chart. Managers must determine the actual problem and avoid looking only at symptoms. By using actual data, as well as individuals' perceptions, the manager will get a clearer picture of the real problem. Managers often leave out this step and jump to conclusions without understanding the root problem. They react on and solve the problem based on those visible symptoms, not the actual root causes of the problem. In other cases, managers are distracted by another problem identified in the data-gathering process and solve it instead of the original problem. Failure to accurately identify the root cause is one of the major reasons why a solution that is tried is unsuccessful. It is often advantageous to invite individuals from outside the laboratory situation to discuss the issues, as they may have insight into the problem and its causes that others within the organization would miss.

Criteria Establishment

Step three in the problem-solving process involves establishing criteria on which potential solutions will be evaluated. Clear specifications of (1) what the decision has to accomplish (this is the most difficult step), (2) what minimum goals must be attained, (3) what objectives the decision has to reach, and (4) what conditions it has to satisfy (boundary conditions) all must be determined. Ideally, based on the definition of the problem and analysis of its cause(s), only one objective should be set that any acceptable solution could attain.

In the case of a turnaround time, considerations may include the following:

1. What criteria are necessary for quality patient care in the turnaround time of a laboratory test? Is 60 minutes soon enough?
2. Does this test result need to be available for physician review in 30 minutes?
3. What data support this need?

By using this information, the laboratory then could set a standard turnaround time against which future turnaround times could be measured for evaluation purposes.

The standard may need to be varied based on the type of laboratory test being performed or the situation of the patient. If the problem is too complex to set only one objective to meet the goal(s) (the desired outcomes), another means for establishing criteria to evaluate proposed solutions is to make a list of "musts" and "wants." "Musts" are those basic requirements without which the solution would be unacceptable. "Wants" are those qualities that are desirable in any solution and should be assessed according to their priority. This type of checklist may help to maximize the effectiveness of any solution without omitting any essential requirements. Constraints or unchangeable factors must also be identified, as these will limit the options. By identifying them early, the manager can avoid solutions that waste time and money.

Alternative Development and Decision Making

Next, the manager must develop appropriate solutions to solve the problem; this is where managerial decision making takes place. The classic model of decision making assumes managers have access to all the information required to reach a decision and that they can make the optimum decision by easily ranking their own preferences among alternatives. However, according to James March,[3] at Stanford University, managers do not consider all the alternatives or consequences and do not evoke all preferences at the same time. Instead of considering all the alternatives simultaneously, decision makers consider only a few and to look at them sequentially. If good alternatives are missed, the resulting decision is poor. It is hard to develop creative alternatives, so managers are encouraged to look for ways to obtain new ideas. Brainstorming is an excellent method to develop a list of potential solutions. From the list of options that emerge, a realistic range of solutions can be developed and the one that best fits the needs selected according to the evaluation criteria set in step 3. Each alternative can be ranked based on its advantages and disadvantages, weaknesses and strengths, and how well it meets the objective. How each alternative satisfies the must and want requirements from step 3 should also be analyzed. According to Stephen Covey,[4] a win-win solution, wherein both parties feel good and feel committed to the decision and action plan, is what should be strived for. To achieve this takes more than time; it takes patience, self-control, and courage balanced with consideration.

Problem Solution and Feedback

The final step in the problem-solving process is to put the solution into place. Often a decision is made and not implemented. Converting the decision into action is the most time-consuming step. First, an action plan must be written that details the steps that need to be taken to implement the solution and the resources required to do it.

Questions to consider are these:

1. Who needs to know of this decision?
2. What action must be taken?
3. Who is to take the action?
4. What does the action have to be so that the people who have to do it can do it?

Criteria to measure, observe, or discern progress toward the objectives and goals—that is, the ultimate desired outcomes—must be set to evaluate the effectiveness of the solution. Feedback must be built into the decision to provide a continuous testing against the actual experience and the expectations that underlie the decision. This "feedback" must test the validity and effectiveness of the decision against the actual course of events. Managers must consider what went right and wrong with the decision and learn for the future. Without feedback, managers never learn from experience and will make the same mistake again.

DECISION-MAKING PROCESS

Decision making is the process by which managers respond to opportunities and threats by analyzing options, and making decisions about goals and courses of action. This process occurs in step 4 of the problem-solving process. It is the most important management skill that an individual who aspires to become a leader can acquire. The speed in which a decision must be made will vary based on the problem to be solved. Effective managers must make quick as well as complicated decisions by drawing on their own experiences, reliable sources of information, good "sounding boards," and a fairly clear sense of purpose. They also must be willing to act and accept necessary risks when making the decision. At times, a manager must make a quick decision such as in the case of a "life and death" or critical situation. The worst case scenario in these cases may be that not making a decision is worse than making a poor decision. These quick decisions are often made on the run, with limited time, limited information, and limited participation of others. At other times, the decision requires more information to be gathered, more input from others, and lots of alternatives generated and evaluated. These complicated decisions come together in bits and pieces over an extended period of months or even years. Usually, many people are involved. The group decision-making process is discussed later in this chapter.

Decision-Making Traps

Even though making decisions is the most important activity that managers engage in, individuals are generally amateurs when it comes to making the right decision. Because of the numerous internal and external influences that exert pressure on an individual, many hidden traps can be found in decision making (see Hammond et al.).[5] A manager should become aware of these perceptual and behavioral decision traps in decision-making situations to actively avoid them.

The first trap, the **anchoring trap,** is an approach that many negotiators use to influence an individual's perception by giving information up front that later affects the decision that is made. "When considering a decision, the mind gives disproportionate weight to the first information it receives. Initial impressions, estimates, or other data anchor subsequent thoughts and judgments." An example of this trap is a sales representative giving a price for a product or new instrument and what the contract for that commodity would be. The manager then comes back with a counteroffer, which is usually somewhat lower than the price originally offered by the company. However, the company has established, upfront, the negotiation table. A manager should be wary of anchors in negotiations.

Individuals instinctively stay with what seems familiar. Thus they look for decisions that involve the least change. This is called the **status-quo trap.** To protect their egos from damage, individuals avoid changing the status quo, even in the face of early predictions that change will be safer. They look for reasons to do nothing. Quite often, in business, making an incorrect change (doing something) tends to be punished much more severely than doing nothing. In all parts of life, people want to avoid rocking the boat. Managers can avoid this trap by first thinking about their objectives and goals when preparing to make a decision. They should review how these objectives and goals are served by the status quo rather than a change and look at each possible change, one at a time, so as not to be overwhelmed and instinctively want to stay "safe" and unchanged.

The **sunk-cost trap** (or the justify-past-actions trap) is the escalation of commitment because of an individual's past decisions, believe they must continue in that direction, although the reason is no longer valid. The more actions that a manager has already taken on behalf of a choice or direction, the more difficult the manager finds it to change direction or make a different choice. Whenever an individual has invested time, money, or other resources in a decision, or whenever their personal reputation is at stake, they find it much more difficult to change their decision or course of action. How can a manager avoid this trap? As Warren Buffet, a successful business investor, once said, "When you find yourself in a hole, the best thing you can do is stop digging." Managers can help themselves and their subordinates to make better decisions by setting an example of admitting mistakes in their choices and changing course. Subordinates will then believe they can do likewise without penalties.

People have a tendency to subconsciously decide what they want to do before they figure out why they want to do it. The **confirming-evidence trap** is a mental bias that leads managers to seek out information to support their existing point of view while avoiding information that contradicts it. This bias affects where they go to collect data to reinforce a current stance or perspective and how they interpret the facts received. It then leads them to give too much weight to supporting information and opinions and too little to those that are conflicting. To avoid this trap, managers should have someone play devil's advocate or build counterarguments themselves. They should not accept evidence confirming their viewpoint without questioning it and should make sure that the people from which they are gaining a perspective can offer independent information and opinions.

The next mental trap, the **framing trap,** deals with how you view your choices or how you frame the questions around the problem. Because the first step in the problem-solving process is identifying and defining the problem, this trap can be especially dangerous. This trap is also perilous, as it can lead to managers bringing other traps into the process. A frame can establish the status quo, introduce an anchor, lead a manager to justify past actions, or highlight confirming evidence. To avoid this trap, a manager should find ways to restate the problem or situation presented to them in their own way and take the opportunity to see it from different sides to envision various outcomes.

The following three traps are based on the ability of a manager to estimate and forecast uncertain events. Managers make decisions under three conditions: (1) certainty—they know the outcome (this never really occurs), (2) uncertainty—they have absolutely no idea what will happen, (3) or risk—they have some degree of understanding in regard to the possible outcomes (most common). By forecasting what might happen, then a manager will have a better chance of making a successful decision.

In the **overconfidence trap,** managers believe they are better at making forecasts or estimates than they actually are. Overly confident about their ability to predict, most managers set too narrow a range of possibilities. Ironically, research has found a positive relationship between overconfidence and task difficulty. In other words, the harder the task, the more people are apt to make decisions with confidence, almost as a self-justification.

Managers can also be overly cautious or prudent in forecasting; this is called the **prudence trap.** When faced with high-stakes decisions, they tend to adjust their estimates or forecasts "just to be on the safe side." A manager will look for the worst-case scenario and make decisions based on this analysis, which can be just as damaging as being overconfident.

The last trap, the **recallability trap,** is an association bias in terms of "it worked before." In this trap, managers get caught using past experiences to forecast the future and become overly influenced by events that left a strong impression on them.

By being aware that these traps can distort their thinking, involving others in the decision-making process, gathering appropriate data, and building checks and balances into their decision-making process, managers can avoid these traps as they make their decisions.

Group Decision-Making Process

"Enlightened leaders and business managers . . . know that when people are meaningfully involved, they willingly commit the best that is in them. Moreover, when people identify their personal goals with the goals of an Organization, they release an enormous amount of energy, creativity, and loyalty" (Covey p. 221).[6] Although managers find that it is often easier to make a decision alone, they also find that decisions made by oneself are often not the best decisions. Therefore, involving other individuals and groups in the decision-making process is best. However, the type of group involvement should be determined by the quality of decision needed, the amount of information available, and the degree of group acceptance needed for success. The amount of subordinate/group involvement in the decision-making process is referred to as *decision participation.* The leader may follow one of four decision making styles when involving the group in the decision (Yuki, 1981).[7]

In the **autocratic style,** the leader makes the decision without consulting with others. The leader may use only the information available at the time or may obtain more information from group members. The role played by team members in making the decision is one of providing the necessary information to the leader rather than generating or evaluating alternative solutions. In the **consultative style,** the leader obtains suggestions and ideas from the team members, but then makes the decision that may or may not reflect the team members' influence. The third participative style, **joint decision,** is also sometimes called the democratic style. The leader shares the problem with the relevant team members as a group. Together they generate and evaluate alternatives and attempt to reach agreement (**consensus**) on a solution. The leader's role is much like that of chairperson. The leader does not try to influence the group to adopt a solution and is willing to accept and implement any solution that has support of the entire group. In the last style, **delegation,** the leader turns over the problem to the group and lets them generate and evaluate alternatives and attempt to reach agreement on a solution without any leader involvement. When they reach agreement, they tell the leader what their solution is and then together begin the process of implementation.

Approaches to problem solving, such as the Shewhart Cycle of Management and Six Sigma, have common roots and overlapping principles. The roots of process improvement can be traced back to Walter Shewhart who developed the concept of Statistical Process Control, to aid a manager in making scientific, efficient, economical decisions. He based this process control on Carl Frederick Gauss' (1777-1855) work. Gauss introduced the concept of the normal curve (i.e. the Gaussian curve). In the 1920's, Shewhart showed that three sigma from the mean is the point where a process requires correction. Six Sigma as a measurement standard can be traced back to this work. Additionally, Shewhart conceived the Shewhart Cycle of Management process, based on the traditional scientific method to examine processes and remove undesirable causes and their effects. This Cycle of Management process also called the Plan-Do-Check (or Study)-Act cycle (PDCA) was later modified and applied by Deming.[8]

Many measurement standards (Cpk, Zero Defects, etc.) later came on the scene but credit for coining the term "Six Sigma" goes to a Motorola engineer named Bill Smith. Six Sigma" is a federally registered trademark of Motorola. The tools of Six Sigma are most often applied within a simple performance improvement model known as Define-Measure-Analyze-Improve-Control, or DMAIC.

Edward Deming[9] applied the problem-solving approach to work processes and team decision making for Japanese companies. He envisioned it as a circular system in which the work and processes are thought of as a continuous cycle, not a linear path with a beginning, middle, and end. There are many overlaps to this model and John Dewey's reflective thinking process. However, the use of problem-solving tools to help group members make decisions is a key part of the Deming group problem-solving approach. A centerpiece of the Deming's vision of the effective team is the use of the consensus method for making key decisions. A consensus requires unity, but not unanimity, and concurrence, but not consistency. A consensus is reached when all members can say they either agree with the decision or have had their "day in court" and were unable to convince the others of their viewpoint. In the final analysis, everyone agrees to support the outcome. The consensus approach is appropriate when (1) there is no clear answer, (2) there is no single expert in the group, (3) a commitment to the decision is essential, and (4) sufficient time is available to allow everyone to have input.

The following section will discuss the Shewhart cycle as a group decision-making model and contrast this cycle with the Six Sigma methodology.

The Shewhart Cycle

The Shewhart Cycle   As common causes of problems are inherent in every process and are not attributable to the worker, only a data-driven, scientific approach that involves participants in the process can identify and eliminate these causes. The **Shewhart cycle** is a continuous, circular process that includes the 4 steps: Plan, Do, Check and Act (Figure 4–1). The next section describes the components of each step.

Step 1: Plan   The team identifies the real problem and spends time defining and analyzing the nature of the problem. They must spend sufficient effort to understand the steps in the process and the causes of the problem. How the problem is defined affects the kinds of solutions that are seen. By describing the process, reviewing available data, and identifying the customers, the team begins to

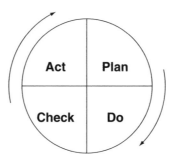

FIGURE 4–1   The Shewhart cycle. The above figure is modified and for public use. *Source: http://138.13.244.106/xpmq/xpmqresources/chapter5handbookA.htm*

understand the process to be studied. Rather than relying on hunches or historical data, the teams develop skills in data collection and analysis to illuminate the root causes of problems and to identify solutions that are meaningful to the customer.

Describe the process.   The process to be studied must be described in a step-wise manner, so that each individual contribution is understood and the resources used are identified.

Example: Laboratory Turnaround Time—Request Receipt

1. *Request received from hospital floor via: telephone call, written communication, computer.*
2. *If the request is from computer system, it can be directly processed.*
3. *If the request is via telephone or written communication, it must be entered into the computer system before it can be processed by the phlebotomist.*
4. *Request sent to phlebotomist to draw.*

Review existing information.   The team must identify potential sources of existing data or information to determine the gaps that need to be filled.

Example: Laboratory Turnaround Time

Information can be gathered from the hospital floor, patient charts, the LIS (laboratory information system), the HIS (hospital information system) and laboratory work logs. Information available might include: number of requests received by laboratory, time of requests sent, method of request transmission, time results returned to patient chart, and time of call from floor.
Potential gaps include:

1. *Personnel time to answer phone calls and send out information.*
2. *How the laboratory handles the requests sent to them.*
3. *The time frame of the responses (turnaround time).*

Identify customers.   Define all of the internal and external customers for a given process. Note: quality should be defined by the needs of the customer.

Example: *Laboratory Turnaround Time*

Internal customers: phlebotomists, receptionists, technicians, technologists
External customers: nursing staff, medical staff, patients

Select appropriate strategies to gather meaningful data.   The team must begin to identify approaches that will allow them to collect data about the outcomes of the current process, the experiences their customers have with the process, and where the problems in that process may exist. Developing surveys of external and internal customers, collecting information from databases, and developing new databases for collection of information are all methods to gather data. The methods used will vary with the process being studied.

Interview customers.   The team surveys the customers and asks them to identify their quality requirements and preferences. This allows the organization to anticipate rather than react to customer needs. The team begins by interviewing their customers, focusing on root causes and barriers to improvement, and basing their decisions and actions on real data. The team members survey customers to provide input to process, to define quality, and to identify concerns about the process.

Example: *Laboratory Turnaround Time*

Interview individual nursing and medical staff about their experiences.
Interview laboratory phlebotomists, technicians, and technologists about their experiences.

Plot process out on a process flow chart.   The process is then tracked on a flowchart form. A flowchart will help to determine the appropriate sequence and to determine what training and resources are necessary and which people need to be involved (Figure 4–2).

Brainstorm problem and produce a fishbone diagram.   Once the process is mapped out, the cause of the problem is then explored through brainstorming and a tool called a fishbone diagram (Figure 4–3). This allows the team to see all of the factors that might affect the process. The *fishbone diagram* (discussed in detail later in this chapter) is an effective method for studying the process and for planning. It is a pictorial list of the factors, with branches representing the main categories of potential causes of problems. Typical categories include people, methods, equipment and materials, and environment.

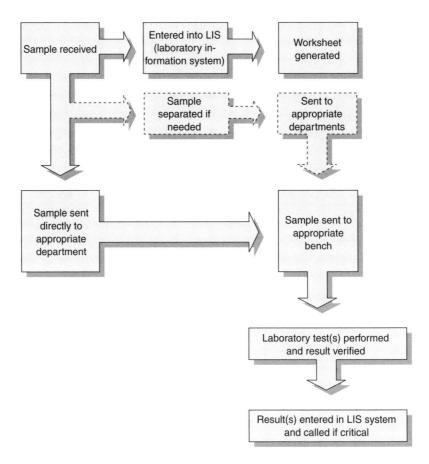

FIGURE 4–2   Example of a process flow chart.

**Collect data on the process.**   Team members gather facts by reviewing exist-ing literature, talking with the customers, and collecting data on the process. Data that is gathered is used as a guide to improvement and diagnosis of the problem, not as an accountability device. The team uses the data to define the problem and understand its root causes. They seek to understand the process and how deci-sions about potential solutions might affect the process.

The team cannot improve a process without data. Data are often numerical, but they might also include characterizations of how a process really works or other kinds of facts. In virtually every process to improve quality, participants learn by using the PDCA cycle that their initial judgments about the nature of the problem and its root causes are, at best, partially supported by the data. Often the data yield surprises.

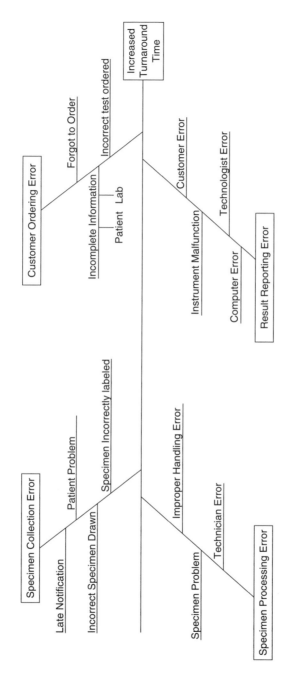

FIGURE 4–3 Laboratory example of a fishbone diagram.

Data on the nature and magnitude of the problem are collected. Then more data are collected to ensure that the cause or causes are the root problem.

Example: Laboratory Turnaround Time

Data that might be collected include:

- *number of requests received by laboratory*
- *time of requests sent*
- *method of request transmission*
- *time results returned to patient chart*
- *time of call from floor requesting results*

Analyze the data.   Data collected may be tallied and analyzed using a chart as shown here. Other tools may also be used to diagram the data (e.g., histograms, pareto charts, scatter diagrams, run charts, statistical process control charts). Scatter diagrams (Figure 4–4) are covered in more detail in the Decision-Making Strategies and Tools section later in this chapter.

Example: Laboratory Turnaround Time

	Reasons for Delays	*Average Time of Delays*	*Average Number of Delays*	*Total*
A	number of requests received by laboratory			
B	time of requests sent			
C	method of request transmission			
D	time results returned to patient chart			
E	time of call from floor requesting results			

Develop a theory or hypothesis.   Team members use the data collected and analyzed to develop a theory or hypothesis about the causes of the problem for process improvement. (If we do such and such, the process will improve in these ways for these reasons.)

Remember, the plan is to fix a process, not the outcomes. A team must be careful about adding steps to a process, as this adds opportunities for new problems. Teams must make each process as simple as possible to improve quality.

> *Example:* **Laboratory Turnaround Time**
>
> ---
>
> *Patient care is being compromised because essential information that should be received by the laboratory is missing. A training session for physicians and nurses should be arranged.*

Step 2: Do   In this step, the team implements the improvement effort they planned using a small-scale test. The individuals responsible for implementation must know what the goal of this change is, must know how it affects the implementation process, and must receive training in the process.

   Test the hypothesis.   In the Do step, the hypothesis that was developed is tried out. A solution is determined and implemented. The team tries out the solution in a limited way to be sure that it works. The question to be asked is: Did the solution work as intended, or does it need revision?

> *Example:* **Laboratory Turnaround Time**
>
> ---
>
> - *Develop and implement a training program for physicians and nurses.*
> - *Track laboratory requests through the process from ordering to reporting out of test results.*
> - *Gather data on turnaround times.*
> - *Send out a follow-up survey to customers.*

Step 3: Check   The results of the improvement effort are measured in this step. The data collected is analyzed and the results studied to see if the process was improved. This gives the team a chance to see if the correct components of the process were measured. It allows team members the opportunity to examine and evaluate any variables that may be present in the process.

   Check by collecting data.   The team tests the hypothesis by collecting data as they did earlier in the process. The results are monitored against the original data to ascertain if the desired outcome is achieved. Data are collected at this stage to be sure that the new process is better than the old one (Figure 4–2).

Step 4: Act   If the results showed the expected improvement, the team should standardize and document all actions with the intention of making the changes permanent. Otherwise, the teams' next step would be to reevaluate by returning to the "plan" step and starting the cycle over with the newly acquired knowledge.

   Implement.   When the team is satisfied with the results, the solution is implemented permanently in all areas where it is relevant.

   Monitor.   Periodically, the process is monitored to ensure that the root cause does not recur and to examine other opportunities for improvement. It is important that the team return to the customers and obtain continuous feedback on the process and how the change is working.

The PDCA cycle enables team members of work groups to identify customer expectations, determine the standards and measurements that will be used to meet these expectations, and continuously evaluate and improve the quality of the work they perform. As issues or problems arise in the application of the process, the systematic problem-solving process ensures the thorough analysis of the problem, the determination of the true cause, and the careful planning and implementation of the optimum solution.

Six Sigma DMAIC Methodology[10]

The Six Sigma DMAIC methodology can also be thought of as a roadmap for problem solving and product/process improvement. DMAIC, as does the PDCA cycle, refers to a data-driven quality strategy for improving processes, and is an integral part of the Six Sigma Quality Initiative. DMAIC is an acronym for five interconnected phases: Define, Measure, Analyze, Improve, and Control. Each step in the cyclical DMAIC Process is required to ensure the best possible results. The first 3 steps of the DMAIC process is encompassed in the splits the Planning step of the PDCA cycle. These process steps include: (1) defining the project goals/customer, (2) measuring the current process performance, and (3) determining the root causes of the problem. Each step is detailed below:

In *Step 1*, defining the project goals and customer (internal and external) deliverables, it is important to first define who customers are, what their requirements are for products and services, and what their expectations are. Then the project boundaries, the stop and start of the process, must be defined. Finally, the process to be improved must be determined by mapping the process flow. *Step 2* measures the process to determine current performance. In step 2, the method to measure the core business process involved is developed. This includes developing a data collection plan for the process, collecting data from many sources to determine types of defects and metrics, and comparing to customer survey results to determine shortfall. *Step 3* analyzes and determines the root cause(s) of the defects. This step includes analyzing the data collected and process map to determine root causes of defects and opportunities for improvement, identifying gaps between current performance and goal performance, prioritizing opportunities to improve, and identifying sources of variation.

Step 4 in the Six Sigma methodology is similar to the "Do" and "Check" steps in the Shewhart cycle. In Step 4 the process is improved by eliminating defects. Creative solutions are used to fix and prevent problems, creating innovative solutions using technology and discipline, and developing and deploying an implementation plan to the targeted process.

Finally, *Step 5*, control future process performance, is basically the "Act" step of the Shewhart cycle. In step 5, the improvements are controlled to keep the process on the new course and to prevent reverting back to the "old way". This step involves the development, documentation and implementation of an ongoing monitoring plan. The improvements are institutionalized through the modification of systems and structures (staffing, training, incentives) in this final step.

Six Sigma uses many of the same tools at the Shewhart Cycle discussed below, but its focus is a more structured application of tools and techniques and tends to be on the financial aspect of the business and the dollars saved through its process improvement. This methodology, when applied on a company-wide scale, becomes part of the culture of the organization.

DECISION-MAKING STRATEGIES AND TOOLS

Data analysis is an essential part of any problem-solving team. Problem areas are identified and useful solutions are determined based on data collected and analyzed. The process can be simplified with the use of several helpful tools. Through the use of such tools, team members can work with their customers through situations or problems that arise. By the team focusing on processes used in a laboratory environment, a system to address a situation or problem can be created that allows everyone involved to feel like they have some control. Further, it is hoped that individuals involved will possess responsibility for the success of the laboratory, as well as for their own role in the process. Eight analytical tools are described next: (1) benchmarking, (2) brainstorming, (3) scatter diagrams, (4) Pareto charts, (5) PMI—plus/minus/interesting, (6) decision trees, (7) fish bone diagram/honeycomb cause and effect, and (8) cost/benefit analysis.

Benchmarking

An organization can determine a measure of its processes against those of recognized leaders in the field and how it measures up to the standard set by those leaders. This process provides an opportunity to identify where improvement will be most beneficial and is called **benchmarking.** Both quantitative and qualitative performance measures can be used to benchmark an organization. Organizations usually establish performance indicators in 4 categories: 1) cost effectiveness, 2) staff productivity, 3) process efficiency, and 4) cycle time. Some examples of performance indicators that benchmarking practitioners can use, depending on the needs of their specific benchmarking task, are found in Table 4–1.

Brainstorming

Brainstorming is a method for developing creative solutions to problems. It works by focusing on a problem and then deliberately coming up with as many unbounded solutions as possible and then pushing the ideas as far as possible. The idea of brainstorming is to generate, clarify, and evaluate a sizable list of ideas, problems, or issues. Brainstorming is a popular technique for enlisting the creative thinking of an individual to meet the purpose of the team. During the brainstorming session there is no criticism of ideas: The idea is to open up as many possibilities as possible and to break down preconceptions about the limits

TABLE 4–1. Performance Indicators

Performance Indicator	Data to Gather and Analyze
Accuracy	Do the performance reports of the laboratory show that tests are performed accurately and precisely?
Responsiveness	Does the laboratory respond to requests from their customers in a timely manner? Do they address potential problems?
Monitoring	Does the laboratory have an ongoing quality improvement program that identifies important problems in patient care?
Accessibility	How accessible is the operation to its clients?
Quality	How often do laboratory reports have to be amended?
Coverage	Does the laboratory provide a comprehensive set of tests?
Timeliness	Are the laboratory results reported in a timely manner? What is the turnaround time?
Cost	Does the reimbursement rate for the tests equal the cost?
Reporting	Are the laboratory results reported correctly and timely?

Adapted from the American Productivity & Quality Center Benchmarking Indicators. http://www.apqc.org

of the problem. Once this has been done, results of the brainstorming session can be analyzed and the best solutions can be explored either using further brainstorming or more conventional solutions.

In the generation phase, the team leader reviews the rules for brainstorming and the team members generate a list of items. The objective is quantity, not quality of ideas. In the clarification phase, the team reviews the list to ensure everyone understands each item. Discussion is scheduled for a later time. In the evaluation phase, the team examines the list to remove duplicative, nonrelevant, or forbidden (on basis of agreed upon ground rules) items.

Scatter Diagrams

A *scatter diagram* is a plot of one variable versus another to see if there is any relationship between the two (e.g., customer turnaround time and time of day). Variable A is plotted on one axis and Variable B is plotted on the other. Different factors can affect process and the people doing the work. The combination of two factors can often have a positive or negative effect on the process. When there is no correlation, no apparent relationship between the two variables is found. If positive correlation is found, there is a defined, predictable relationship between the two variables. An increase in one variable is accompanied by a predictable increase in the other variable. On the other hand, although there is a defined, predictable relationship between the two variables, in negative correlation each increase in one variable is accompanied by a predictable decrease in the other variable (Figure 4–4).

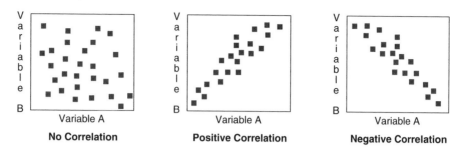

FIGURE 4–4   **Example of scatter diagrams.**

Pareto Charts

Pareto charts help to identify major factors and distinguish between the "vital few" causes and the potentially less significant ones. They are used to rank order causes from most to least significant. Such a graphic technique is based on the Pareto principle, which states that just a few of the causes often account for most of the effect. It is often referred to as the 80-20 rule (80% of the problems can be attributed to 20% of the causes). The Pareto diagram displays, in decreasing order, the relative contribution of each cause to the total problem. Relative contribution may be based on the number of occurrences, the cost associated with each cause, or another measure of impact on the problem (Figure 4–5).

PMI—Plus/Minus/Interesting

PMI stands for *'plus/minus/interesting.'* It is a valuable development (by Edward de Bono) of the pros and cons technique used for centuries. PMI is a basic decision-making tool. When you are facing a difficult decision, simply create a table with the categories *Plus, Minus,* and *Interesting.* In the column underneath the Plus heading, write down all the positive points of taking the action. Underneath the Minus heading, write down all the negative effects. In the Interesting column, write down the extended implications of taking the action, whether positive or negative.

Scoring your PMI table.   You may be able to make a decision from the table alone. Alternatively, consider each of the points you have written down and assign a positive or negative score to each appropriately. The scores you assign can be entirely subjective. Once you have done this, add up the score. A strongly positive score indicates that an action should be taken; a strongly negative score indicates that it should be avoided (Table 4–2).

Decision Trees

Management invariably encounters situations in which uncomfortable decisions must be made. In some cases, the difficulty may be that, although certain alternative choices are clear, the consequences of these choices are not readily apparent.

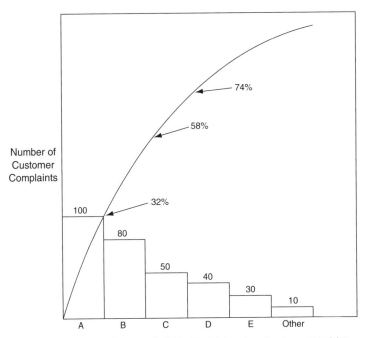

Deficiencies A through C account for 74% of the total number of customer complaints.

FIGURE 4–5   Pareto Chart.

TABLE 4–2.   Example of a Plus/Minus/Interesting Table Used in Decision Making

Should that laboratory send a test out to be performed at another laboratory?

Plus	Minus	Interesting	Total
Less expensive (+5)	High turnaround time (−6)	Newer technology (+1)	
High volume (+3)	Less exposure for MT students (−3)	Learn more about new technology in-house (+2)	
Chance of sample misplacement greater (+5)	Less technologists needed (−3)	More difficult to get sample to laboratory (−4)	
	Loss of technologist's expertise (−3)		
Totals + 13	−15	−1	−3

Total = −3—It would be best to keep the test in-house.

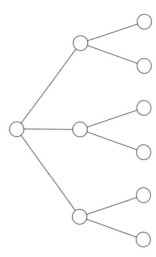

FIGURE 4–6   Decision tree.

One possible tool for a manager in such a situation is decision tree analysis. A *decision tree* is a graphic diagram consisting of nodes and branches. The nodes are of two types. The first is a rectangle that represents the decision to be made. The branches emanating from decision nodes are the alternative choices with which the manager is faced. One one alternative can be implemented. The second type of node is a circle. Circles represent chance nodes. That is, the alternatives emanating from chance nodes have some element of uncertainty as to whether or not they will occur. The primary benefit of a decision tree is that it provides a visual representation of the choices facing the manager (Figure 4–6).

Fish Bone/Honeycomb Cause and Effect

A fishbone diagram (Figure 4–7) systematically analyzes cause-and-effect relationships and identifies potential root causes of a problem. Cause-and-effect or fishbone diagrams are used to display the relationships between a given effect and its potential causes. Such a graphic technique is used to sort out and relate the interactions among the factors affecting a process. A well-detailed cause-and-effect diagram is shaped like a fishbone.

Cost-Benefit Analysis

Cost/benefit analysis refers to the several approaches for determining and comparing the forward looking, incremental costs, benefits, and values of solution alternatives. It determines whether the results of a particular course of action are of

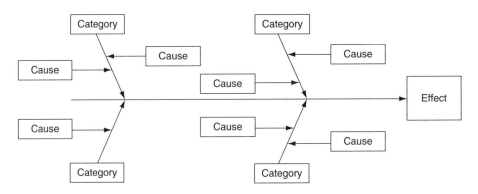

FIGURE 4–7   **Fishbone/Honeycomb Cause and Effect.**

sufficient benefit to justify the cost of taking the action. Ideally, precise, in-depth economic analyses should be performed by examining the cash flow impact of each alternative, taking into account the time value of money. However, less rigorous evaluations may be appropriate if there are no significant amounts of up-front investment and/or ongoing cash outflows involved.

These are just a few of the many analytical tools available to teams and managers to detail out processes to make an informed decision. The value of the tools lies in the ability of the team to look at various pieces of data in different perspectives and frames of reference. It helps the team members to move from their departmental biases to a more neutral point of view; however, it is also important for the team to not focus so much on the use of these tools that it delays their decision making.

SUMMARY

Problem solving and decision making are important functions of a laboratory manager to ensure both the smooth operation of the laboratory and quality patient care. By using John Dewey's reflective thinking process, managers should identify the problem, analyze it using data gathered, establish criteria for making a decision and develop alternatives, and finally implement the solution. By following this process, they can avoid the many traps, both internal and external, that exist in the decision-making step of the problem-solving process. Involving individuals in the problem-solving process can be important to the buy-in of the final decision. Using a systematic problem solving process, such as the PDCA, and analysis tools, such as scatter diagrams and Pareto charts on the data gathered, ensures the thorough analysis of customer expectations and concerns with a detailed view of the entire problem.

SUGGESTED PROBLEM-BASED LEARNING ACTIVITIES
Chapter 4: Managerial Problem Solving and Decision Making

Instructions: Use Internet resources, books, articles, colleagues, etc., to present solutions to the problems listed below. There is no one correct solution to any problem.

Note to Instructor: Students in class may be divided into groups and given the problem-based learning activity to discuss and solve. Once the group has reached consensus as to a solution, the group may present it to the other students in the class. This activity will provide all students with information regarding solutions to the problem.

Problem #1
Suppose you are a laboratory director and one of your supervisors resigns. Create a work group to share supervisory responsibilities over that laboratory section until a new individual can be hired and trained.

Problem #2
Imagine yourself as a laboratory supervisor or manager. How would you delegate authority? How would you organize this process?

Problem #3
Create a transition team to implement a change in laboratory operations. Identify and clarify the roles of the individuals on the team.

REFERENCES

1. Dewey, J. *Problem Solving Tasks (Reflective Problem-solving) How We Think.* Boston: D.C. Heath and Company, 1933.
2. Hersey P, Blanchard K. *Management of Organizational Behavior.* Prentice Hall, Inc. 8th Edition. Englewood Cliffs, NY., 2000.
3. James G. March, a pioneering and respected expert on decision making at Stanford University, Jack Steele Parker Professor of International Management, Emeritus.
4. Covey SR. *Principle-Centered Leadership.* Simon & Schuster. NewYork, NY., 1992.
5. Hammond JS, Keeney RL, Raiffa H. The Hidden Traps in Decision Making. *Harvard Business Review.* Sept-Oct, 1998.
6. Covey SR. *Principle-Centered Leadership.* Simon & Schuster. NewYork, NY., 1992.
7. Yukl GA.: *Leadership in Organizations.* Prentice-Hall, Inc., Englewood Cliffs, NJ., 2005.
8. Six Sigma *http://www.isixsigma.com/*

9. Deming WE: *Out of the Crisis*. The MIT Press; 1st edition. 2000.
10. Brue G: *Six Sigma for Managers*. Mcgraw-HillCompanies, Inc. NJ. 2005.
11. Higgins L, Hack B: Measurement in the 21st Century. American Productivity & Quality Center. http://www.apqc.org. 2004.

Bibliography

Birnbaum R, Deshotels J: Has the Academy Adopted *TQM*? *Planning for Higher Education*. 1999; 28: 29-37.

Brue G: *Six Sigma for Managers*. McGraw-Hill Companies, Inc. NJ. 2005.

Chaffee EE, Sherr LA: *Quality: Transforming Postsecondary Education*. Washington DC, The George Washington University, 1992.

Chaffee EE: Assessing Impact: Evidence and Action. Presentations from the AAHE Conference on Assessment & Quality; Miami Beach, FL., June: 11–15, 1997.

Coate E.: The Introduction of Total Quality Management at Oregon State University. *Higher Education*, 1993; 25: 303-320.

Covey SR: *Principle-Centered Leadership*. Simon & Schuster. New York, NY., 1992.

Covey SR: *The 8th Habit: From Effectiveness to Greatness*. Simon & Schuster. New York, NY., 2004.

Dewey J: *Problem Solving Tasks (Reflective Problem-solving) How We Think*. Boston, D.C. Heath and Company, 1933.

Grant LF, Kelley JH, Northington L, Barlow D: Using TQM/CQI Processes To Guide Development of Independent and Collaborative Learning in Two Levels of Baccalaureate Nursing Students. *Journal of Nursing Education*, 2002; 41: 537–40.

Hammond JS, Keeney RL, Raiffa H. The Hidden Traps in Decision Making. Clinical Laboratory Management Review 1999 January/February, p. 40.

Helms MM, Williams AB, Nixon JC: TQM Principles and Their Relevance to Higher Education: The Question of Tenure and Post-Tenure Review. *International Journal of Educational Management*. 2001; 15: 322–331.

Hersey P, Blanchard K, Johnson D: *Management of Organizational Behavior*, 8th Ed. Prentice Hall Inc. Englewood Cliffs, NJ., 2000.

Masters RJ, Leiker, L: Total quality management in higher education: applying Deming's fourteen points. *CUPA Journal* 1992; Summer: 27–31.

Munoz MA: Total Quality Management and the Higher Education Environment: Impact on Educational Leadership Theory and Practice. 1999; Eric Document ED462880.

Patterson M, Baker D, Gable C, et al: Faculty research productivity in allied health settings: A TQM approach. *J Allied Health* 1993; Summer: 249–261.

Richardson WC: Introduction to the final draft report of the advisory panel for allied health. *J Allied Health* 1992; Fall: 25–28.

Seymour D, Chaffee EE: TQM for student outcomes assessment. *AGB Reports* 1992; January/February: 26–30.

Streibel BJ, Joiner BL, Scholtes PR: *The Team Handbook.* Joiner/Oriel, Inc., Madison, WI., 2003.

Vazzana G, Elfrink J, Bachmann DP: A Longitudinal Study of Total Quality Management Processes in Business Colleges. *Journal of Education for Business* 2000; 76: 69–74.

Soetaert E: Quality in the Classroom: Classroom Assessment Techniques as TQM. *New Directions for Teaching and Learning.* 1998; 75: 47–55.

Yukl GA: *Leadership in Organizations.* Prentice-Hall, Inc, Englewood Cliffs, NJ., 2005.

Internet References

American Productivity & Quality Center
  http://infoweb.magi.com/~riqn/benchr.html

Decision Tree
  http://www.eskimo.com/~mighetto/lstree.htm

Six Sigma
  http://www.isixsigma.com/

Problem Solving
  http://en.wikipedia.org.wiki/Problem_solving

Problem Solving and Decision Making
  http://ollie.dcccd.edu/MGMT1374/book_contents/2planning/prob_solvg/prob_solv.htm

Managing people is one of the key responsibilities of laboratory managers. The ability to understand and follow human resource guidelines and regulations, as well as to perform job analyses, write job descriptions, and manage work groups, is critical to this end. Laboratory managers must also participate in performance evaluation and professional development issues with their employees. An introduction to the basic aspects of education and training also assists laboratory managers to achieve good human resource skills.

Section II consists of four chapters based on human resource issues. Because of the overlap of select terms and concepts in each of the topics covered, discussions of them occur in multiple chapters, where appropriate.

Section II Contents:

Human Resource Guidelines and Regulations

CHRISTINE V. WALTERS, MAS, JD, SPHR

Chapter Outline

Objectives

Following successful completion of this chapter, the learner will be able to:

1. List and define at least two key legal issues and at least one proactive measure an employer may take in the area of recruitment.
2. List and define at least two key legal issues and at least one proactive measure an employer may take in the area of compensation.
3. List and define at least two key legal issues and at least one proactive measure an employer may take in the area of leave benefits.
4. List and define at least two key legal issues and at least one proactive measure an employer may take in the area of employee/labor relations.
5. List and define at least two key legal issues and at least one proactive measure an employer may take in the area of termination.
6. Accurately describe the minimum legal duty imposed on an employer for each of these areas.
7. Compare and contrast various approaches to managing conflicts in each of the areas covered in this chapter.

Key Terms

Affirmative Action

Age Discrimination in
  Employment Act (ADEA)

Americans with Disabilities Act
  (ADA)

Bona Fide Occupational
  Qualifications (BFOQ)

Equal Employment Opportunity
  Commission (EEOC)

Equal Pay Act (EPA)

Fair Labor Standards Act of 1938
  (FLSA)

Family and Medical Leave Act
  of 1993 (FMLA)

Title VII of the Civil Rights Act
  of 1964

Unlawful Harassment

INTRODUCTION

Human resource management (HRM) is an element critical to the successful operation of any department in any industry. Managers, directors, and supervisors who are not familiar with the basic elements of HRM serve as a potential liability for their own organization, rather than an asset, and are likely to find themselves embroiled in costly litigation. This chapter is intended to provide an overview of the fundamental concepts of HRM in five basic areas: recruitment, compensation, leave benefits, employee relations, and termination. Case studies and subsequent discussions are incorporated into this chapter as appropriate to illustrate key points. It is not intended to serve as nor constitute legal advice. Managers should always contact their human resources practitioner, or legal counsel, before making any decision that may adversely affect any employment relationship. Other chapters in Section II of this text will provide readers with more detailed information about these and other areas involved in HRM. This chapter is intended to familiarize those responsible for the supervisory duties within a department or laboratory with the issues that are most frequently problematic to employers.

RECRUITMENT

Success in any business requires success in competition. Thus, every company within various industries strives to recruit and retain the most highly qualified personnel. Companies are constantly challenged to create new and better services, programs, and benefits with which to entice the most qualified candidates to work for their organization. In the excitement of that competitive spirit, however, many managers have not been provided the opportunity to learn the basics of the recruitment process. What questions may properly be asked in an employment interview? What information should be divulged when answering a call for an employment reference? If a candidate for employment discloses the existence of a disability or need for a religious accommodation, how should you respond? Understanding the basic requirements of the recruitment process is key to creating a high quality, stable workforce.

Table 5–1 lists federal laws that most frequently affect the employment relationship, the number of employees an organization must employ before each law is applicable, and some websites of the federal agencies that regulate the particular statute.

Affirmative Action

Executive Order 11246 (Order), entitled "Equal Employment Opportunity," was issued by President Lyndon Johnson on September 24, 1965. This order, generally known as *Affirmative Action*, prohibits federal contractors, subcontractors, and federally assisted construction contractors and subcontractors (contractors), who conduct more than $10,000 in government business in 1 year from discriminating in employment decisions on the basis of race, color, religion, sex, or national origin. Certain government contractors or first-tier subcontractors with 50 or more employees and $50,000 or more in government contracts are required to develop and maintain a written affirmative action plan (AAP). In November 2000, the Office of Federal Contract Compliance Program, of the Department of Labor, published a rule that clarified that, except in limited circumstances, the contractor must maintain a separate plan for each of its establishments. Contrary to popular belief, affirmative action is not a quota system or a system that gives preference to certain candidates. Affirmative action does require an employer to measure and assess three areas that may be envisioned as concentric circles (Figure 5–1).

For example, an employer is not required to hire a member of a minority group or a female when a more qualified candidate is available. Affirmative action is a commitment by the employer to proactively reach out into various employment pools and continue to seek the most qualified candidate but from a variety of sources, rather than from the same sources the employer has always used such as the local newspaper or community or local colleges and universities.

TABLE 5–1.   Federal Laws That Most Frequently Affect the Employment Relationship

Federal Law	Covered Employers	Website (where applicable)
Americans with Disabilities Act (ADA), 1990	Employers with 25 or more employees	http://www.eeoc.gov/policy/ada.html
Age Discrimination in Employment Act (ADEA), 1967	Employers with 20 or more employees	http://www.eeoc.gov/policy/adea.html
Civil Rights Act of 1991	Employers with 15 or more employees	http://www.eeoc.gov/policy/cra91.html
Drug Free Workplace Act, 1988	Organizations with federal contracts of $100,000 or more and all individual, federal contractors and grantees	http://www.dol.gov/elaws/drugfree.htm
Equal Pay Act, 1963	same as FLSA	http://www.eeoc.gov/policy/epa.html
Executive Order 11246 (Equal Employment Opportunity)	certain federal contractors and subcontractors	http://www.dol.gov/dol/esa/public/regs/compliance/ofccp/fs11246.htm
Fair Credit Reporting Act	All	http://www.ftc.gov/os/statutes/fcrajump.htm
Fair Labor Standards Act (FLSA)	Almost all	http://www.dol.gov/esa/whd/flsa/
Family and Medical Leave Act (FMLA)	Employers with 50 or more employees	http://www.dol.gov/esa/whd/fmla/
Immigration Reform and Control Act of 1990 (IRCA)	All	http://www.dol.gov/esa/regs/compliance/ofccp/ca_irca.htm
Occupational Safety and Health Act (OSHA)	Employers with 2 or more employees (exclusive of self-employed)	http://www.osha.gov/
Title VII, Civil Rights Act of 1964	Employers with 15 or more employees	http://www.eeoc.gov/policy/
Uniformed Services Employment and Re-employment Rights Act (USERRA), 1994	All	http://www.dol.gov/elaws/vets/userra.asp/

The outermost circle represents the applicant pool, that is, the pool of all quali-fied candidates in the employer's geographic labor market. This information is available through federal, state, and local departments of labor. The second circle represents the pool of candidates who actually apply for employment with any particular company. Employers obligated to maintain an affirmative action plan must track all applications received, including the race and gender of applicants

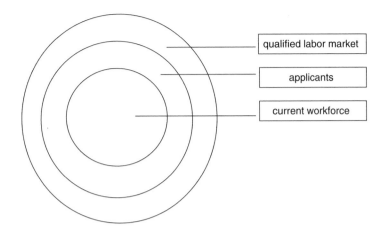

FIGURE 5–1 **Three areas of assessment required by Affirmative Action.**

and the position(s) for which they have applied. Currently this information must be tracked for all applicants, as the employer defines an applicant. In March 2004, a number of federal agencies published proposed regulations that would limit or clarify the definition of an E-applicant, that is one who applies for employment through electronic means such as the internet. The third circle represents the employees who are employed by the company. This data should be tracked through an internal human resources information system (HRIS). If any of the numbers in these three groups are statistically disparate from the general labor market, the employer should audit the company's outreach, recruitment, and hiring practices to ensure those practices are not having an adverse impact on women, minorities, persons with disabilities, or protected veterans.

Many employers maintain voluntary affirmative action plans or programs, even though they are not required to do so under the Order. Affirmative action programs have faced many legal challenges in the last decade. It is currently recommended that voluntary affirmative action programs or plans be implemented only to remedy a history of past discrimination. Programs or plans used as a proactive measure to enhance diversity within an organization have come under legal scrutiny in the last several years.

Position Descriptions

The recruitment process should begin with the writing of the job description. The best job description lists the **essential functions** of the job, defined as those that are most important and/or performed with the greatest frequency of all required tasks within a job. The job description should also include a listing of the requirements with regard to education and experience. Although an employer may want or prefer candidates with a college degree for a particular position, it is important to list only those factors that are *bona fide occupational qualifications (BFOQ)*. An employer may limit employment in a particular job to persons of a particular sex, religion, or national origin if the employer can show that sex, religion, or national origin is an actual qualification for performing the job. For example, although a clinical laboratory scientist may need a specialized degree or training to conduct certain laboratory tests, it is likely that comparable education, although helpful, is not required for a person to successfully perform the duties of a laboratory assistant. A sample job description is provided in Table 5–2.

After the job description is completed, the employer will need to attach an appropriate pay or salary range to that job. It is generally the duty of the human resources department to conduct market surveys and ensure their compensation structure is both internally equitable as well as market competitive. Maintaining internal equity requires comparing the current wages paid to each person currently employed within a particular job classification with regard to a number of factors such as each incumbent's level of education, years of experience in the field, and years of experience in the job with that employer. Hiring a new candidate at a rate of pay higher than current incumbents with comparable education and experience in the field may require an upward wage adjustment for every other worker in that job classification. If this is done, it can be very costly to the employer and must be weighed against the return on the investment of bringing in that one new candidate. If the candidate is hired at the higher rate, and no adjustment is made, the likely result is not just a reduction in employee morale and resentment toward the new worker but potential claims of wage discrimination. Additional information on and samples of job/position descriptions are located in Chapter 6.

Equal Pay Act

The *Equal Pay Act (EPA),* which is part of the Fair Labor Standards Act of 1938 and is administered and enforced by the EEOC, prohibits wage discrimination between men and women in the same establishment who are performing similar work under similar working conditions. For example, imagine that a healthcare clinic has just opened a new cancer research center. The market is competitive in this area, and the clinic finds that it cannot hire a highly qualified clinical laboratory scientist for less than $25.00 per hour. Several candidates apply and a male is selected and paid the appropriate rate. In the Department of Histology, however, a female scientist is paid only $20.00 an hour. The work the two scientists perform is similar as are their working conditions. In this case, while there is clearly a difference between the wage being paid to the male and female scientists, it most likely would not be a violation of the EPA, as the higher rate is (1) driven by the market demand based on the area of research and (2) would be paid to any incumbent in the cancer research laboratory, male or female. If, however, market data did not support that the higher rate was required or competitive in the area of cancer research, or if it was discovered that female scientists in the new cancer research center were paid less than $25.00 per hour, the employer may be found guilty of wage discrimination and violation of the EPA. It is also important to remember that wage discrimination is blind to gender. A male employee may bring charges of wage discrimination just as well as a female. A male scientist working in a predominantly female work environment should not receive a lower wage than his female counterparts just because he is more easily recruited.

TABLE 5–2. Sample Job Description

Position Title: Laboratory Technician
Job Group: Laboratory-Technical   Pay Grade: ___   Position #___

Summary of Duties
Following routine protocols under the close supervision of a faculty investigator or a senior technician, performs laboratory tests utilizing requisite laboratory equipment and instruments, making minor adjustments as required. Typically works with biohazardous and/or radioactive materials. Responsible for laboratory maintenance, preparing solutions and media, and ordering supplies. May be responsible for care of laboratory animals.

Essential Job Functions
- Performs laboratory tests and/or experiments that may include various assays, specialized techniques such as electrophoresis and basic tissue culture, following established procedures or protocols.
- Operates requisite laboratory equipment and instruments, records data, maintains and makes minor adjustments to equipment.
- Uses universal safety precautions to protect self and co-workers from biohazardous materials, including blood-borne pathogens.
- Complies with biohazard/radiation safety standards through proper handling of potentially hazardous chemical and biological agents and/or radiation sources in the workplace.
- Completes annual university biohazard/universal precaution/radiation safety training, as appropriate.
- Prepares sterile media such as agar in plates, jars, or test tubes for use in growing bacterial cultures.
- Prepares solutions, reagents, and stains following standard laboratory formulas and procedures.
- Uses sterile techniques to avoid contaminating laboratory experiments.
- Prepares, cleans, sterilizes, and maintains laboratory equipment, glassware, and instruments used in research experiments.
- Monitors inventory levels, orders materials and supplies in accordance with established policies and procedures, counts orders on receipt.

Scope of Responsibility
Knows the informal policies, procedures, and practices necessary to conduct the normal function of a specific section, unit, or work area. Is aware of the role of the position and its potential impact on the working unit.

Decision Making
Carries out duties and responsibilities with limited supervision. Makes decisions and establishes work priorities on essentially procedure-oriented operations.

Authority
Does not direct the activities of staff or a function.

Communication
Exchanges routine information in an appropriate manner requiring good oral and written communication skills.

(continued)

TABLE 5–2. Sample Job Description *(continued)*

Education
Associate degree in medical laboratory science or a laboratory science from an accredited institution.

Experience
Gained through college level classwork in the sciences or summer employment. Biological science coursework or experience in a biological laboratory is preferred.

Certification
MLT(ASCP) or CLT(NCA) or equivalent.

Physical Requirements
• Work produced is subject to precise measures of quantity and quality
• Work environment may include areas of unpleasant extremes of cold or heat
• Biohazardous conditions such as the risk of radiation exposure, fumes or airborne particles, and/or toxic or caustic chemicals may be present in this work environment, which mandates attention to safety considerations
• Near vision to see objects clearly within 20 inches
• Sharp focus to adjust vision when doing close work that changes in distance from eyes
• Full spectrum vision to identify and distinguish color
• Finger dexterity required to manipulate objects with fingers rather than with whole hand(s) or arm(s), for example, using a keyboard
• Handling by seizing, holding, grasping, turning or otherwise working with the hand or hands, but without finger dexterity
• Sitting in a normal seated position for extended periods
• Occasionally lifting, carrying objects weighing 10 lb or less
• Occasionally pushing, pulling objects weighing 30 lb or less
• Ability to move about

This description is a general statement of required major duties and responsibilities performed on a regular and continuous basis. It does not exclude other duties as assigned.

Interviewing

One of the greatest pitfalls in recruitment is interviewing. Although human resource professionals are usually trained in current employment practices, including how to develop interviewing questionnaires and templates and what questions are not appropriate to ask, front line supervisors and managers often do not receive this training. As a result, and with no bad intent, they may ask questions that are at best offensive and at worst unlawful. Table 5–3 lists questions that should be avoided during the interview process and removed from job applications. Keep in mind that many states and local jurisdictions provide legal protections for members of certain classes that go beyond those provided by federal law, such as marital status or sexual orientation.

The Americans with Disabilities Act is covered in more detail later, but it is worth noting here that an employer has a duty to provide a reasonable accommodation for a job applicant as well as employees. For example, some companies

TABLE 5–3. Questions to Avoid During the Interview Process

What is your date of birth?
When did you graduate from high school?
Are you married?
How many days did you miss from work last year?
Are you currently taking any prescription medication?
Do you currently have or have you any history of a disability?
What is your country of national origin?
Are you a U.S. citizen?
Have you ever been arrested?
Have you ever filed a claim for workers' compensation?

have a rule that all applications for employment are to be completed in the human resources department. An employer may have to grant an exception to that rule as a reasonable accommodation for a candidate with a visual impairment who arrives in the human resource office and asks to take the application home to use a reading device to complete the application. Learners are encouraged to read Chapters 6 and 7 for more information on conducting job analyses and interviews, as well as related issues of evaluating an employee's performance of assigned duties and responsibilities.

COMPENSATION

The *Fair Labor Standards Act of 1938 (FLSA)* is the federal law that defines the minimum wage, overtime, and other requirements related to how certain employees are to be paid. The term *nonexempt* refers to employees who are to be paid for every hour in which the employee performs work for, or is under the control of, the employer. With few exceptions, the FLSA also requires that nonexempt employees receive wages at the rate of 1.5 times the employee's regular rate of pay for any hours worked beyond 40 hours in 1 work week. Note that there are limited exceptions for companies in some industries, such as health care, that have established an 80-hour work week. These situations should be evaluated on a case-by-case basis as well as in conjunction with state laws that may impose greater requirements. This law can be quite complex and its interpretation convoluted, but if a supervisor follows a few basic rules, complications should be easily avoided.

Some employees are exempt from the provisions of the FLSA and are, thus, termed, "exempt" employees. Generally, these employees are classified as executive, administrative, or professional. A number of parameters must be used in determining whether any particular job should be classified as exempt or nonexempt. Because these exemptions are narrowly defined, employers should carefully check the exact terms and conditions for classification and work in conjunction with the company's human resources department and compensation experts to ensure proper classification. Improperly classifying a nonexempt employee as exempt, as well as any other violation of the FLSA, can have serious financial consequences as a result of fines or penalties imposed by the Department of Labor. These fines may be imposed against an individual supervisor as well as the company, in amounts up to $10,000, in addition to civil money penalties plus damages for back pay, liquidated damages, and more.

Many companies have rules that overtime must be approved in advance of being worked. What if the employee is very dedicated to the job and chooses to come in early, performs work, and tells the supervisor that the company need not pay the employee for this extra time because the employee understands that permission was not granted in advance? Does the employer have to pay the employee for the extra time worked? What if an employee continues to work through his or her lunch period to catch up on some work? Does the employer have to pay the employee for what would otherwise be an unpaid lunch period? The answer is yes in both cases. Even if the work is performed without the permission or knowledge of the employer, the employee is still due appropriate compensation. The employer may, however, limit the compensation that is due under the FLSA by granting the nonexempt employee some time off later in the same work week to avoid incurring hours worked in excess of 40 in that work week.

Employers may also fail to properly pay nonexempt employees when an employee is on the employer's premises during his or her scheduled shift but not performing work.

Case Study: Three Scenarios Involving Compensation

An employee in Laboratory A is scheduled to work from 8:00 AM to 4:30 PM, with one break for lunch from 12:00 to 1:00 PM. The employee accurately records her arrival at work at 8:00 AM. The employee then walks to the company's cafe, gets breakfast, and returns 15 minutes later and begins working. Is the employer obligated to pay the employee for the period covered from 8:00 AM to 8:15 AM?

An employee arrives to work at 8:00 AM and is scheduled to conduct blood specimen testing. The equipment, however, is not working and cannot be repaired until at least 9:30 AM. In the interim, the supervisor instructs the employee to stay in the department until the repair specialist arrives. While waiting, the employee does some studying for a course he is taking at the local, community college. Is the employer obligated to pay the employee for the time the employee studies?

An employee drives into the employer's parking lot at 7:58 AM. He is scheduled to work from 8:00 AM to 4:30 PM. To avoid recording a late time of arrival for work, the employee parks his car outside the door, walks into his department, and records an 8:00 AM arrival time and then leaves to park his car, returning to the department at 8:10 AM. Is the employer obligated to pay for the period from 8:00 AM to 8:10 AM?

The intent of the FLSA, as drafted more than 65 years ago, was to provide compensation for an employee who performs work or remains under the employer's control. Thus, in the first and third scenarios the answer is No. The employer is obligated to compensate employees only for the time they performed work in the laboratory, not for the time spent eating breakfast or parking the car. Keep an eye out for the common practice of nonexempt employees who eat lunch at their desk while working. If a nonexempt employee is not relieved of his or her duties during a scheduled, unpaid meal period, then the employer owes that employee compensation for the time worked, even if while simultaneously eating lunch. In the second scenario, even though no work was performed, the reason for the work stopping was beyond the employee's control. In addition, he remained under the control of the employer until the equipment was repaired. As a result, the employer may be obligated to pay that employee for that idle time. A proactive manager will find other work an employee may perform during down time.

Another common practice in which many employers engage is the granting of compensatory time off from work for nonexempt employees in lieu of overtime wages. At this time, the FLSA generally prohibits private (nongovernmental) employers from granting nonexempt employees compensatory time off from work. For example, imagine that you have a research grant due this Friday. You need your laboratory assistant to work some overtime to help get some last minute administrative details put together. When you convey this news to the employee, he says that would be fine because he would also like to take off early one day next week to take care of some personal business. If you and the employee both agree to this arrangement, can you grant the employee the compensatory time off from work next week in exchange for the additional hours worked this week? The answer is, No. To do so would be a violation of the FLSA. Note that legislation has been proposed for a number of years to permit this type of voluntary arrangement if the employer and employee both agree. As of this writing, those efforts have been unsuccessful.

Compensatory time off from work is also a strategy that employers use with exempt employees with the intent of enhancing the flexibility of work schedules. The new federal regulations that became effective in August 2004 expressly permit the additional payment so long as the exempt employee is still paid the required minimum salary on a salary basis.

LEAVE BENEFITS

While the overall administrative oversight of leave benefits (e.g., sick leave, vacation, personal, military) is generally regulated by the human resources department, problems most frequently arise at the departmental level when a request for some form of leave is initially denied or misapplied by a manager or supervisor. For the purpose of this discussion, the leave benefits covered are presented under two categories: Family and Medical Leave Act and Military and Other Leave.

Family and Medical Leave Act

The *Family and Medical Leave Act of 1993 (FMLA)* provides eligible employees with up to 12 weeks of leave (paid or unpaid) for the employee's own serious health condition, for the care of an immediate family member who has a serious health condition (spouse, child, parent), and for the care of the employee's child following birth or adoption. The FMLA is applicable to any employer in the private sector who is engaged in commerce or in any industry or activity affecting commerce, and who has 50 or more employees each working day during at least 20 calendar weeks or more in the current or preceding calendar year. In addition, all public agencies (state and local government) and local education agencies (schools) are covered. These employers do not need to meet the 50 employee requirement. The FMLA guarantees the employee the right to return to the same or comparable position he had when the leave commenced, upon his or her return to work. A comparable position is one that provides the employee with the same wages, hours, and conditions of employment as the position originally held.

An eligible employee is one who has worked for the employer for at least 12 months (not necessarily consecutively) and at least 1,250 hours in the last 12 months. The employee must work at a worksite with at least 50 employees employed within 75 miles of that site. Although there is more than one definition of what conditions constitute a serious health condition, and they are quite detailed, the general definitions are those conditions that require inpatient care or continuing treatment by a health care provider. The nuances of administrating leave under the FMLA are very broad and easily warrant a chapter unto themselves. Here, we cover those areas of the FMLA that most often result in misinterpretation or misapplication.

Case Study: Leave Benefits

An employee calls in on Monday and tells you that he will be absent that day. On Tuesday, the employee calls in again and tells you that he is very sick and will be out for at least three more days, if not the entire week. The following Monday, you have not heard back from the employee so you call him at home. He says that he saw a physician on Friday afternoon and has been conditionally diagnosed with pneumonia, is scheduled for diagnostic testing, and will be out at least until the test results come back at the end of the week. The following Monday, following a two-week absence, the employee returns to work. What should you do? What portion of the absence, if any, may be applied to FMLA?

The U.S. Department of Labor administers the FMLA and has published interpretive guidelines that require an employer to give an employee notice that an absence is being counted towards FML within at least two business days of learning that the employee may have a qualifying event under the Act. In this case, the employer learned this on the first Tuesday, the employee's second day of absence from work. What happens if the employer knew that the leave may have qualified under FMLA, failed to give the employee proper notice, and the employee has returned to work? The leave may be designated retroactively but some penalty may apply, so held the U.S. Supreme Court in March 2002.

It is also important to note that while the FMLA provides employees the right to unpaid leave, the employer is permitted to run paid leave benefits, such as sick leave, vacation pay, workers' compensation and other benefits concurrently with FML. This is a sound business practice to prevent employees from taking up to 12 weeks of unpaid leave and returning to work with full, paid leave banks.

Military and Other Leave

Employers have certain duties to provide some limited benefits and protections to employees who take time off from work to perform a variety of social obligations, such as those required for military service, including weekend reservists units. Separate federal laws cover nearly all employers, including federal contractors. The law provides employees and candidates with certain rights to be free from discrimination based on their military obligations, including a conditional right to return to the same or a comparable position when they return from military service, as granted under the Uniformed Services Employment and Reemployment Rights Act (USERRA).

Employers should also become familiar with the laws in their state and local jurisdictions. Many provide further protections for employees taking leave to vote, respond to a subpoena for jury duty, or to serve as a witness at a trial. For example, Maryland law requires employers to grant employees at least two consecutive hours off from work while the polls are open to vote on election day.

EMPLOYEE RELATIONS

The arena of employment legislation and litigation is replete with challenges to employers' practices relating to a myriad of issues under the law. Federal, state, and local administrative agencies such as the *Equal Employment Opportunity Commission (EEOC)* and its counterparts are continually challenged to meet the demands of burgeoning case loads alleging discrimination in employment based on a person's membership in a legally protected class. Although the 1990s brought the enactment of several pieces of federal legislation imposing additional duties on employers, Title VII remains the most commonly cited law under which persons file charges with the EEOC. During fiscal year 2004, Title VII charges accounted for the greatest precentage of charges received by the EEOC, as compared to any other single statute.

Title VII of the Civil Rights Act of 1964

The *Title VII of the Civil Rights Act of 1964,* prohibits discrimination based on race, color, creed, religion, national origin, and sex. Keep in mind that a plaintiff may file a claim of discrimination alleging discrimination under more than one federal statute as well as more than one protected class. The burden of proof in such cases rests first with the person bringing the charge to show that (1) he belongs to a protected class; (2) he was qualified for a job; (3) though qualified, some adverse employment action was taken against him (fired, not hired, demoted, etc.); and (4) thereafter the employer continued to seek applicants with the plaintiff's qualifications. If the plaintiff is able to establish each of these threshold elements, the burden then shifts to the employer to show a legitimate, nondiscriminatory reason for taking the adverse employment action. If the employer can do so, then the plaintiff is afforded one more opportunity to show that the reason given by the employer is a pretext and not the real reason for the decision. On June 12, 2000, the Supreme Court held that a plaintiff was not required to provide any evidence that the real reason for the adverse action was based on some unlawful, discriminatory intent, but only that the reason given by the employer was not true. The Court held that so long as the plaintiff was able to rebut the reason the employer gave as pretextual, then it may be appropriate for a jury to infer that the employer's motive was unlawful discrimination.

Case Study: Employee Relations—Civil Rights

A private laboratory has contracts with several companies to conduct "for cause" testing of employees whom the employer suspects have reported to work under the influence of drugs or alcohol. To ensure the donor does not tamper with the urine sample, employees must be monitored when giving a sample. The laboratory has a technician who currently conducts these tests. They have run into a problem, however. The clinical laboratory technician is male. Although employees sent for testing are permitted to give a urine specimen behind a curtain, many female employees refuse to do so with the male laboratory technician in the room. On these occasions, the laboratory has to call a female laboratory technician from another area to oversee the specimen collection process.

Would the laboratory be able to lawfully advertise for only female applicants for this position to monitor female donors? The answer is "Yes." When the work being performed may be reasonably perceived as private or personal in nature (security guards conducting searches of persons, video monitors in department store dressing rooms), then gender may be considered a BFOQ. It is important to note, however, that the courts have held that race may never be used as a BFOQ.

Unlawful Harassment

No issue under Title VII has received more attention over the last decade than issues related to unlawful harassment. From 1986 to 1993, the Supreme Court heard two landmark cases that laid the foundation for sexual harassment litigation under Title VII. From March 1998 to May 1998, however, the Court heard three cases (plus two under another federal statute) that further refined the definition and liability standards for unlawful harassment. The EEOC then followed suit and published new guidelines in June 1999 stating that *unlawful harassment* includes behaviors "based on race, color, sex (whether or not of a sexual nature), religion, national origin, protected activity, age, or disability. Thus, employers should establish anti-harassment policies and complaint procedures covering *all* forms of unlawful harassment."

Both the definition and liability standards for employers have changed a great deal. It is important that managers and supervisors understand the new duties and responsibilities that have been imposed on employers as a result of these decisions.

The Supreme Court has declared that the distinction between the former classifications of quid pro quo sexual harassment and hostile environment claims is of "limited utility." In cases in which an employee alleges some tangible economic harm (e.g., lost job, demotion, reduction of overtime or compensation), the employer may be held liable or strictly liable, meaning the employer will have no opportunity to put forward a defense. Only in the case of an allegation of harassment with no tangible economic harm may the employer be permitted to put forward an affirmative defense. That affirmative defense is basically a three-prong defense that requires the employer to show: (1) that the employer took reasonable care to prevent the harassment from occurring, (2) that the employer took reasonable care to promptly correct the harassment, and (3) the employee unreasonably failed to pursue these preventive or corrective measures or otherwise avoid harm. If the employer can meet all three elements, the company may escape liability for a claim of unlawful harassment. As a result, it is imperative that employers provide and document thorough training for managers and employees on unlawful harassment prevention, multiple resources for reporting complaints, and respond promptly to any questions, concerns, or complaints related to unlawful harassment.

In addition, the demographic landscape of harassment claims has changed quite dramatically after 9/11. In the year following the 9/11 attacks, the percentage increase in the number of claims of religious discrimination and harassment that were filed with the U.S. Equal Employment Opportunity Commission (EEOC) were more than double the preceding year. From 2000 to 2001, claims increased about 9.7%; from 2001–2002 the same claims increased at a rate of nearly 21%. They became so prevalent the EEOC named them "Post-9/11" and/or "Backlash" cases. Thus, employers are wise to follow the EEOC's guidance and develop policies and training programs that prohibit all forms of unlawful harassment, not just sexual.

Age Discrimination in Employment Act

The *Age Discrimination in Employment Act (ADEA),* passed in 1967, prohibits discrimination against any person 40 years old or older. Clinical laboratory managers and supervisors should also note that courts have held that even if both persons are 40 years old or older (a candidate not hired and the candidate hired, for example) the employer may still be guilty of age discrimination by not hiring the older worker. For example, if there are two applicants for a position, one is 42 years old and the other is 52, the 52-year-old candidate may have a prima facie case of age discrimination if she can present some evidence that the employer did not hire her because she was older than the other candidate, even though the other candidate was also over 40 years old.

It is important to check with your human resources department or legal counsel, as many states also have laws that prohibit discrimination against persons of any age, including those less than 40 years old.

Americans with Disabilities Act (ADA)

Case Study #1: Employee Relations—ADA

A clinical laboratory has a vacancy for a medical transcriptionist. The job requires candidates to be able to type at least 60 words per minute with an error rate of no more than 5%. Candidate A has more than 10 years in medical transcription, types 65 words per minute with a 2% error rate. She also has a very strong work record; however, she has been diagnosed with strong indications of carpel tunnel syndrome in her right wrist. To limit the tingling sensation and pain she occasionally experiences, she wears a wrist brace that extends over the lower portion of her hand on both sides and is visible even when she wears long sleeves. Candidate A applies in person for the job. She completes the application and takes a typing test. Impressed with her application, resume, and score on the typing test, the recruiter offers to immediately interview Candidate A for the position. One week later, Candidate A calls the employer to determine her status for employment. The recruiter tells her that, although she was highly qualified for the position, another candidate, whose qualifications were equally impressive, was selected. Candidate A has now filed a charge of discrimination with the EEOC alleging discrimination based on both perceived and present disability. Assuming Candidate A did have qualifications equal to those of the person hired for the job, did the employer discriminate against Candidate A based on a real or perceived disability?

The *Americans with Disabilities Act (ADA)* was passed in 1990 and prohibits discrimination based on a number of classifications of disabilities: a person who presently has a disability, has a past history of a disability, is perceived to have a disability, or associates with a person who has a disability. The Act defines a disability as any physical or mental impairment that substantially limits a major life activity. Major life activities are defined as, among other things, walking, talking, maintaining active employment, and conducting daily hygiene. The Act requires an employer to provide a qualified candidate or employee with a **reasonable accommodation.** A qualified candidate or employee is one who can perform the essential functions of the job with or without a reasonable accommodation. The employer does not, however, have to provide the candidate or employee with the best accommodation or one preferred by the candidate or employee.

Case Study #2: Employee Relations—ADA

A laboratory's busiest day is Monday. An employee tells his supervisor that he is currently undergoing medical treatment for a serious health condition. The treatment includes dialysis, which can only be conducted on Mondays and will require him to be absent from work for the entire day. The employee is asking to have his job reduced to a part-time position, Tuesday through Friday, at least until the treatment is completed. At this time, his doctor projects the treatments will continue for at least 12 weeks. The supervisor knows that he cannot properly run the laboratory with one fewer person every Monday. Laboratory testing and results will be delayed, affecting patient care. The supervisor also knows there is a vacant position in Laboratory B that can accommodate the employee's request. Transferring the employee to Laboratory B would enable the supervisor to hire at least a temporary, full-time replacement.

Can the supervisor transfer the employee to work in Laboratory B part-time and hire a full-time replacement, at least temporarily? The answer is most likely, "Yes." The scenario actually involves the potential application of two federal laws. If the employee is eligible for Family and Medical Leave (FML), that law permits an employer to at least temporarily transfer an employee to another, comparable position, while taking intermittent FML. Under the ADA, the employer would also be providing the employee with a reasonable accommodation, assuming the condition qualifies as a disability under the ADA, although not the accommodation preferred by the employee. Note, however, if the employee requested a transfer to Laboratory B as a reasonable accommodation for a disability, the employer may be required to grant the request, even if a more qualified candidate is available for the job. In addition, keep in mind that if using the remedial device, such as medication, results in some other condition that substantially limit a major life activity, such as an inability to stay awake at work, then the employee may fall back under the purview and protection of the ADA.

In 1998, the Supreme Court of the United States answered another critical question. Is a person with a disability (high blood pressure or poor eyesight) who is no longer substantially limited in a major life activity when he uses a remedial device (medication or contact lenses), still covered under the ADA? The Supreme Court held that such persons were not intended to be and were not covered by the Act. Thus, if a candidate or employee is able to use a remedial device or measure so that he is no longer substantially limited in a major life activity, then that person is not covered by the ADA. Keep in mind that this would likely *not* include an amputee, for example, who wears a prosthetic leg so that he can walk and ambulate. Even with the prosthetic leg, he may still not be able to engage in some major life activities that many of us take for granted, such as running, jumping, walking or standing for extended periods. In addition, keep in mind that if using the remedial device, such as medication, results in some other condition that substantially limit a major life activity, such as an inability to stay awake at work, then the employee may fall back under the purview and protection of the ADA.

TERMINATION

A common basis of the employment relationships is the **at-will employment doctrine.** This doctrine maintains that the employment relationship is terminable at the will of either party. An employee may leave his or her job, at any time, for any reason. Likewise, an employer may terminate the employment relationship at any time for any reason, including no reason. The limitation is that an employer may not terminate the employment relationship for an unlawful (discriminatory) reason.

Often, however, employers limit this relationship either intentionally through the use of written employment contracts or, unintentionally, through the creation of employment policies, practices, or statements inadvertently made during the interview process which are later construed to create an employment contract.

All policies, procedures, and handbooks should be reviewed and approved by your human resources department and general counsel before being published and distributed to employees or candidates for employment.

When it comes to terminating the employment relationship, a myriad of claims can arise including invasion of privacy, breach of contract, wrongful discharge, and more. Here are five tips to follow. Each tip addresses one of five elements, often referred to as the elements of **just cause.** Although they are not generally required absent a collective bargaining (union) agreement or other written contract, they serve as a reasonable foundation by which to assess the thoroughness of your reasons for discharging any employee.

1. Forewarning: Can you show that the employee in question has received some notice, either through instruction, coaching, a policy manual, or training, regarding the standard or expectation that he has failed to meet? Is this an assumption on your part, or do you have documentation to show that the employee received such notice?
2. Proper investigation: Have you spoken to all parties you can reasonably be expected to have knowledge regarding the information that has led to your decision to discharge? Most important, have you spoken to the employee to get his or her side of the story? Even if you believe there is no reasonable explanation the employee could provide, it is still imperative to give the employee that opportunity to present his or her case.
3. Evidence: Can you show that the information on which you are basing your decision to terminate is factual and not just perception or hearsay? Are there records to support your findings? If there are no tangible records, are there witnesses who are willing to give either a verbal or written statement supporting your decision? Are these witnesses credible?
4. Lack of discrimination: An employer should determine whether any single decision to discharge is consistent with comparable scenarios and past practice. If another employee engaged in the same wrongful conduct in another department and was *not* discharged, the employer should be able to justify why discharge may be appropriate in one department and not another. For example, lateness or absenteeism may be a much more serious offense in a critical care unit, owing to the potential, negative impact to patient care than it would in the office of volunteer services or gift shop.
5. Penalty meets the offense: Better known as the punishment fits the crime, it is important to assess whether the employee's behavior is salvageable and might be corrected with a lesser penalty. Discharge is often perceived by

arbitrators and courts as economic capital punishment and a measure of last resort. If it is reasonable that the employee might modify his or her behavior with a disciplinary suspension, consider that in lieu of discharge. Very serious or repeated infractions, however, deserve concomitant sanctions.

Managers should also become familiar with the basics of labor law and employees' rights under the National Labor Relations Act. One example was recently illustrated by a decision of the National Labor Relations Board in July 2000, which held that if a manager or supervisor interviews an employee as part of an investigation that may lead to disciplinary action of the employee being interviewed and the employee states that he or she does not want to meet with the management without a representative, the manager must grant the employee's request before continuing with the interview.

SUMMARY

The employment relationship can be as rewarding as it is fraught with pitfalls for liability. It has been the goal of this chapter to provide clinical laboratory managers and supervisors with some of the basics of the employment relationship so they may proactively identify issues in the workplace that have the potential to disrupt business operations and begin generating alternatives for avoiding a problem, rather than trying to negotiate the settlement of a problem after it has arisen.

The best manager and administrator need not be an expert in any of these areas but will be familiar with the basic concepts. They are then able to serve as a resource to the organization in seeking more information and asking questions before making any decision that affects any employee in the organization.

SUGGESTED PROBLEM-BASED LEARNING ACTIVITIES
Chapter 5: Human Resource Guidelines and Regulations

Instructions: Use Internet resources, books, articles, colleagues, etc., to present solutions to the problems listed below. There is no one correct solution to any problem.

Note to Instructor: Students in class may be divided into groups and given the problem-based learning activity to discuss and solve. Once the group has reached a consensus as to a solution, the group may present it to the other students in the class. This activity will provide all students with information regarding solutions to the problem.

Problem #1
Suppose your department has shown a 25% turnover rate. As manager you must develop a plan to encourage employee retention. In your plan, identify factors associated with excessive turnover.

Problem #2
Identify and define motivational techniques used in your institution to foster effective team interaction.

Problem #3
Suppose you are a laboratory manager and have an employee who is habitually late to work. Develop an action plan to remedy this behavior.

BIBLIOGRAPHY

Alaimo M: An unexpected problem surfaces for employers conducting third-party harassment investigations. *National Personnel Law Update.* Miller, Canfield, Paddock & Stone; Detroit, MI., July 1999.

Black HC: *Black's Law Dictionary*, 6th ed. West Publishing Co., St. Paul, MN., 1990.

Goring DC: Private problem, public solution: affirmative action in the 21st century. *Akron Law Review* 33 Akron L. Rev. 209, 2000.

Leonard B: Relieving FMLA headaches. *HR Magazine,* July, 1999, p. 41.

Mauro T: Direct proof of intent not necessary in job discrimination suits. *The Legal Intelligencer* NATIONAL NEWS June 13, 2000, p. 4.

Poe AC: Make foresight 20/20. *HR Magazine*, February, 2000, p. 74.

Internet Resources

Department of Labor: Small Business Handbook
   http://www.dol.gov/osbp/sbrefa/ main.htm

Equal Employment Opportunity Commission: Charge Statistics FY 1992 Through FY 2004
   http://www.eeoc.gov/stats/charges.html.

Equal Employment Opportunity Commission: Enforcement Guidance: Vicarious Employer Liability for Unlawful Harassment by Supervisors
   http://www.eeoc.gov/ policy/docs/harassment.html

Equal Employment Opportunity Commission: Revised Enforcement Guidance: Reasonable Accommodation and Undue Hardship Under the Americans with Disabilities Act, October 2002
   http://www.eeoc.gov/policy/docs/accommodation .html

HR Tools
   http://www.hrtools.com

6

Job Analysis, Work Descriptions and Work Groups

JANET HALL, MS, CC(NRCC)

Chapter Outline

Objectives

Following successful completion of this chapter, the learner will be able to:

1. Describe the importance of a clear, detailed job description.
2. Describe how job descriptions are developed.

3. List the components of a job description.
4. Describe the process of worker selection.
5. Describe the key components of evaluating performance.
6. Describe the difference between criteria-based and competency-based performance evaluations.
7. Describe the basic components of a work group.
8. Describe the dynamics of work groups.

Key Terms

Competency-Based
  Performance Evaluation
Criteria-Based Performance
  Evaluation

Job Analysis
Job Description
Performance Evaluation
Work Groups

Case Study: Job Analysis, Work Descriptions and Work Groups

Katie has recently accepted a position as laboratory supervisor at a large suburban hospital. Although she is thrilled with her new position and working environment, Katie's laboratory manager has indicated that there is a major conflict in her laboratory that she needs to resolve as quickly as possible. The employees whom Katie supervises have been working as an efficient team for more than five years. In the past few months, however, turnaround time for laboratory tests has increased and the laboratory has been filled with tension and resentment toward Helen, a medical technologist, who joined the team approximately six months previously. Helen is an experienced technologist with exceptional knowledge and skills. She is energetic, hardworking and she possesses a positive attitude. Katie and Helen enjoy a good working relationship. Helen's co-workers, however, have complained that Helen tries to "stick her nose into everyone else's job" and that she slows the output of the other staff members with her unwanted involvement.

Issues and Questions to Consider

1. *How can Katie use her knowledge of the development of work groups to analyze the interpersonal dynamics of the work group under her supervision?*
2. *How can Katie use job analysis and existing job descriptions to improve the productivity of the work group and reduce the tension among its members?*
3. *In particular, what approach could Katie use to retain Helen's enthusiasm and commitment to the laboratory while curtailing Helen's negative effect on turnaround time for laboratory testing?*

INTRODUCTION

Effective management requires the thoughtful analysis and measurement of **job** tasks and the careful evaluation of how employees perform those tasks to achieve the goals of the organization. To accomplish this, a job analysis should be performed to determine exactly what management expects from the employee. A job analysis is an evaluation and documentation of the tasks, conditions, requirements, and authority arrangements of a working situation. A job/work description is defined as a written document describing the tasks, expectations, reporting relationships, and other information relative to the employment of an individual. Ideally the job description should be a concise yet comprehensive summary of the findings of the job analysis. Too often, however, because of time constraints or lack of experience, managers write job descriptions based on historical documents or on a quick analysis of the current situation.

Managers are often faced with selecting individuals who meet the criteria determined from a job analysis and subsequent job description to fill open positions. A good understanding of the selection process is critical for a manager to successfully fill such job openings. Once an individual is hired, managers continue to monitor the employee through performance evaluations that may be competency or criteria-based. Further, managers may elect to use the assistance of their employees in the formation of work groups to accomplish designated tasks.

This chapter is designed to first introduce the learner to the specifics of conducting a thorough job analysis and creating an appropriate job description. An in-depth discussion of the selection process that includes job application, regulatory and internal criteria (see Chapter 5 for additional regulatory information) and conducting an effective and legal interview are then presented. Then an overview of the performance evaluation aspect of a laboratory manager's job is presented including a discussion of the two types of such evaluations, competency-based and criteria-based (see Chapter 7 for more information on performance evaluation). The final section is an introduction to the principle and uses of work groups.

JOB ANALYSIS

Job analysis may be done either formally or informally. Most often it is done informally, with a very general knowledge of the expectations of the employee and the working relationships of the employee with fellow employees and with management. Although an informal analysis is frequently adequate, it is not the best way to approach the issue. A formal job analysis involves observation and measurement of tasks and relationships with others and a thorough documentation of the information gathered.

When performing a job analysis, many facets must be considered (Table 6–1).

1. *Working conditions* should be analyzed. Working conditions include the physical environment in which the employee performs the work (e.g., temperature, lighting, noise level, physical requirements such as whether or not the employee is seated or standing and for what percentage of the time, requirements for lifting, whether or not the employee is working alone or with other employees).

2. *Task Analysis:* The actual tasks being performed should be evaluated to determine the amount of time required to perform them and whether there are specific requirements for space, equipment, etc.

TABLE 6–1. Factors Considered in a Job Analysis

- Working conditions
- Task analysis
- Technology
- Scope of labor
- Legal issues
- Interaction with co-workers

3. *Technology:* The instrumentation or other equipment, including computers, used in the performance of the job should be listed along with any special requirements or skills needed to operate them.

4. *Scope of labor:* The level of employee who can or should be performing the task set should be evaluated. The availability in the marketplace of persons with these specific qualifications should be assessed. It may be necessary to adjust the skill level to the availability of the required employees.

5. *Legal issues:* The legal requirements for specific licensures or training should be included.

6. *Interaction with coworkers:* The method and extent of the interaction of the employee should be evaluated both in terms of efficiencies and ensuring that the skill mix and communications with co-workers is adequate.

Although the items to be evaluated may be the same, the analysis of every job will be unique based on its individual characteristics and requirements.

The job analysis can be accomplished by one or multiple individuals and can involve a number of approaches. Most frequently it is performed by the Department of Human Resources of the institution, only because they have the skills, knowledge, and experience of having done it in many settings. The specific criteria used vary widely, but are consistent at least in content and scope. Occasionally an industrial engineer may be engaged to do the analysis. The focus of the engineer is in ergonomics and motion, and they are most valuable when developing positions in a new environment. Another resource, at least in classifying the job, is the Department of Transportation's coding system. Their system assigns a 9-digit code based on the type of occupation, the functional level of difficulty with respect to data, people and things, and other criteria. Although it is useful academically, it is not particularly useful when the analysis is used to develop a job description.

JOB DESCRIPTION

After performing the job analysis, a *job description* is developed. The purpose of the job description is twofold. First, it documents the characteristics of the job and the requirements of the candidates. Equally important, it acts as a measure against which employee performance can be assessed.

The job description, also referred to as a work or position description, should be concise, yet thorough. One large healthcare organization has a one-line job description for each of its positions. Although this approach is indeed concise, it does not lend itself to clarity or to giving the confidence to both management and staff that they know what is expected and what will be used to determine whether the employee is meeting job expectations. The description should contain measurable criteria to be used in the performance evaluation. Ideally the job description document should be the evaluation tool.

The format of the job description varies widely, but in general it should address a number of facts, nine of which are described here (Table 6–2).

1. *Job title and classification:* The specific title of the position should be stated (e.g., Medical Technologist II). This title includes the name of the position and the level of the position within that category (II).

2. *Exempt status:* The description should indicate whether the employee is exempt (salaried) or nonexempt (hourly).

3. *Education/experience:* The description should indicate the specific level or range of education required to perform the job. It may be stated in terms of "required" or "preferred" or a combination of the two. The same is true of experience (e.g., a minimum number of years of experience in the same or relation position).

4. *Knowledge:* The description should spell out the specific skills required to perform the job. These skills may be broad (knowledge of medical terminology) or very specific (experience with Analyzer X required). Generally it is better to be less specific, as equipment changes over time while basic skill sets do not. The degree of specificity is determined by a number of factors including the size of the facility and the scope of the job.

5. *Duties:* The description should list specific duties and tasks to be performed. The extent of detail will depend on the complexity of the job and the number of tasks to be performed. This area of the description lends itself to quantification of performance of the specific tasks when doing a performance appraisal.

6. *Interactions*: The description should indicate with whom the employee will have interaction, whether daily or periodic. Examples are nursing, admitting department, and housekeeping.

TABLE 6–2. Format for a Job Description

- Job title and classification
- Exempt status
- Education/experience
- Knowledge
- Duties
- Interactions
- Safety
- Reporting lines
- Approvals

7. *Safety:* The description should clearly indicate what possible exposures the employee may encounter and classify the employee as a "contact" (likely to come into contact with hazardous materials) or "noncontact."

8. *Reporting Lines:* The description should indicate the line of authority and where the employee falls in that line. The employee may only report upwards (e.g., "reports to the Supervisor of the Chemistry Laboratory") and/or may have other employees as direct reports to them ("oversees technologists and technicians in the Chemistry Laboratory.")

9. *Approvals:* The description should be reviewed and have approval signatures of the person who wrote the description, the Laboratory Manager, and the executive to whom the Laboratory Manager reports. It is also helpful to have the Human Resources Department sign to indicate their review and approval of the contents and intent of the description.

Once formulated and approved, the job description should be reviewed periodically (at least annually) to be certain that it continues to reflect the job, as it exists in real time. This is particularly important if it is to be used as an evaluation tool in addition to a simple description. Appendix 6–A on p. 121 contains an example of a job description for a medical technologist/clinical laboratory scientist in a community-based hospital.

Selection Process

Once the job is analyzed and documented and the description is developed, it is time to hire the best person. With the pool of qualified personnel shrinking rapidly, it becomes even more important to carefully hire and retain people who both "fit" the institution and who can grow and develop to the benefit of both the employee and the institution. Turnover in the healthcare market has always been problematic, as has the perception of limited chance for advancement. These factors make it even more critical to hire with care and then bend over backwards to create job satisfaction so that employees will stay.

The Job Application

Once the job has been "posted," either within the institution or in print or electronic media outside the institution, the first step in the hiring process is the job application. The format of the **job application** is not accidental. A number of regulations require the asking of certain questions, while others forbid the asking of other questions. Appendix 6-B on pp. 127–129 is an example of a typical job application form.

The provisions of Title VII of the Civil Rights Act enacted by Congress in 1964 are the basis of many of the hiring practices used by employers. Title VII forbids employers of more than 15 persons to discriminate against anyone on the basis of race, color, religion, sex, or national origin. The original Title VII law was expanded to include persons with disabilities, Vietnam veterans, and persons between 40 and 70 years old. For these reasons job applications do not request information about these.

Regulatory and Internal Criteria

Once the application is in hand, regulatory and internal criteria must be met.

    1. *Regulatory criteria:* As indicated by the job description, the applicant requires a certain level of education or a certification. The Clinical Laboratory Improvement Amendment of 1988 (CLIA 88) cites specific educational and certification requirements for different levels of employees. In addition, there may be local or state requirements that must be met, or the hiring institution may have its own more stringent criteria based on its individual needs.

    2. *Internal criteria:* Without violating the equal rights provisions, the hiring institution may have written or unwritten criteria related to the particular dynamics of a work group or individual characteristics that are deemed necessary to succeed in the position.

    The next step in the process is to review applications received and narrow the field to a handful of candidates who appear to be most qualified for the job. This process is sometimes handled by the human resources department, at least for screening purposes. If this is the policy, the appropriate laboratory manager/supervisor should then review those applications that have survived the initial "cut" and schedule interviews with as many candidates as necessary, but preferably not more than five.

Interviewing

A formal or informal **interview** is the next step. The interviews may be done by a group of persons who will be working closely with the candidate, or by one or more individual interviews. How this is handled may depend on availability of interviewers and/or past history and/or personal preference. Whatever method is chosen, it is important to keep questions asked as consistent as possible to be able to accurately evaluate the candidates in relation to each other. Developing a list of questions that is reviewed by all interviewers and asked of all candidates works well and allows for such consistency. Questions may be specific or part of a behavioral interview during which the candidate is asked more about how they would react in certain situations rather than direct questions about skills. The behavioral assessment is more commonly used for managerial positions than the specific skills questions, which are used for more technical types of positions. Table 6–3 shows examples of questions that may be asked. Table 6–4 outlines questions that **cannot** be asked during an interview.

    Finally, there should be some type of objective rating tool indicating specific characteristics/qualifications and a quantifiable rating scheme so that a total number of "points" can be assigned to each candidate. Table 6–5 is an example of such a scale. A combination of a quantifiable rating tool and a more subjective, narrative evaluation may also be used with the understanding that the selection

TABLE 6–3. Commonly Made Inquiries During a Job Interview

1. Tell me about your educational background.
2. What experiences led you to choose your career path?
3. How has your previous work experience prepared you for this job?
4. Tell me about your most significant accomplishments.
5. What type of problems have you solved in accomplishing your work assignments?
6. What has been your current job's biggest challenge?
7. Describe the most common problems you encounter at your (previous/current) job.
8. What happens when two priorities compete for your time?
9. Describe two things that motivate you at work.
10. How do you determine if you are successful?

result may not be totally quantifiable. Once the selection is made, the employee is offered a position. If the employee accepts the position, thus completing the **hiring**/selection process, a start date is determined.

PERFORMANCE EVALUATION

Evaluation of job performance is a task that few managers relish, but it is extremely important to employees and can be made reasonably painless by following a few simple guidelines. *Performance evaluation* really starts during the

TABLE 6–4. Things That Cannot Be Asked During a Job Interview

Generally any questions designed to elicit information as to race, color, age, sex, religion, handicap, or arrest and court records unless based on a documented occupational qualification should not be asked. Inappropriate questions include these:

- Questions about the applicant's name that would indicate applicant's lineage, ancestry, national origin, or descent or marital status.
- Questions about whether an applicant is married, single, divorced, or engaged and questions regarding number and age of children, potential children, or child care arrangements.
- Questions regarding age or date of birth. The Age Discrimination in Employment Act of 1967 forbids discrimination against persons between the ages of 40 and 70 years old.
- Questions regarding the nature or severity of any handicap. The Rehabilitation Act of 1973 forbids employers from asking job applicants general questions about whether they are handicapped.
- Questions regarding the applicant's sex, race, birthplace or origin of parents, spouse, or other relatives.
- Questions regarding applicant's religious denomination or affiliation, church, parish, pastor, or religious holidays observed.
- Questions relating to arrests or convictions of applicant.

TABLE 6–5. Sample Interview Rating Scale

INTERVIEW EVALUATION FORM

Candidate Name: _____

Rate the candidate on the criteria below using a scale of 0 to 5, with 0 indicating that the candidate cannot be rated on the specific attribute, 1 indicating the lowest score and 5 indicating the highest possible.

Evaluative Criteria	**Ranking**	**Comments**
Educational Background		
Work Experience		
Research/Professional Activities		
Laboratory Experience		
Communication Skills		
Interpersonal Skills		
Overall Rating		

Comments:

_____

_____

_____

_____

Interviewer Signature	Date

orientation period, when a trainer is teaching the new employee the details of the job and continues to a more formal stage at the end of the probationary period when a formal performance appraisal is completed and documented. Two types of performance evaluation are defined and discussed in this section: competency-based and criteria-based.

Competency-Based Versus Criteria-Based Evaluations

Competency-based performance evaluations are helpful during the orientation period because they require the new employee to actually perform tasks while being observed so that the trainer knows that they are performing them to documented standards. Competency-based performance evaluation is an evaluation based on a limited number of specifically defined tasks that are taught and assessed by direct observation during the orientation period and periodically thereafter. The number of tasks assessed during orientation is considerably greater than those done, for example, at an annual performance appraisal, because all of the tasks are new to the new employee. Observing the new employee as he or she is being trained and documenting on an orientation checklist the satisfactory completion of a learned task assures both the trainer and trainee that the task has been completed successfully. The hard copy documentation serves as proof to inspectors that the individual was, indeed, evaluated on specific tasks and that the individual was deemed proficient at those tasks. The orientation checklist should include a list of specific tasks, the date they were certified/completed, and the signature or initials of the person documenting the training. The checklist, once completed, should be kept indefinitely in the employee's personnel file.

A second means of performance appraisal is the *criteria-based performance evaluations*. This method uses an evaluation based on rating the performance of the employee on specifically defined criteria such as knowledge, judgment, attendance, reliability, and interactions with fellow employees. Ideally the checklist of criteria to be considered will be a part of the job description. In addition to the checklist, however, is a series of standards and criteria used to determine the rating given on the evaluation. For example, for rating attendance, the laboratory may use the standards listed in Table 6–6.

The standards are objective and measurable and leave no doubt from the records about the performance of the employee. Both the employee and the employer have documented proof of why a particular rating was given.

Many institutions have adopted an evaluation process that is a hybrid of the criteria-based and competency-based methods. Frequently these have measurable standards for each task, one of which is that all competencies were performed at an acceptable level. In addition, there may be a place for narrative comments by the employer and by the employee.

Some institutions have adopted a policy of 360-degree evaluations for managers, where both the person to whom the manager reports and those who report to the manager complete the evaluation form either together or separately. There are pros and cons for the 360-degree evaluation. Sometimes the input from those being managed is more narrative than quantifiable, but the employees feel that they have some input into the evaluation. The most important feature is that input from those who are managed be strictly confidential so that there is no opportunity for biasing the manager's opinions toward the employee.

However they are handled, performance evaluations should not draw any surprises for the employee. Monitoring of performance is an ongoing process, not a once a year event. Communication must be fostered so that both the employee and the manager are aware at all times of the level of performance being achieved.

TABLE 6–6.   **Rating Standards for Attendance**

Exceeds expectations	No unexcused absences. No more than 2 sick frequencies with a total of 3 days used.
Meets expectations	One unexcused absence. No more than 4 sick frequencies with a total of 7 days used.
Does not meet expectations	More than 1 unexcused absence. Greater than 4 sick frequencies with a total of 8 days used.

WORK GROUPS

Most laboratories are staffed by employees with diverse skill sets and capabilities. This is true because there are many different types of tasks that make up the operation of a laboratory. In a very small laboratory, a few employees with similar, broad skill sets will operate the laboratory. In most laboratories, however, the work is broken down into tasks that require different levels of skills. For example, phlebotomists collect the specimens and deliver them to the laboratory. They use a different set of skills from the processing people who receive the specimens, log them in, and prepare them for analysis. Another group includes the medical technologists who analyze the specimens and report the results. Yet another group may be clerical and handle reporting and results distribution. The smooth operation of the laboratory requires that all of these employees with different skill sets work closely together to accomplish the tasks required to get a result back to the patient's caregiver.

Work groups may be formal or informal. Formal work groups are usually assigned to a particular area to perform different pieces of the process. Staffing and scheduling define these work groups. Informal work groups tend to develop within these groups based on the personalities and priorities of the persons in the groups. Certain role expectations are gained in formal groups and are defined by the task sets of the individual members. Other role expectations develop over time in the informal work groups, but are just as important to the way in which the group functions as is the formal definition of the group.

Work groups tend to take on personalities of their own. Some are efficient and operate smoothly; others are disjointed and dysfunctional. Taking the same group of people from one work site to another, even though the surroundings and tasks may be different, does not generally change how well the group works together. There is a certain bonding that occurs among members, and, indeed, the dynamic of the group does tend to change. Groups go through developmental stages (Table 6–7). When a new employee enters the group, the balance achieved in the old group shifts to accommodate the particular skills and personality traits of the new member. The group first goes through a forming stage. It is a tentative time when the members are getting to know one another, the "pecking order" may be established, and mutual accommodation of tasks and priorities takes place. The group then enters a storming stage, where any imbalances come to the forefront and must be resolved. Some groups never get beyond the storming stage, and the manager needs to either step in and smooth out the process or rearrange the group by adding or deleting members to strike a balance. During the

TABLE 6–7. Developmental Stages of Work Groups

- Forming stage
- Storming stage
- Norming stage
- Performing stage

third stage, the norming stage, members have come to agreement on how things are done and who does them and a general leveling off occurs. Finally, the group may reach the performing stage, where all members are comfortable with the dynamics and are productive and happy.

Turnover, which is an ongoing problem in healthcare, has a profound effect on the efficient functioning of work groups. Each time a member leaves and is replaced, the group starts over at the forming stage and must progress through the other stages before it again becomes an efficient work organization. The task of the manager is to expedite this process through open communication and fostering of good relationships among employees so that the time required to reach the performing stage is as short as possible.

Changing the structure and tasks of work groups is sometimes a lesson in management by trial and error. Generally the formal groups will remain relatively stable unless process problems indicate that the group needs to restructure. It is the influence of the informal groups, however, that usually causes problems that must be addressed by the manager. Two or more individuals, for example, may attempt to undermine the integration of another individual, either openly or convertly.

The most effective way to manage work groups is to have clear guidelines for employees as to what is expected, select employees carefully, have a quantifiable and reasonable evaluation process in place, and communicate openly with employees at all levels.

SUMMARY

Effective management requires the thoughtful analysis and measurement of job tasks and the careful evaluation of how employees perform those tasks to achieve the goals of the organization. A job analysis is an evaluation and documentation of the tasks, conditions, requirements, and authority arrangements of a working situation. The factors assessed in performing a job analysis include the working conditions, tasks, technology, scope of labor, legal issues, and interactions with co-workers that affect a particular position. After performing the job analysis a job description is developed. The purpose of the job description is twofold. First, it documents the characteristics of the job and the requirements of the candidates. Equally important, it acts as a measure against which employee performance can be assessed. Once formulated and approved, the job description should be reviewed periodically (at least annually) to be certain that it continues to reflect the job, as it exists in real time. A number of regulations, established by the provisions of Title VII of the Civil Rights Act, govern the interview and selection process. In addition, the hiring institution will develop internal criteria, in accordance with equal rights provisions, to guide the selection and hiring processes. Developing a list of questions before the interview to be asked of all candidates and reviewed by all interviewers works well and allows for such consistency. There should be some type of objective rating tool indicating specific characteristics/qualifications and a quantifiable rating scheme so that a total number of "points" can be assigned to each candidate. Performance evaluation really starts during the orientation period, when a trainer is teaching the new employee the details of the job and continues to a more formal stage at the end of the probationary period when a formal performance appraisal is done and documented. Competency-based performance evaluations are helpful during the orientation period because they require the new employee to actually perform tasks while being observed so that the trainer knows that they are performing them to documented standards. A second means of performance appraisal is the criteria-based performance appraisal. This method uses an evaluation based on rating the performance of the employee on specifically defined criteria such as knowledge, judgment, attendance, reliability, and interactions with fellow employees. Ideally the checklist of criteria to be considered will be a part of the job description. Monitoring performance is an ongoing process, not a once a year event.

Work groups may be formal or informal. Certain role expectations are gained in formal groups and are defined by the task sets of individual members. Other role expectations develop over time in the informal work groups, but are just as important to the way in which the group functions as is the formal definition of the group. The most effective way to manage work groups is to have clear guidelines for employees as to what is expected, select employees carefully, have a quantifiable and reasonable evaluation process in place, and communicate openly with employees at all levels.

SUGGESTED PROBLEM-BASED LEARNING ACTIVITIES
Chapter 6: Job Analysis, Work Descriptions and Work Groups

Instructions:	Use Internet resources, books, articles, colleagues, etc., to present solutions to the problems listed below. There is no one correct solution to any problem.
Note to Instructor:	Students in class may be divided into groups and given the problem-based learning activity to discuss and solve. Once the group has reached consensus as to a solution, the group may present it to the other students in the class. This activity will provide all students with information regarding solutions to the problem.

Problem #1
Suppose the medical director of your institution has requested a STAT laboratory to be placed in the emergency department. You have been charged with researching and reporting on your recommended plan of actions to make this request a reality. Include the aspects of job analysis, work descriptions, and work groups into your plan.

Problem #2
Select a position in the laboratory and write an appropriate job description and corresponding work description for this position.

Problem #3
Suppose the night shift personnel have quit and as laboratory manager, you must devise a plan of action to provide coverage of this shift until a replacement has been

hired and trained. (Learners are encouraged to review Chapter 14 of this text for additional information helpful in devising your plan.) Indicate provisions in your plan for incorporating work groups, a thorough shift job analysis, and revised work descriptions for the open night shift positions.

BIBLIOGRAPHY

Bacal, Robert: Manager's Guide to Performance Reviews. McGraw Hill, New York, 2004.

Belker LB: *The First-Time Manager.* AMACOM, New York, NY., 1997.

Bozzo, P: *Cost Effective Laboratory Management.* Lippincott Williams and Wilkins, Philadelphia, PA., 1998.

Brannick, M.T., Levine, E.L.: Job Analysis: Methods, Research, and Applications for Human Resources Management in the New Millennium. Sage Publications, Thousand Oaks, CA., 2002.

Cohen EG: *Designing Groupwork.* Teachers College Press Columbia, New York, NY., 1994.

DeMarco T, Lister T: *Peopleware: Productive Projects and Teams,* 2nd ed. Dorset House, New York, NY., 2000.

Grote, D.: The Performance Appraisal Question and Answer Book A Survival Guide for Managers. AMACOM, 2002.

Mathis RL, Mathis L, Jackson JH: *Human Resource Management.* South-Western Publishing Company, Cincinnati, OH., 2000.

Nigon DL: *Clinical Laboratory Mangement, Leadership Pinciples for the 21st Century.* McGraw-Hill Health Professions Division, New York, NY., 2000.

Rees F: *How to Lead Work Teams: Facilitation Skills,* 2nd ed. Jossey-Bass Inc, New York, NY., 2001.

Travers EM: *Clinical Laboratory Management.* Lippincott Williams and Wilkins, Philadelphia, PA., 1996.

Turner, M.: Groups at Work: Theory and Research (The Applied Social Reserach Series). Lawrence Erlbaum Associates, Inc., Mahwah, NJ., 2001.

Varnadoe LA: *Medical Laboratory Management and Supervision.* F.A. Davis Company, Philadelphia, PA., 1996.

Veruki: *The 250 Job Interview Questions: You'll Most Likely Be Asked . . . and the Answers That Will Get You Hired!* Adams Media Corporation, Avon, 1999.

Internet Resources

Descriptions Next
    http://www.descriptionsnext.com
HR Guide to the Internet: *Job Analysis:* Overview
    http://www.hr-guide.com
Performance Evaluation Information
    http://hrsg.ca
TeamBuilding
    http://www.teamtechnology.com

APPENDIX 6–A: SAMPLE JOB DESCRIPTION

STATE CLASSIFICATION JOB DESCRIPTION

Salary Group B3   Class No. 4400

MEDICAL TECHNOLOGIST I

GENERAL DESCRIPTION

Performs entry-level clinical laboratory work. Work involves performing medical testing procedures and reporting the results to the appropriate medical authority for evaluation, diagnosis, or
treatment. Works under close supervision with minimal latitude for the use of initiative and independent judgment.

EXAMPLES OF WORK PERFORMED

Performs newborn screening procedures such as neonatal T4, TSH, and similar tests.

Performs serological tests for medical screening such as RPR, rubella, and similar tests.

Performs erythrocyte protoporphyrin screening assay.

Performs diagnostic procedures in urinalysis and in hematology.

Performs identification procedures on samples submitted for parasite, fungal, and mycobacterial
studies.

Reads bacterial bioassay inhibition test plates.

May conduct bronchospirometric studies to determine lung function.

May analyze blood and gas samples; evaluates and reports findings.

May plan, arrange, and assist with cardiac catheterizations.

Performs related work as assigned.

GENERAL QUALIFICATION GUIDELINES

Experience and Education

Experience in clinical laboratory work. Graduation from an accredited four-year college or university with major course work in the natural sciences or a related field is generally preferred. Experience and education may be substituted for one another.

Knowledge, Skills, and Abilities

Knowledge of medical technology concepts and practices, clinical laboratory methods and procedures, and quality assurance methodologies.

Skill in the use of laboratory equipment.

Ability to conduct clinical laboratory tests to determine deterioration or change in reagents or
equipment which might influence test results; and to keep abreast of new testing techniques and
procedures.

Registration, Certification, or Licensure

Must be registered as a Medical Technologist or a Clinical Laboratory Scientist.

APPENDIX 6–B

PLEASE TYPE OR PRINT

Administrative Services

OFFICE OF HUMAN SERVICES
737 WEST LOMBARD STREET
BALTIMORE, MARYLAND 21201
AN EQUAL OPPORTUNITY / AFFIRMATIVE ACTION / ADA EMPLOYER
JOBLINE (410) 706-5JOB

APPLICATION FOR EMPLOYMENT

INDICATE POSITION(S) AND POSITION NUMBER(S) APPLIED FOR:

_____

_____

_____

_____

| LAST NAME | FIRST | MIDDLE | **FOR OFFICE OF HUMAN RESOURCES MANAGEMENT USE ONLY** |

POSITIONS QUALIFIED FOR:

STREET ADDRESS

1. _____

| CITY | STATE | ZIP CODE |

2. _____

| SOCIAL SECURITY NO. | PHONE NUMBERS |

3. _____

HOME: ( )

4. _____

ARE YOU CURRENTLY AUTHORIZED TO WORK FOR ALL EMPLOYERS IN THE UNITED STATES ON A FULL TIME BASIS?
☐ YES ☐ NO
OR ONLY FOR YOUR CURRENT EMPLOYER?
☐ YES ☐ NO

BUSINESS: ( )

OTHER: ( )

5. _____

☐ INTERNAL
☐ EXTERNAL

EMPLOYMENT RECORD BEGIN WITH YOUR CURRENT OR MOST RECENT POSITION AND WORK BACKWARD. INCLUDE ALL PERTINENT MILITARY AND VOLUNTEER WORK WHICH WILL BE CREDITED AS PAID EXPERIENCE. INCOMPLETE APPLICATIONS MAY NOT BE ACCEPTED. ANY OTHER SURNAME DIFFERENT FROM ABOVE SHOULD BE INDICATED NEXT TO THE APPROPRIATE EMPLOYER.

Employer

DATES EMPLOYED
FROM   TO

Your Duties and Responsibilities:

Street Address   City   State   Zip Code

MO YR   MO YR

Telephone ( )

Last Position Held

First Position Held

BASE SALARY

Name and Title of Supervisor

Reason for Leaving   Explain

Did You Work Full-Time? ☐ Yes ☐ No

☐ Resignation
☐ Layoff
☐ Termination
☐ If Still Employed, Why Leaving?

FIRST   LAST

$ $

If "No," Percent of Time Worked: _____ %

Number of Employees Supervised: _____

Employer

DATES EMPLOYED
FROM   TO

Your Duties and Responsibilities:

Street Address   City   State   Zip Code

MO YR   MO YR

Telephone ( )

Last Position Held

First Position Held

BASE SALARY

Name and Title of Supervisor

Reason for Leaving   Explain

Did You Work Full-Time? ☐ Yes ☐ No

☐ Resignation
☐ Layoff
☐ Termination
☐ If Still Employed, Why Leaving?

FIRST   LAST

$ $

If "No," Percent of Time Worked: _____ %

Number of Employees Supervised: _____

Employer

DATES EMPLOYED
FROM   TO

Your Duties and Responsibilities:

Street Address   City   State   Zip Code

MO YR   MO YR

Telephone ( )

Last Position Held

First Position Held

BASE SALARY

Name and Title of Supervisor

Reason for Leaving   Explain

Did You Work Full-Time? ☐ Yes ☐ No

☐ Resignation
☐ Layoff
☐ Termination
☐ If Still Employed, Why Leaving?

FIRST   LAST

$ $

If "No," Percent of Time Worked: _____ %

Number of Employees Supervised: _____

11.00041 (Rev. 5/95)

CONTINUATION SHEETS AVAILABLE
UMAB IS A DRUG FREE, NON-SMOKING ENVIRONMENT

(Courtesy of University of Maryland.)

Schools	Name and Address of School	Dates		Number of Years and Credit Hours Completed	Major or Type of Program	Type of Degree or Certification and Date Received
		From	To			
High School or Grade School						
College						
Graduate School						
Vocational / Business School						

DO YOU POSSESS ANY OF THE FOLLOWING SKILLS? CHECK "YES" OR "NO."

Data Entry	☐ Yes ☐ No	Legal Terminology	☐ Yes ☐ No	Shorthand	☐ Yes ☐ No
Word Processing	☐ Yes ☐ No	Medical Terminology	☐ Yes ☐ No	Typing	☐ Yes ☐ No
Machine Transcription	☐ Yes ☐ No	Scientific Terminology	☐ Yes ☐ No	Approximate Typing Speed _____	

LIST ADDITIONAL SPECIAL QUALIFICATIONS AND SKILLS (E.G. OFFICE MACHINES / COMPUTER EQUIPMENT OPERATED, SOFTWARE PACKAGES USED, FOREIGN LANGUAGES SPOKEN, LABORATORY EQUIPMENT USED, ETC.)

IF THE POSITION(S) YOU ARE APPLYING FOR REQUIRES A LICENSE (INCLUDING DRIVER'S LICENSE), CERTIFICATION OR OTHER AUTHORIZATION TO PRACTICE A TRADE OR PROFESSION, COMPLETE THIS SECTION.

Type / Class	License Number	Expiration Date	Granted By (Board or Commission)	State

U.S. Military Service	Date of Entrance	Date of Discharge

IF YOUR ANSWER IS "YES" TO ANY OF THE FOLLOWING QUESTIONS, EXPLAIN IN BOX TO RIGHT. PLEASE NOTE THAT "YES" ANSWERS TO ANY OF THESE QUESTIONS DO NOT AUTOMATICALLY DISQUALIFY YOU FROM EMPLOYMENT.

a. Have you ever worked for the State of Maryland or the University of Maryland? ☐ Yes ☐ No

b. Have you been interviewed for a position with the University of Maryland at Baltimore within the last twelve months? ☐ Yes ☐ No

c. Have you ever been convicted in court for anything other than a minor traffic violation? (Please be advised that we may check records through the Criminal Justice Information System Central Repository). ☐ Yes ☐ No

d. Are you under 18 years of age? ☐ Yes ☐ No

e. Have you been discharged from military service within the past 90 days? ☐ Yes ☐ No

MAY WE CONTACT YOUR PRESENT EMPLOYER? IF "NO," PLEASE EXPLAIN. ☐ Yes ☐ No
YOUR FORMER EMPLOYERS / SCHOOLS WILL BE CONTACTED FOR REFERENCES.

PLEASE INDICATE AVAILABILITY BY CHECKING ONE OR MORE OF THE FOLLOWING:
☐ Full-Time ☐ Day Hours Only
☐ Part-Time ☐ Any Hours Considered

APPLICANTS WITH DISABILITIES REQUIRING ACCOMMODATIONS SHOULD CONTACT THE EMPLOYMENT DIVISION AT (410) 706-7171 OR MD RELAY SERVICE 1-800-735-2258.

"UNDER MARYLAND LAW AN EMPLOYER MAY NOT REQUIRE OR DEMAND ANY APPLICANT FOR EMPLOYMENT OR PROSPECTIVE EMPLOYMENT OR ANY EMPLOYEE TO SUBMIT TO OR TAKE A POLYGRAPH, LIE DETECTOR OR SIMILAR TEST OR EXAMINATION AS A CONDITION OF EMPLOYMENT OR CONTINUED EMPLOYMENT. ANY EMPLOYER WHO VIOLATES THIS PROVISION IS GUILTY OF A MISDEMEANOR AND SUBJECT TO A FINE NOT TO EXCEED $100."
This provision does not apply to applicants for law enforcement positions pursuant to Labor and Employment Article, Section 3-702 (b) (Annotated Code of Maryland).

I certify that all information on this application is accurate and complete and recognize that it is subject to verification. I also understand that any offers of employment and / or continuance thereof may be contingent upon its accuracy and completeness. I understand that I may be required to pass a physical examination upon an offer of employment.

Signature of Applicant	Date

THE UNIVERSITY OF MARYLAND AT BALTIMORE IS AN EQUAL OPPORTUNITY/AFFIRMATIVE ACTION EMPLOYER

Performance Evaluation and Development

LANI BAROVICH, MS
DENISE M. HARMENING, PhD, MT(ASCP), CLS(NCA)

Chapter Outline

OBJECTIVES

Following successful completion of this chapter, the learner will be able to:

1. Promote two-way communications between the supervisor and employee regarding employee's job performance.
2. Provide an opportunity for increased job effectiveness and development.
3. Demonstrate an understanding for promoting a win-win relationship with the employee.
4. Apply skills in:
   - Communications
   - Feedback
   - Guidance
   - Evaluation
   - Development planning
5. Develop a performance development evaluation approach using basic principles of professional development.
6. Describe and demonstrate the importance of learning, independent thinking, and sharing expertise for individual pride in performance and development.
7. Demonstrate the comfortable use of the evaluation model developed to support basic principles of professional development and evaluation.

Key Terms

Collaborative Management
Competency Modeling
Feedback Skills

Performance Development
Performance Objectives
Task/Production Management

Case Study: Performance Evaluation and Professional Development

Thomas Hancock has been the administrator of the clinical laboratories of a large urban hospital for many years. He excels at fiscal management and he has been successful in acquiring a state-of-the-art laboratory information system to increase efficiency in the laboratories. However, he is reluctant to hold department meetings or provide feedback to staff. Staff evaluations are seldom completed and his department team is unmotivated.

Mr. Hancock primarily communicates to his staff through memos. All processes must be handled according to his rules and he is unwilling to accept input from others. No one is allowed to make decisions on their own (no matter how small). When a staff member does something Mr. Hancock does not like he sends a memo to everyone pointing out the problem and how it should have been handled. The result is that everyone thinks he/she made the mistake and yet they are not really sure what is wrong.

Staff members are given job/position descriptions when they are hired, but they have not been reviewed or updated in several years. Therefore they do not clearly define the core responsibilities, making individuals feel frustrated because many of their accomplish-ments are not recognized or rewarded. Each year, cost of living allowances (COLAs) and a merit pool increase ranging from 2–5% are provided. Mr. Hancock gives everyone the same rating and the same increase because he prefers not to differentiate between his out-standing and average performers. The individuals needing improvement in their perfor-mance usually end up in the employee relations department with a grievance that is resolved on the side of the employee because there is no record of disciplinary action taken by Mr. Hancock.

Mr. Hancock's turnover in the laboratories is high. Staffing analysis shows that the top performers leave at a consistent rate while average performers stay longer. Staff stated that they felt unappreciated as well as distrustful of their supervisor and others in the de-partment. The hospital's top management is concerned about the turnover and the high costs associated with recruiting qualified clinical laboratory professionals.

Issues and Questions to Consider

Using the models described in Performance Evaluation and Professional Development chapter answer the following:

1. *Is Mr. Hancock using management by task/production or collaboration? Describe ex-amples of his management characteristics.*
2. *Describe how Mr. Hancock could create an atmosphere of growth and learning and decrease turnover of his top performers.*
3. *How can Mr. Hancock improve department communications and trust?*
4. *What first step is necessary for effective performance evaluation? Why?*
5. *How can Mr. Hancock effectively reward his top performers and improve perfor-mance for those whose work is below standards?*

INTRODUCTION

Most managers shrink from their most important task—managing the perfor-mance of others. Opposition to performance evaluation is not new. Seventeen hundred years ago the following observation was recorded about a man ap-pointed to evaluate the performance of the imperial family in China's Wei dy-nasty: "The Imperial Rater seldom rates men according to their merits, but always according to his likes and dislikes."

Performance evaluation is a time-consuming but important aspect of labo-ratory management, but most employees and managers often dread it. Trying to develop and establish a fair, just, and equitable evaluation process, which is also a positive experience for both the employee and the supervisor, is a chal-lenging task. By establishing a performance development program, the evalua-tion process can be turned into a "win-win" situation for both the employees and the managers by becoming a tool for professional development. A clear un-derstanding of performance development, including its benefits and how it works, is essential for both employees and supervisors. The employee in con-sultation with his or her supervisor should establish performance expectations and measurements at the beginning of the process. The supervisor or manager should guide employees in recognizing and developing the competencies required to meet the organizational or laboratory's objectives. A successful performance development program and subsequent evaluation must have input from the employee.

In this chapter on performance evaluation and professional development, we hope to provide a new approach to the process. We begin with building relationships and mastering feedback skills. Our focus is on self-evaluation and development with management feedback. This approach provides for collaboration and partnership in the performance evaluation process for professional development and a win-win relationship.

MANAGEMENT TOOLS FOR PAINLESS PERFORMANCE EVALUATIONS AND PERFORMANCE DEVELOPMENT

Performance development is an ongoing two-way process for communicating about the employee's job performance and helping them achieve excellence in their position and job satisfaction. It involves many processes: goal setting, feedback, guidance, motivation, evaluation, and development planning. It is an ongoing process that both supervisors and employees actively use throughout the year.

Research on human personality suggests that individuals need to be treated with civility and respect. They want opportunities to feel independent and competent. They actively desire to pursue goals to which they are committed. However, most organizations manage individuals using *task/production management.* Research on production management indicates its characteristics, which are production/task-oriented, tend to create situations in which the individual feels submissive, passive, and dependent. For consistency task/production management does not encourage individuals to use the abilities they believe to be important or develop them. Activities are not aimed at the individual's needs but at the manager and organization's, thus creating frustration, resentment, and underproduction. This chapter presents an approach to managing people developed by Dr. Phillip L. Hunsaker and Dr. Anthony J. Alessandra.

The *collaborative management* philosophy incorporates the belief that individuals participate in this type of management because they feel appreciated and understood. They are not being forced to comply by a mandate from their supervisor. The collaborative management process must be built around trust. Trust requires openness and honesty on the part of both the supervisor and the employee. A successful win-win relationship is built on trust. If there is trust the employee will collaborate because he or she feels understood by the supervisor and the supervisor understands the problems. The employee wants to make decisions to solve problems. Table 7–1 explains the difference between production/task management and collaborative management.

TABLE 7–1. Comparison of Task/Production Management (left column) and Collaborative Management (right column)

• Creates power base	• Creates trust relationship
• Identifies problem	• Defines problem solution
• Provides plan for employee	• Develops action plan together
• Threat—if you don't do it	• Supports risks taking
• Oversees—punishment/reward	• Coaches and follow-up

Adapted from Hunsaker PL, Alessandra AJ: Building productive managerial relationships. In *The Art of Managing People,* 10th ed. Prentice-Hall, Englewood Cliffs, NJ, 1980.

PRINCIPLES OF COLLABORATIVE MANAGEMENT

The four basic principles of collaborative management are trust, understanding, independence, and solutions (Table 7–2). By using these principles you can (1) increase job effectiveness and improve performance and (2) create an atmosphere of growth and learning for professional development. Actions always speak louder than words. Therefore, you must be willing to trust your employees and give them opportunities for independence and collaboration. Remember you cannot succeed with these principles unless you are willing to trust your employees. This means you must be open and honest, and your employee must feel he or she can be open and honest with you. You can then form a trust-bond relationship. This relationship provides the foundation for collaborative management.

Five-step performance development process   To move successfully into collaborative management we recommend a five-step process to establish an effective relationship for joint problem solving. Keep in mind actions speak louder than words. If you are not willing to trust your employees and develop a partnership then you cannot be successful in the 21st Century—the Information Age. Our new world of constant change requires teams, collaboration, and partnership. Learning collaborative management techniques will ensure successful out-

TABLE 7–2. Four Basic Principles of Collaborative Management

Trust	Relationship between employee and manager that requires openness and honesty.
Understanding	Individuals perform because they feel understood by the manager and understand the problem.
Independence	Individuals resent being manipulated, controlled, or persuaded into making a decision even if that was the decision they would eventually have made. They need the right to make their own decisions.
Solutions	Management should not solve the employee's problems. They will resent this. Rather, point out problems and ask for solutions.

comes with many of your relationships. The 5 steps recommended to establish an effective relationship for joint problem solving are identified and described as follows:

1. *Trust:* Mutual respect and understanding is prerequisite for joint problem solving. Collaboration and teamwork cannot happen unless a firm trust relationship is developed with the employee. Employees want a supervisor who they feel understands and cares about them. They prefer a supervisor they know they can rely on. They need to know that the manager is interested in their personal needs, career goals, and continual growth and development. They need to know they can take risks, which will help in their personal and professional development.

2. *Problem solving:* The manager can promote trust by being involved in problem solving with the employee. The manager must continually review personal and task goals and provide praise as often as possible. He or she must also guide and coach the subordinate when there is a problem to be solved or a plan correction to be made to successfully accomplish goals. The success of this activity hinges on effective information sharing and information-gathering skills.

3. *Action Plans:* The major role of the manager is to listen "actively" and ask questions. Direct the action planning process toward personal and professional goals as well as business objectives. The new action plan should be mutually beneficial toward improved performance and development with clearly stated measurable outcomes.

4. *Implementation:* Subordinates become committed to plans when they are allowed to have a major role in determining goals and objectives of a plan of action.

5. *Feedback:* The supervisor must continually seek feedback from the subordinate and provide support in order to monitor the plan and desired results. The supervisor uses *feedback skills* by responding quickly with praise when results are positive and to situations needing plan corrections before they become a problem.

Understanding People

Managers cannot promote professional development unless they understand people. They need to be aware of the importance of recognizing differences both in learning and behavioral styles. Awareness can help keep tensions at a minimum. Managers can enhance their knowledge of these learning concepts.

Learn How to Learn.   Successful managers are distinguished by their ability to adapt and master change within the organization. This affects their jobs and career demands. All individuals have unique ways of learning, with both strong and weak points. It is important for managers to be aware of their own and subordinates' learning styles and the alternatives made available. Personal and team development can then proceed in the most efficient and effective manner.

Keep Tension at a Minimum.   Individuals have different behavioral styles and process information in different ways, which often creates tension. The collaborative manager must be able to perceive these differences and adapt to them to use employees' abilities most effectively. Trust decreases when tension increases. It is important to recognize difference in order to maintain a balance.

Interactive Communication Skills

Communication skills need continual learning. It is the single most important skill we often fail to master both personally and professionally. This section provides an overview and framework for improving communication skills that will assist managers in the evaluation and professional development process.

Questioning:

> *"Would you tell me, please, which way I ought to go from here?"*
> *"That depends a good deal on where you want to get to," said the Cat.*
> *"I don't much care where—" said Alice.*
> *"Then it doesn't matter which way you go," said the Cat.*
>
> *Alice in Wonderland, Lewis Carroll*

How to ask questions requires practice. To coach the employee successfully the manager must have the ability to ask the right question at the right time. This is critical for the development of collaboration and teamwork. Getting people to "open up" and discover things for themselves is an art. Questions are used to:

1. Gather information.
2. Understand perspectives and frame of reference.
3. Provide information. For example, did you know there is a training program to develop computer skills?
4. Obtain participation.
5. Clarify understanding.
6. Receive opinions and suggestions. This provides an opportunity for positive feedback and building trust.
7. Create consensus to reach agreement or discover differences.

Listening: The supervisor must attempt to be objective to be successful at listening. Listening is not simply hearing. It requires emotional, intellectual, and physical input in search of truly hearing what is being said. The listener must concentrate and physically demonstrate sensitivity by showing various physical changes so that the person speaking feels that he or she is being heard. Managers who are poor listeners will miss messages and opportunities and, perhaps, address the wrong problem. More important the manager who is a poor listener will create distrust.

Barriers to effective listening are the following:

1. No motivation
2. Lack of attention

3. Poor attitude
4. Lack of awareness of good listening skills
5. Inappropriate setting
6. Emotions
7. Prejudices

Image:

First impressions are lasting impressions and the most important.

How others see you often determines how you will be treated. By projecting an image that is professional, authoritative, knowledgeable, successful, and enthusiastic, managers are more likely to be trusted by those they supervise. It is important to develop an image and style that promote trust. To accomplish this goal the manger must pay attention to the following:

1. Body language. How you walk—erect and strong; shake hands—firm; eye contact—direct when appropriate (always consider culture preferences); approachable (smile or pleasant expression).
2. Clothing—neat and professional.
3. Demonstrate competencies with respect to knowledge, skills, and ability regarding the field of expertise.
4. Flexibility—requires recognizing differences and willingness to accommodate individual preferences when appropriate. The manager will need to sometimes negotiate and ensure that everybody wins. He or she must be understanding, reasonable, and tactful.
5. Positive/enthusiastic—look for the opportunities. Recognize and praise accomplishments frequently.

Voice tones:

People usually choose the meaning of what is said rather than how it is said.

The exact words said with a different vocal emphasis can have significantly different meanings. To communicate effectively the manager must be aware of not only the way to say things but also of the vocal intonations of others. This is how to gather more information, meaning, and feeling from the words spoken. How the manager uses his or her voice will help or hurt the development of trust. Build trust with voice tones by:

1. Projecting in a strong and confident resonance.
2. Speaking clearly.
3. Demonstrating enthusiasm through the use of pitch, volume, and inflection.
4. Never speaking in monotones.
5. Using a natural rather than "put-on" voice.
6. Speaking slowly or rapidly depending on the subject and emphasis desired (always pay attention to facial expressions).

How to Develop Feedback Skills

Most managers, even experienced ones, dislike conducting performance evaluations because they wish to avoid:

- Conflict
- Taking responsibility for their evaluation of another person's performance
- Giving feedback

Few managers know how to give and receive feedback well. Nevertheless, managers must learn how to give feedback to maximize employees' performance. Managers need to think differently about giving feedback. They need to shift their focus from feedback avoidance to feedback skill development. They must practice how to:

- Establish clear and agreed to goals, expectations, and measurable outcomes.
- Meet on a regular basis to discuss progress.
- Request feedback from the employee on their support.

Key Principles

- *Feedback needs both manager and employee.* A two-way conversation must take place in which both parties speak openly and listen to each other's points of view. When we engage in conversation we create the opportunity to build collaboration and trust.
- *Feedback must provide for individual focus.* The manager must create a process that allows both the manager and employee to share individual points of view. When each person brings his or her professional history and value system into the conversation, the results can be much richer.
- *Feedback must begin with what's working.* Managers must always begin by focusing on the positive. How can we do more of the good that is happening? Always be forward focused. When the manager begins with the positive, it sets the stage for good feedback. The manager will not be effective unless he or she genuinely wants to help the employee to be successful.

Managers can put those three principles into action by addressing four key elements when they prepare for performance evaluations: observe, assess, look at performance results, and develop a plan of action (Table 7–3).

TABLE 7–3. **Key Elements in Preparing for Performance Evaluations**

- **Observe**—review core responsibilities, goals, and accomplishments
- **Assess**—what are the results of established measurable outcomes
- **Results**—success or failure
- **Develop**—plan of action

TABLE 7–4. Principles of Performance Development

Clearly define objectives and clearly outline the performance assessment process.

- Clearly define how the employee's work contributes to the overall goals and subsequent success of the laboratory/institution.
- Provide timely and accurate feedback throughout the assessment period (usually a year).
- Provide direction, guidance, and support to employees throughout the assessment period.
- Conduct occasional performance review discussions with written documentation at least two to three times a year.
- Provide recognition and reward linked to excellent performance.

Performance Evaluation and Performance Development Approach for "New Age" Employees

The primary responsibility of all managers is mentoring and providing opportunities for growth and development of their staff. The performance evaluation is the tool for documenting collaborative plans for development. The process provides an opportunity to reflect on the past year and reward the employee for contributions to the organization. It is an opportunity to talk about strengths and what is working. It is the supervisor's responsibility to support the employee with positive feedback and encourage open communications. Employees take pride in their work and want to feel appreciated and respected. A formal process (performance evaluation) offers the opportunity to show appreciation and/or indicate which activities need improvement. One of the many supervisor responsibilites consists of helping employees contribute to the overall department and/or facility goals through accomplishing specifically defined *performance objectives.* These performance objectives should be kept in mind as the manager completes the evaluation. This evaluation is a critical part of performance development. Employees will be more motivated and much more productive, producing a higher quantity and quality of work when certain principles are followed (Table 7–4).

A well-planned performance development program should provide supervisors and employees with a tool to improve performance and enhance laboratory/institutional effectiveness. By motivating and directing employees' efforts and providing adequate resources, a performance development program can help the laboratory and institution achieve their long-range goals and foster improved ongoing communication between supervisors and employees.

PERFORMANCE EVALUATION AND PERFORMANCE DEVELOPMENT GUIDELINES

Step One: Preparation for Process

1. Ensure that an updated job/position description and resume are included when the self-evaluation form is submitted to the employee.

2. Review previous goals and feedback meetings, which have taken place during the year.
3. As soon as the employee has completed the self-evaluation compare notes from previous meetings and compare evaluation of goals.
4. Schedule a mutually agreed to meeting date for the evaluation well in advance to provide the employee time to prepare.

Step Two: Interview Preparation

1. Conduct the interview in a private atmosphere. Sometimes a "neutral" site may be helpful.
2. Consider personal biases and don't allow them to influence the evaluation.
3. Consider the whole period of evaluation, not just the employee's performance at the end of the period.
4. Use the feedback tools and keep the interview a two-way feedback discussion.
5. Avoid these tendencies:
   - *Consistent leniency:* Tendency to "go easy on people" to be nice to everyone.
   - *Consistent severity:* Tendency to "be too hard on people" to uphold high standards.
   - *Central tendency:* Tendency to rate almost everyone as average on nearly every goal/standard/competency instead of being more realistic in judgment.
   - *Prejudice:* Tendency to allow a personal feeling toward the person being rated to influence judgment, including biases that relate to age, sex, race, nationality, or other non-job-related factors.
   - *Other tendencies:* (1) Overlooking problems outside the staff member's control; (2) Blaming the person's "personality;" (3) Allowing the last evaluation to influence thinking on this evaluation; do not be trapped into thinking that you have to give a rating of outstanding because you have in the past; (4) Giving high ratings to those who appear to be most active rather than those who are most productive (Table 7–5).

TABLE 7–5. Factors Important in Establishing Clear Performance Objectives and Expectations

- Define an updated, current, and accurate job description.
- Define reasonable and attainable expectations.
- Define relevance and importance of the expectations to successful performance of the job.
- Expectations should support and relate to the unit/team or laboratory department.
- Skills of the employee should match expectations (if not, an action plan should be established to acquire skills).
- Define examples of behavior/results for each performance factor.

TABLE 7–6. Rating Scale

Outstanding
Above Standards
Meets Standards
Below Standards
Unsatisfactory

An important area in the performance development program is the rating scale that should be clearly defined and reviewed with the employee during the performance development cycle phase. Table 7–6 gives an example of a rating scale. Definitions and examples of the rating scale should be provided to the employee in clear understandable language. These definitions should serve as guidelines that can be used to measure the level of each employee's performance. Table 7–7 gives some selected examples for each level of rating, but does not represent the comprehensive list available.

Step Three: Interview

1. A performance evaluation interview is central to the process. It is a formal discussion between the manager and staff member to evaluate how the staff member is performing in terms of accomplishments, responsibilities, and outcomes, as well as how the staff member can perform more effectively in the future.

2. The purpose of this meeting is to (a) discuss the staff member's self-assessment, (b) give the manager's own assessment, and (c) plan for the next period. The performance evaluation meeting provides both the manager and staff member the opportunity to give and receive feedback on performance. How well the manager uses that opportunity depends in large part on excellent feedback and communication skills.

3. Here are a few tips on how to begin the interview. Make every effort to begin the interview on the right foot, putting the staff member at ease with a friendly and open introduction. The initial few minutes have a great impact on the outcome of the interview.

- Explain the purpose of the performance evaluation.
- Let the staff member discuss his or her self-evaluation first.
- Ask the staff member to discuss, clarify, or elaborate on the information given on the form prepared. This is especially important if the staff member's self-evaluation is dramatically different from the evaluation.
- Tell the staff member what you agree with first and then what you disagree with. Finally, bring up areas that the staff member has not discussed that are important.
- Avoid criticizing personality traits.
- Be objective: talk about measurable, observable behaviors or results.

4. Use effective communication skills

- Listen for emotional and logical content.

TABLE 7–7. Rating Scale Explanation

Outstanding:
- Performance that exceeds expectations, performing duties above and beyond those of his or her regular job.
- An employee who has taken the initiative to develop new strategies that have benefited the success of the laboratory and/or institution.
- An employee who has improved the work environment by anticipating problems and planning for their solution.
- An employee who creatively designed or developed innovative approaches to achieving success in the workplace.

Above Standards:
- An employee who has shown one or more examples of having the ability to work at a level that exceeds his or her regular job-related duties.
- An employee who continues to show growth and a willingness to improve performance.
- Employee demonstrates unusual proficiency in performing difficult and complex aspects of the job competently and thoroughly, including extra and unique tasks assigned.

Meets Standards:
- Employee's performance meets the criteria and standards of job performance for practically all aspects of the job.
- Performance is steady and reliable and is maintained with a minimum of supervision.
- An employee who regularly performs his or her job functions with reliability and competence.

Below Standards:
- Performance that is in need of improvement in one or more areas related to job duties and responsibilities.
- Performance meets some requirements of the position but does not consistently meet the key, most important duties, responsibilities, requirements, and expectations of the job.
- Occasionally meets the performance expectations, but requires development.

Unsatisfactory:
- Fails to meet expectations and assignments were frequently completed at an unacceptable level of performance.
- Quality of work is poor and requires an unreasonable amount of supervision.
- Consistently fails to meet deadlines and standards of accuracy.

- Listen attentively.
- Allow time for discussion.
- Coach rather than criticize.
- Ask for clarification of points you do not understand.
- Say what you think the speaker is feeling.
- Be supportive.
- Observe nonverbal cues.
- Avoid defensiveness.
- Emphasize mutual problem solving.
- Summarize and give feedback.
  5. Praise
     - Be specific.

- Be direct.
- Praise often.
6. Use constructive criticism
   - Be specific.
   - Define desired outcomes.
   - Offer suggestions about how to achieve desired outcomes.
   - Encourage the staff member by expressing faith that he or she can change.
   - Listen attentively to the staff member's response.
7. Before closing, review the interview to make sure
   - You have made clear the points you wanted to cover.
   - The staff member has expressed his or her ideas thoroughly.
   - You have learned about the staff member's motivations and concerns on the job.
   - The staff member understands your expectations and how you evaluated his or her overall performance.
   - Goals have been set and prioritized or activities defined.
   - An action plan has been cooperatively developed and is mutually supported.

Step Four: Feedback

1. Follow-up with feedback. The performance appraisal process does not end with the evaluation interview. Continue to give feedback consistently throughout the next appraisal period.

2. Feedback consistent with day-to-day information exchange that you share with the staff member. These comments are usually unplanned and spontaneous, yet should always be clearly stated.

3. To be an effective reinforcer, feedback, whether positive or negative, must occur soon after a behavior.

4. Do not defer dealing with unpleasant issues until the next performance evaluation session. They should be addressed as they occur, which requires direct confrontation.

Step Five: Mentoring

1. Remove roadblocks to productivity. There are a variety of ways to help support the staff member's work more efficiently and effectively. A large part of improving performance and professional development is a state of mind—a way of doing things better and emphasizing continual improvement.

2. The following are suggestions for removing roadblocks to improve performance and increase opportunities:
   - Make necessary resources available.
   - Open channels of communication.
   - Be flexible with action plan revisions.
   - Give staff members information they may need to be effective.
   - Provide support for risk taking.
   - Give recognition of progress on an ongoing basis.

- Acknowledge achievements departmentally.
- Provide constructive feedback when appropriate.

COMPETENCY MODELING

A current hot topic for performance development and evaluation is *competency modeling.* The idea for testing for competence was first proposed in the early 1970s by David McClelland, a former Harvard psychologist. McClelland was asked by the U.S. Foreign Service to find new research methods that could predict human performance and reduce the bias of traditional intelligence and aptitude testing. There is a great deal of confusion surrounding this concept since it began 25 years ago. This is due to evolution and original ideas. The definitions of competency, core competency, and competency model follow:

- **Competency:** The knowledge, skill, ability, or characteristic associated with high performance on a job, such as problem solving, analytical thinking, or leadership. Some definitions of a competency include motives, beliefs, and values.
- **Core competency:** Organizational capabilities or strengths—what an organization does best. A core competency might be product development or customer service.
- **Competency model:** A performance evaluation design that uses core competencies (organizational capabilities or strengths, that is, what an organization does best). Examples of such model formats are located later in this chapter.

To construct the appropriate competency model one of the following tools must be used for building the model:

- *Job-analysis interviews:* The interviews can be conducted in person, or in focus groups. Interviews are the best method of data collection.
- *Questionnaires:* Normally used when there are many employees to be interviewed. It is critical, however, to have appropriate questions, a sufficient sample returned, and results analyzed for accuracy.
- *Competency-model formats:* Some models use statistical data to describe the competency requirements in specific detail and use less detail in the competency descriptions. Others reverse the balance.

The competency model for a manager or supervisor might be to identify success factors (competencies), provide a behavioral description of each one, rank-order the factors by criticality, and establish a proficiency level for each factor (Table 7–8). Success factors might include managing change, setting a vision, sharing information, and supporting teams.

Competency models must be governed by the collective wisdom of the people that need and build them. The decision to use a particular type of competency model should be determined by the desired applications.

If competency modeling is used, the self-appraisal form should be adjusted by replacing core responsibility with core competency or competency. An example of a self-appraisal form is included in Appendix 7–A on pp. 148–151.

TABLE 7–8. Sample Competency Model for a Systems Engineer

Technical Cluster	Proficiency Ratings

Systems Architecture

Ability to design complex software applications, establish protocols, and create prototypes.

0- Is not able to perform basic tasks.
1- Understands basic principles; can perform tasks with assistance or direction.
2- Performs routine tasks with reliable results; works with minimal supervision.
3- Performs complex and multiple tasks; can coach or teach others.
4- Considered an expert in this task; can describe, teach, and lead others.

Data Migration

Ability to establish the necessary platform requirements to efficiently and completely coordinate data transfer.

0- Is not able to perform basic tasks.
1- Understands basic principles; can perform tasks with assistance or direction.
2- Performs routine tasks with reliable results; works with minimal supervision.
3- Performs complex and multiple tasks; can coach or teach others.
4- Considered an expert in this task; can describe, teach, and lead others.

Documentation

Ability to prepare comprehensive and complete documentation including specifications, flow diagrams, process control, and budgets.

0- Is not able to perform basic tasks.
1- Understands basic principles; can perform tasks with assistance or direction.
2- Performs routine tasks with reliable results; works with minimal supervision.
3- Performs complex and multiple tasks; can coach or teach others.
4- Considered an expert in this task; can describe, teach and lead others.

Summary

The performance development program can be an excellent tool for professional development of both employees and supervisors. By using this program, employees can be introduced to the basic principles of professional development, which are built on the foundation of a commitment to learning, independent thinking, a willingness to share expertise, and the development of professional pride. Specific performance and measurable results are used to establish a common understanding of the employees' performance strengths and weaknesses. Performance discussions are based on previously agreed to, job-related factors important to the overall success on the job. Performance discussions are highly individualized and reflect employees' unique goals, abilities, and development needs. The performance management program guides the employee in analyzing his or her own performance and with the support from the supervisor, the employee can both understand strengths and define improvement needs. The performance discussion should be based on the entire review period and not on just recent performance. All the meetings should incorporate constructive criticism and focus on how to improve performance rather than reiterating past failures or shortcomings. Using a well-planned and implemented performance development program should allow the employee to address professional issues, interpersonal skills, career planning, goal setting, and foster pride and recognition of the employees' strengths and contributions to the laboratory/institution.

SUGGESTED PROBLEM-BASED LEARNING ACTIVITIES
Chapter 7: Performance Evaluation and Professional Development

Instructions: Use Internet resources, books, articles, colleagues, etc., to present solutions to the problems listed below. There is no one correct solution to any problem.

Note to instructor: Students in class may be divided into groups and given the problem-based learning activity to discuss and solve. Once the group has reached consensus as to a solution, the group may present it to the other students in the class. This activity will provide all students with information regarding solutions to the problem.

Problem #1
Suppose a minority employee feels that he or she was not promoted based on their minority status. As manager, how do you handle this situation?

Problem #2
Design a performance appraisal and supporting documents to be used in your laboratory.

Problem #3
Create a problem employee and prepare a plan of action for correcting the issues relating to this problem behavior.

BIBLIOGRAPHY

Bridges, W: Managing Transitions. Harper Collins Publishers, New York, New York, 1991.

Butteriss, M: Re-Inventing HR Changing Roles To Create The High-Performance Organization, John Wiley & Sons Canada Limited, Etobicoke, Ontario, 1998.

Chang RY, De Young P: *Measuring Organizational Improvement Impact.* Richard Chang Associates, Inc. Publications Division, Irvine, California, 1995.

Citrin, JM, Smith RA: The Five Patterns of Extraordinary Careers: The Guide for Achieving Success and Satisfaction, Crown Business, New York, New York, 2003.

Conger, JA: Learning To Lead. Jossey-Bass Publishers, San Francisco, California 1992.

Covey, SR: Principle Centered Leadership. Summit Books, New York, New York, 1991.

Dichter, E: Motivating Human Behavior. McGraw-Hill Book Company, New York, New York, 1971.

Dotlich DL, Cairo, PC: Action Coaching. Jossey-Bass Publishers, San Francisco, California, 1999.

Fisher, R, Ury, W: Getting To Yes. Penguin Books, New York, New York, 1992.

Gilbert, TF: Measuring Potential For Performance Improvement. Lakewood Publications, Minneapolis, Minnesota, 2003.

Jones, JE, Bearley, WL: 360 Degree Feedback. HRD Press, Amherst, MA. & Lakewood Publications, 1996.

Kravetz, DJ: The Directory For Building Competencies. Kravetz Associates, Bartlett, Illinois, 1995.

Krugg D: *Enlightened Leadership.* Enlightened Leadership International, Inc. Englewood, CO., 1998.

Neal JE: *Effective Phrases for Performance Appraisals: A Guide to Successful Evaluations*, 9th ed. Neal Publications, 2000.

Nigon DL: *Clinical Laboratory Management, Leadership Principles for the 21st Century.* McGraw-Hill Health Professions Division, New York, 2000.

Rummler, GA: Performance Is The Purpose. Lakewood Publications, Minneapolis, Minnesota, 2002.

Simmons, A: When Performance Reviews Fail, September 2004, T+D Magazine.

Tjosvold, D: Learning To Manage Conflict. Lexington Books, New York, New York, 1993.

Varnadoe LA: *Medical Laboratory Management and Supervision.* F.A. Davis, Philadelphia, PA., 1996.

Internet Resources

How To Do An Employee Appraisal
http://www.visitorinfo.com/gallery/howapp.htm

HR Guide to the Internet: *Personnel Section*
http://www.hr-guide.com

Human Resources Development Information at the Human Resources Learning Center
http://www.human-resources.org

Institute for Professional Development
http://www.ipd.org

McNamara, Ph.D., C: Performance Management: Performance Appraisal (Generic to Performance Management)
http://www.managementhelp.org/perf_mng/appraisl.htm

Pam Pohly's Net Guide: Toolbox for Health Managers & Administrators
http:// www.pohly.com

Powerful Tools For Positive Performance. American Productivity & Quality Center, Houston, Texas
www.apqc.org

TAPPED IN
http://www.tappedin.org

APPENDIX 7–A

SECTION IV

SAMPLE/SELF-APPRAISAL

Employee Name: _____

Project/Location: _____ *Supervisor:* _____

Period Covered: From: _____ *To:* _____

1. *Attached is the most recent description for your position. Does this description accurately reflect your current duties and responsibilities?* _____Yes   _____No

2. *Based on your position description, indicate your core responsibilities and what was accomplished during the year. Each of us should include responsibilities relating to customer service, whether external or internal customers. If you had objectives from the prior evaluation period, indicate where objectives were accomplished and where they were not met. You may also want to include any special projects or assignments that were outside of your normal day-to-day responsibilities or other major accomplishments.*

Core Responsibilities	Accomplishments

Supervisor's Remarks:

If Appropriate:

Special Assignments/ Objectives From the Prior Year	Target Date	Accomplishments

Supervisor's Remarks:

(continued)

3. *What are the strengths of your performance? How would you improve the way you perform your responsibilities? Consider the performance factors indicated in the introduction and any others you feel appropriate in your response. These may include:*

Commitment To Excellence	*Human Relations Skills*
Job Knowledge	*Communication (Listening as*
Customer Knowledge	*well as Expressing)*
Administrative Capabilities	*Initiative and Independent Action*
Decision Making	*Managing Resources*
Teamwork	*Contributions to Stated Goals*
Problem Solving	*Professional Behavior*

Supervisor's Remarks:

---

4. *What significant difficulties did you encounter in your position during the appraisal period? Include difficulties that were within and outside your control. What assistance from the organization or your supervisor would be helpful to you in meeting these challenges in the future?*

5. *What additional responsibilities would you recommend for yourself? Are there aspects of your position you would like to change or improve? What actions are you currently taking or planning to take to further develop your skills and potential in this position? What actions can your supervisor, co-workers or company take to assist you?*

6. *In preparation for your upcoming discussion with your supervisor, list at least three possible performance objectives for yourself for the coming year. (Because each position has different responsibilities the number of objectives will vary depending on the position.) Please list them in order of priority, beginning with your highest priorities.*

   These objectives should be related to the key responsibilities of your position and, as much as possible, to the mission and plans of your department and the organization. Consider the corporate objectives and the objectives of your customers, and how your objectives relate to them. Focus on long-term objectives as well as short-term. Each of us should include specific objectives relating to customer service and how to improve quality service.

   Objectives should include continuous improvement and/or growth in a position rather than simply a continuation of current responsibilities and how you carry them out. What can be improved? How can quality be assured? How can we assist the customer further?

   If improvements are needed in particular areas of your performance, develop objectives for those improvements. Be as specific as possible.

Objectives may involve acquiring new knowledge and skills, improvements in activities in which you are already involved, and new activities and projects. Objectives should be specific, measurable in terms of quantity or quality, useful and attainable (although significant effort may be required).

Briefly describe each objective, include a timetable, and any resources or training you might need in order to achieve your objectives.

Objective I:

Timetable:

Resources or Training Necessary:

Objective 2:

Timetable:

Resources or Training Necessary:

Objective 3:

Timetable:

Resources or Training Necessary:

Objective 4:

Timetable:

Resources or Training Necessary:

Objective 5:

Timetable:

Resources or Training Necessary:

(continued)

Feel Free to attach additional sheets as necessary.
Please feel free to include any additional comments or suggestions you care to make.

_____   _____

Employee's Signature   *Date*

_____   _____   _____

Supervisor's Signature   *Date*   *Date of Appraisal*
                                                              Discussion

SUPERVISOR'S SUMMARY

Provide an overall summary of the meeting with the employee. Include discussion of any areas of disagreement between yourself and the employee. You may want to describe the strengths of the employee's performance. Please indicate if any improvements are needed for satisfactory performance.

Indicate overall description of the employee's performance:

　　　_____　*Unsatisfactory/Needs Significant Improvement*
　　　_____　*Below Standards*
　　　_____　*Meets Standards*
　　　_____　*Above Standards*
　　　_____　*Outstanding*

_____   _____

Supervisor's Signature   *Date*

_____   _____

Manager's Signature   *Date*

_____   _____

Employee's Signature   *Date*

Education and Training: Practical Tips For Educators and Trainers

DENISE M. HARMENING, PhD, MT(ASCP), CLS(NCA)

Chapter Outline

Objectives
Key Terms
Case Study
Introduction
Domains and Levels of Learning
Applications of Instructional Objectives
   as Learning Outcomes
Assigning Taxonomy Levels to
   Educational Objectives

Matching the Level of Instruction to the
   Needs of the Learner and the Task
Summary
Suggested Problem-Based Learning
   Activities
Bibliography
Internet Resources

Objectives

Following successful completion of this chapter, the learner should be able to:

1. List and define the three domains of learning.
2. List Bloom's taxonomy levels.

3. Apply Bloom's taxonomy levels to the construction of behavioral objectives.
4. Assign taxonomy levels to the educational objectives.
5. Define learning outcomes.

Key Terms

Affective Domain

Cognitive Domain

Instructional/Educational Objectives

Learning Outcome

Psychomotor Domain

Taxonomy Levels

Case Study: Education and Training

You are a manager of a laboratory at a large university-based hospital in an academic health center. You have received complaints from your employees that "Mary" is not a team player. You have observed that Mary prefers to work alone and is not receptive to training student interns. At times, she can be abrasive toward others; however, she is extremely knowledgeable and her work is meticulous and accurate. She is never late and has never used sick time in her 5-year tenure with your department. Your counseling meeting with Mary reveals that she is intimidated by the prospect of training student interns because she has no background or experience in providing instruction.

Issues and Questions to Consider

1. *Evaluate Mary's potential as an instructor in your laboratory. Assess both her strengths and weaknesses.*
2. *How would you approach facilitating Mary's participation in the clinical training of student interns?*
3. *At the most basic level what would Mary need to know to match the level of instruction to the needs of the learner?*
4. *How would Mary develop specific learning objectives for the student interns?*
6. *What would Mary need to do to ensure that the learning outcomes were met?*

INTRODUCTION

In a teaching hospital, many individuals are required to provide instruction as part of their job without any formal training in education. One of their most difficult tasks is planning for instruction and matching the level of instruction to the needs of the learner. For example, training objectives for laboratory technicians who have two years of college education should be at a different level than technologists who have four years of college. **Training** at a specialist level would require an even higher level of complexity. Regardless of the level of instruction, it has been well established that the educational process of teaching and learning are significantly enhanced if both the teacher and learner have a clear definition of the expected *learning outcome* for the instructional task; however, several

TABLE 8–1.   The Three Domains of Learning

Domain	Definition
Cognitive	Acquiring and applying knowledge
Psychomotor	Ability to perform tasks or skills
Affective	Attitudes or feelings

differences exist in expectations for learning outcomes. For example, in some cases the learner is expected to acquire or apply knowledge; in other situations, the learner is expected to develop a skill or demonstrate proficiency. In still other instances, the outcome requires the learner to acquire an appropriate attitude or work ethic toward a task. These different educational outcomes define what is commonly known as the three "domains of learning" (Table 8–1).

DOMAINS AND LEVELS OF LEARNING

This chapter provides the learner with an overview of the domains and levels of learning followed by an in-depth discussion of the design and application of instructional objectives as learning outcomes. In addition, the chapter also describes the process of assigning learning levels to instructional objectives, as well as matching the level of instruction to the needs of the learner and the task.

The different levels of learning or *taxonomy levels* describe how a learner may progress from beginner to expert in each domain of learning. The main purpose of the taxonomy levels is to aid the instructor in defining the different learning outcomes. By using taxonomy levels, specific learning objectives can be developed starting with a basic level and progressing to increasing levels of difficulty in all three domains of learning (Table 8–2).

The taxonomy level for the *cognitive domain* is probably the most recognized and well used of those currently developed. This taxonomy level was formulated in 1958 by a committee headed by Dr. Benjamin Bloom and is now commonly referred to as Bloom's taxonomy levels. Table 8–3 lists and defines the six taxonomy levels of the cognitive domain.

TABLE 8–2.   Taxonomy Levels of the Three Domains Of Learning

Cognitive	Psychomotor	Affective
Levels of Understanding	*Levels of PsychomotorDevelopment*	*Levels of Feeling*
1. Knowledge	1. Reflex movements	1. Receiving
2. Comprehension	2. Basic fundamental movements	2. Responding
3. Application	3. Perceptual abilities	3. Valuing
4. Analysis	4. Physical abilities	4. Organization
5. Synthesis	5. Skilled movements	5. Characterization
6. Evaluation	6. Non-discursive movement	

TABLE 8–3. Bloom's Taxonomy Levels

1. **KNOWLEDGE: (Recall) The remembering of previously learned material.** This may involve the recall of material ranging from specific facts to complete theories, but all that is required is the bringing to mind of the appropriate information. Knowledge is defined as the remembering of previously learned material.
2. **COMPREHENSION: (Understanding) The ability to grasp the meaning of material.** This may be shown by translating the material from one form to another (words to numbers), by interpreting material (explaining or summarizing), and by estimating future trends (predicting consequences or effects). Comprehension is defined as the ability to grasp the meaning of material. These learning outcomes go one step beyond the simple remembering of material and represent the lowest level of understanding.
3. **APPLICATION: The ability to use the learned material in new and concrete situations.** This may include such things as rules, methods, concepts, principles, laws, and theories. Application refers to the ability to use learned material in new and concrete situations. Learning outcomes in this area require a higher level of understanding than those under comprehension.
4. **ANALYSIS: The ability to break down learned material into its component parts so that its organizational structure can be understood.** This may include identification of the parts, analysis of the relationship between the parts, and recognition of the organizational principles involved. Analysis refers to the ability to break down material into its component parts so that its organizational structure may be understood. Learning outcomes here represent a higher intellectual level than comprehension and application because they require an understanding of both the content and the structural form of the material.
5. **SYNTHESIS: The ability to put parts together to form a new whole.** This area stresses creative behaviors with emphasis on formulation of *new* patterns or structures. Synthesis refers to the ability to put parts together to form a new whole. This may involve the production of a unique communication (theme or speech), a plan of operations (research proposal), or a set of abstract relations (scheme for classifying information). Learning outcomes in this area stress creative behaviors, with major emphasis on the formulation of new patterns or structures.
6. **EVALUATION: The ability to judge the value of material for a given purpose.** Judgments are based on definite criteria. These may be internal criteria (organization) or external criteria (relevance to the purpose), and the student may determine the criteria or be given them. Evaluation is concerned with the ability to judge the value of material (statement, novel, poem, research report) for a given purpose. Learning outcomes in this area are highest in the cognitive hierarchy because they contain elements of all of the other categories, plus conscious value judgments based on clearly defined criteria.

If objectives in the cognitive domain are well written, the intended learning outcomes should be clear and easy to measure through testing. A major problem experienced by educators in this domain is that the six levels overlap, creating some confusion related to the correct level in which to place the objective. As a result, Bloom et al. have listed a number of verbs that can be used in writing objectives. The intended purpose of this list is to facilitate the selection of the correct verb in writing the instructional objective. The taxonomy level is defined by the verb. Table 8–4 lists the verbs (behavioral terms) and instructional objectives of the various taxonomy levels of the cognitive domain.

TABLE 8–4. Verbs (Behavioral Terms) and Instructional Objectives of the Taxonomy Levels of the Cognitive Domain

Taxonomy Level	Verbs (Behavioral Terms)	Instructional Objectives
Knowledge	Defines, describes, labels, identifies, matches, names, states, selects	*Know* terms, facts, methods, procedures, concepts, principles
Comprehensive	Explains, estimates, infers, distinguishes, defends, converts, generalizes, gives examples, summarizes, paraphrases, rewrites	*Understand* facts and *principles, interpret* charts and graphs, *translate* verbal to mathematical formulas, *estimate* future consequences inferred from data
Application	Changes, calculates, demonstrates, discovers, manipulates, modifies, operates, predicts, prepares, produces, relates, shows, solves, uses	*Applies* concepts and principles to new situations, *applies* laws and theories to practical situations, *solve* mathematical problems, *constructs* charts or graphs
Analysis	Breaks down, diagrams, differentiates, distinguishes, identifies, illustrates, infers, outlines, points out, relates, selects, separates, subdivides	*Recognizes* unstated assumptions, *evaluates* relevancy of the data, *distinguishes* between facts and inferences
Synthesis	Categorizes, combines, complies, composes, creates, designs, generates, modifies	*Proposes* or *plans* a new entity, *integrates* learning from different parts to solve a problem, formulates a new concept
Evaluation	Appraises, compares, concludes, criticizes, justifies, interprets, explains, supports, describes	*Judges* the value of written material, and the value of work by use of internal criteria or external standards of excellence

Many educators and trainers find these verbs helpful. Irrespective of the verb used, however, one should keep in mind the intent of the objective regardless of experience in writing objectives. The verb used for the intended learning outcome may be interpreted differently by the learner. For example, the verb *illustrate* in an objective may be intended to have the learning outcome be a drawing or diagram of a complex structure, but the learner may interpret this verb to mean that he or she must point out something to satisfy the learning objective. The best way to learn to use Bloom's taxonomy levels is to provide some examples (see next section).

In practice, the taxonomy levels of the cognitive domain are by far the most widely used; however, the psychomotor and affective domains are not well used in educational settings.

The ***psychomotor domain*** can be well used in the laboratory training area to define the level of competency expected of a learner in performing a variety of

TABLE 8–5. Examples Of Immunohematology Clinical Educational Objectives

On completion of the immunohematology rotation the student will be able to meet the following objectives within acceptable limits as determined by the clinical faculty.
1. Evaluate quality control in the immunohematology laboratory and formulate a logical course of action when reagent controls fall outside normal limits.
2. Perform ABO and Rh grouping including weak D (formerly Du) status on designated patients and donor units.
3. Describe the principle and applications of direct antiglobulin testing and include the follow-up testing of positive direct antiglobulin tests.
4. Perform antibody screening and identification procedures and select any of the following special techniques that may be useful for investigating antibody problems:

• Elution	• Adsorption
• Enzyme treatment	• Temperature manipulation
• Enhancement media	• Neutralization (optional)

5. List the federal, state, and peer review agencies and committees that monitor blood banks and transfusion services.
6. Compare and contrast the following adverse reactions to transfusion in regard to cause, classic signs and symptoms, recommendations for future transfusion, and serologic investigation (if applicable).
   - Immediate hemolytic
   - Delayed hemolytic
   - Febrile nonhemolytic
   - Urticarial
   - Anaphylactic
   - Bacterial
7. Formulate a strategy for troubleshooting basic problems in technique and procedure.
8. Exhibit professional attributes and attitudes and maintain professional standards when interacting with professionals within the laboratory and the healthcare facility.

tasks, for example, performing tests with a 100% accuracy or operating instrumentation. Once the objectives are written for this domain, the learning outcomes are relatively easy to measure. Measurement may require a checklist of steps to be completed for a procedure or performance of the task with 100% accuracy. Practical examinations are frequently used to assess objectives written in the psychomotor domain.

The *affective domain* can be helpful in defining learning expectations for students with respect to work ethic, initiative, interpersonal skills with co-workers, patient confidentiality of laboratory results, and professional interaction with other individuals on the healthcare team. The major problem experienced by most educators or trainers is that objectives in this domain are difficult to write and even more difficult to measure objectively and quantitatively.

The National Accrediting Agency for Clinical Laboratory Science (NAACLS) currently requires that clinical and didactic educational objectives be written in all three domains. The didactic training should involve more cognitive learning objectives and the clinical setting more psychomotor. Table 8–5 lists examples of clinical educational objectives for the blood bank laboratory rotations of the

University of Maryland School of Medicine's Medical Technology program. The reader should quickly review this list and classify the domain of learning for each objective.

APPLICATION OF INSTRUCTIONAL OBJECTIVES AS LEARNING OUTCOMES

Instructional/educational objectives may be written in many different formats. It is important to use instructional objectives to balance the level of instruction with the needs of the learner. Achieving this balance with clearly written objectives will provide the basis for the measurable outcome assessment. One of the most common errors in writing objectives is to state the objective in a manner that focuses attention on the teaching activity rather than the learning outcome, for example, to demonstrate to students how to use a cell washer. Can this be measured as a learning outcome for the student? Actually, the educator has achieved this objective once the demonstration is completed. A better way to write this objective is in terms of the type of learning outcomes we expect. After the teacher's demonstration, the objectives may be written as follows: After observing the demonstration, the learner will be able to:

(Cognitive)	**1.**	Describe the steps of proper operation of the blood bank cell washer.
(Cognitive)	**2.**	List the precautions necessary when using the cell washer.
(Cognitive)	**3.**	List the steps for calibration of the cell washer.
(Psycho-motor)	**4.**	Demonstrate skill by using the cell washer with acceptable performance for five patient samples.

Instructional objectives written in this format place the focus on the student and the type of knowledge and proficiency required as a result of the learning experience. A shift in focus from the learning process to the learning outcomes clarifies the intent of the instruction and sets the stage for evaluation of that instruction. The verbs *describe, list,* and *demonstrate* are specific types of behavior that indicate how the student shows that he or she has learned. Furthermore, these objectives are easily measured. It is important to be able to distinguish between stating objectives in terms of what will be taught and learning outcomes expected from students.

Read the following two objectives and decide which one is stated as an expected learning outcome.

The learner will be able to:

1. Instill an appreciation for the different types of transfusion reactions.
2. List and define the different types of transfusion reactions.

Clearly, the second objective specifies how a student will demonstrate learning after the instructional period. Note the second objective begins with a verb that implies an activity (which can be measured) on the part of the student. An educational objective should clearly indicate the intent of the instruction in terms of the type of behavior ("list and define") that the student is expected to demonstrate.

The verb in the first objective, *instills,* implies that the *teacher,* not the student, is engaged in the activity, and the objective cannot be appropriately measured. Stating educational or instructional objectives as learning outcomes contributes to the instructional process by:

1. Providing direction for the educator/trainer.
2. Conveying clearly the instructional intent to others.
3. Providing a guide for instructional content, teaching methods, and materials to be used during instruction.
4. Providing a guide for constructing tests and other methods of evaluation of student competency.

A common error made in teaching is neglecting to use the educational objectives to construct tests. As a result the student does not know what is important and is not guided or focussed in the learning process; consequently, the test may not be a valid measure of the student's knowledge or proficiency.

Another common error in writing objectives is stating the objective in terms of the learning process instead of the learning outcome. Which of the following objectives is stated as an instructional/learning outcome?

The learner will be able to:

1. Gain knowledge of antigen-antibody reactions
2. Apply the basic principles of antigen-antibody reactions in performing ABO typing

The second objective clearly indicates what the student can do at the end of instruction. The first objective focuses on the "gaining of knowledge" (the learning process) rather than the type of behavior that provides evidence of the expected outcome of the learning experience.

These errors of stating objectives in terms of the teacher's performance and the learning process can be avoided by focusing on the type of student performance expected (learning outcome) at the end of instruction. To summarize, instructional/educational objectives should be concise, clear statements that define instructional intent in terms of the desired learning outcomes.

ASSIGNING TAXONOMY LEVELS TO EDUCATIONAL OBJECTIVES

One of the most difficult tasks is selecting the proper taxonomy level for the objective in the domain of learning. NAACLS requires, as a part of their accreditation process, that Medical Technology/Clinical Laboratory Science programs use objectives in various taxonomy levels and that examination questions assign taxonomy levels. The reader should refer to Table 8–3, which lists and defines Bloom's taxonomy levels, before working through the following examples:

Level 1, *knowledge,* involves recall, the remembering of previously learned material. This simplest level of learning requires basic memorization of information that may range from simple facts to complex principles or theories.

Example

The student will be able to list the hemoglobin/hematocrit required for the donation of blood.

Level 2, *comprehension,* is the ability to grasp the meaning of the material or information. This usually requires interpretation of information to indicate learning.

Example

The student will be able to interpret the ABO group from the serologic reactions listed for each patient.

Level 3, *application,* requires the ability to use the learned material in new and defined situations.

Example

The student will be able to calculate the number of platelet units needed to increase a patient's platelet count from 10,000 to 50,000.

Level 4, *analysis,* requires using the first three levels of knowledge, comprehension, and application previously described. It represents the ability to break down learned material into component parts so that the overall structure or organization can be understood. The level requires the learner to demonstrate insight in selecting the most significant parts of the material, identifying important components, and understanding relationships. The learner must be able to distinguish relevant from nonrelevant information, distinguish facts from assumptions, and identify the underlying principles of the concepts.

Example

The student will be able to select the appropriate product for transfusion after review and interpretation of the patient's clinical history and laboratory results.

Level 5, *synthesis,* is the ability to put parts or components together to form a new whole. This level requires the learner to combine elements to form something new through some creative or intuitive process. The learner is expected to develop an original application of the material learned.

Example

The student will be able to design a protocol for the investigation of hemolytic transfusion reactions in a 350-bed community hospital.

Level 6, *evaluation,* is the ability to judge the value of material for a given purpose. This is the highest level of understanding and requires the learner to use all five taxonomy levels in forming an assessment or judgment. This level usually involves the use of values and value judgments. Evaluation implies the determination of the value or quality of information in making a judgment that is usually based on appropriate established criteria. Evaluation involves making judgments based on factual information or values.

Example

Using the criteria for "ruling-out," the student will determine the appropriate "selective cells" to identify the patient's antibody(ies).

By now, it is apparent that trying to use all six taxonomy levels, which greatly overlap, for writing educational objectives is not only burdensome, but impractical for our field. As a result, most educators use the abbreviated version of taxonomy levels published by the American Society for Clinical Pathology (ASCP) (Table 8–6). In practice these three levels are used to assign taxonomy levels for test questions used for the certifying examinations given by the ASCP Board of Registry. In addition Standard 9A, of the NAACLS self-study process also requires assignment of taxonomy levels for test questions used in Medical Technology programs.

In the cognitive domain of learning, the Bloom's taxonomy levels can be correlated with the ASCP levels by arbitrarily assigning: knowledge as taxonomy level 1;

TABLE 8–6. **ASCP Taxonomy Levels**

TAXONOMY 1 – *Recall:* Ability to recall or recognize previously learned (memorized) knowledge ranging from specific facts to complete theories.

TAXONOMY 2 – *Interpretive Skills:* Ability to use recalled knowledge to interpret or apply verbal, numeric, or visual data.

TAXONOMY 3 – *Problem Solving:* Ability to use recalled knowledge and the interpretation/application of distinct criteria to resolve a problem or situation and/or make an appropriate decision.

---

comprehension and application as level 2; and analysis, synthesis, and evaluation as level 3.

MATCHING THE LEVEL OF INSTRUCTION TO THE NEEDS OF THE LEARNER AND THE TASK

The final component in planning for clinical instruction is to match the level of instruction to the needs of the learner. Clinical laboratory instructors must possess the ability to train individuals at several different levels of education and to ensure that the training received at each is appropriate to the tasks. Clinical rotational training is especially difficult for both the student and the clinical instructor because of variations that exist among laboratories. Numerous factors

TABLE 8–7. Examples of Consensus Results: Immunohematology/Blood Bank

Knowledge	Ability
A—Specimen collection, labeling, storage, and preparation	A—None required
B—Immunologic genetic theory	B—Has observed
C—Principles of methods including recognition and resolution of common problems	C—Has performed satisfactorily on practice specimens; may require additional experience
D—Disease manifestation/clinical correlations	D—Proficient; able to perform in job setting after usual employee orientation
E—Differentiates/resolves technical, instrument, physiologic causes of problems or unexpected test results	

Competencies	Knowledge		Ability	
	MT	MLT	MT	MLT
ABO blood typing	A, B, C, D, E	A, B, C, D, E	D	D
Rh blood grouping	A, B, C, D, E	A, B, C, D, E	D	D
Kell/Kidd Duffy systems	A, B, C, D, E	A, C, D	C	C
Miscellaneous blood group systems	None	None	A	A
Antibody screen	A, B, C, D, E	A, B, C, D	D	D
Antibody identification	A, B, C, D, E	A, B, C, D	D	C
Antibody titering	A, B, C, D, E	A, C	C	B
Elutions	A, B, C, D, E	A, C	C	B
Cold antibody workup using IgG AHG	A, B, C, D, E	C	C	A
Antibody removal by ZZAP	A, C	None	A	A
HLA testing	B, C, D	None	A	A

affect the student's clinical rotation experience, including the type and size of the laboratory, geographic region, urban versus rural setting, patient population, and knowledge and expertise of laboratory clinical instructors. Too often, clinical training is tied to the resources available within the laboratory rather than to the knowledge and proficiency needs of the learner. Furthermore, the clinical instructor is faced with the ongoing debate regarding which tasks should be associated with technologists at the various levels of education. For example, a clinical laboratory instructor employed in a large, urban, teaching hospital affiliated with a School of Medicine presented a student with a patient sample containing four unknown antibodies, one of which was anti-G. If one were to match the needs of the learner with this antibody exercise, what would be the appropriate educational level of the student, MLT, MT, or Specialist? Believe it or not, this sample was presented to an undergraduate MT student, and the clinical instructor firmly believed that MTs should be proficient in performing specialized antibody techniques. The confusion with regard to matching the level of instruction to the needs of the learner is understandable when clinical educators lack appropriate information on which to base their clinical instruction.

An excellent resource for clinical instructors is the report from the ASCP-AMS Educators Consensus Conference held in Albuquerque, New Mexico, in March 1995. Entitled, *Technical Curricula for MT and MLT Programs,* the report delineates the knowledge and abilities expected of career-entry graduates.

Table 8–7 further summarizes the knowledge and ability associated with immunohematology/blood bank procedures and tests as required at various learner levels. The ability to perform specialized high-frequency/low-frequency antibody techniques is not considered appropriate at the medical technologist level, but rather should be an integral part of the training at the specialist level.

SUMMARY

Clinical training is a vital component of the student's total educational experience. Armed with the resources and knowledge of what to teach, how to construct behavioral objectives and measurable learning outcomes, as well as how to match the level of instruction to the needs of the learner, the clinical laboratory instructor becomes a highly effective partner in training and mentoring the next generation of clinical laboratory science professionals.

SUGGESTED PROBLEM-BASED LEARNING ACTIVITIES
Chapter 8: Education and Training

Instructions: Use Internet resources, books, articles, colleagues, etc., to present solutions to the problems listed below. There is no one correct solution to any problem.

Note to Instructor: Students in class may be divided into groups and given the problem-based learning activity to discuss and solve. Once the group has reached consensus as to a solution, the group may present it to the other students in the class. This activity will provide all students with information regarding solutions to the problem.

Problem #1
Develop a training program for employees/students.

Problem #2
How do you, as a technologist, develop skills to train students or new employees?

Problem #3
Develop a tool to assess annual employee competence.

BIBLIOGRAPHY

Acharya, C: Students' Learning Styles and Their Implications for Teachers. *CDTL Brief* 2002 Vol. 5 No. 6; 1–3.

Bloom BS et al: *Taxonomy of Educational Objectives, The Classification of Educational Goals, Handbook I: Cognitive Domain,* David McKray Company, Inc, New York, 1956.

Gronlund N: *Preparing Criterion-Referenced Tests for Classroom Instruction,* MacMillan Co, New York, 1973.

Gronlund N: *Stating Behavioral Objectives for Classroom Instruction,* MacMillan Co, New York, 1970.

Harmening D et al: Defining the roles of medical technologists and medical laboratory technicians. *Lab Med* 1995; 26(3):175–8.

Krathwohl DR et al: *Taxonomy of Educational Objectives: The Classification of Educational Goals, Handbook II: Affective Domain,* David McKray Company, Inc, New York, 1964.

Lehmann C, Leiken A: Time to change medical technology education. *Med Lab Observer,* 1996; 63–65.

Leino-Kilpi H: The use of curriculum objectives in nursing education. *J Adva Nurs,* 1993; 18(3):465–70.

Miller T, Brelade S: 101 Tips for Trainers, Pearson Education Company, London, England, 1997.

Murdock J, Neafsey PJ: Self-efficacy measurements: an approach for predicting practice outcomes in continuing education? *J Cont Educ Nurs* 1995; 26(4): 158–65.

Sollosy D: Categorizing Questions by Taxonomy. Workshop for Canadian Association of Medical Laboratory Educators, Halifax, Nova Scotia, June, 1993.

Stoker D, Hull C: Teaching and Learning in Practice. *Nursing Times* 1994; 90(12): i–viii.

Synder J et al: Developing medical laboratory curricula: a systematic approach to consensus. *Lab Med* 1995; 26(9):576–80.

Technical Curricula for MT and MLT Programs. A Report from the ASCP-AMS Educator's Consensus Conference, Reengineering the Curriculum for the 21st Century for MTs and MLTs. Albuquerque, NM., March 2–3, 1995.

Wolgin F: Assessing learning outcomes. *J Nursing Staff Development* 1992; 8(3): 139–40.

Internet Resources

Center for Research on Learning and Teaching University of Michigan
http://www.crlt.umich.edu/
New Horizons for Learning
http://www.newhorizons.org/
Inclusive Teaching
http://depts.washington.edu/cidrweb/inclusive/
Benjamin Bloom's Taxonomy of Learning Domains - Cognitive, Affective, Psychomotor Domains - design and evaluation toolkit for training and learning
http://www.businessballs.com/bloomstaxonomyoflearningdomains.htm
The Encyclopedia of Educational Technology. A publication of San Diego State University, Department of Education
http://coe.sdsu.edu/eet/articles/BloomsLD/index.htm

Changes in the healthcare industry have resulted in the laboratory operating more like a business. Businesses have a bottom-line goal to ensure profitability and survival of the organization. This mindset has forced laboratory managers to increase their awareness of and focus on the financial management side of their positions.

Section III includes four chapters designed to provide a basic introduction to the financial side of management. Numerous business and financial terms are covered as appropriate for the topic; some are covered in more than one chapter because they overlap in the world of financial management. Reinforcement of these terms and concepts is intended to assist the learner in understanding financial management and its interrelationships.

Section III Contents:

9

Fundamentals of Financial Management

JAN R. HEIER, DBA, CPA
PAUL A. GRIFFEY, MBA, MT(ASCP)

Chapter Outline

Objectives

Following successful completion of this chapter, the learner should be able to:

1. Discuss the importance of financial management in the healthcare industry.
2. Identify the different types of organizational business operations.
3. Identify and interpret basic financial statements.
4. Compare and contrast financial and managerial accounting.

5. Recognize revenues and expenses involved with laboratory operations.
6. Explain basic performance tools and ratios used by management in forecasting performance and in the decision making process.
7. Briefly discuss budgeting and the way it relates to revenue and expense management.
8. Explain how to use a Cost-Volume-Profit Analysis.
9. Understand the behavior of laboratory costs.
10. Explain the costs associated with laboratory testing.
11. Explain how to analyze laboratory costs.
12. Explain how to derive and use "cost per test."

Key Terms

Assets	Liabilities
Balance Sheet	Liquidity Ratios
Break-even Analysis	Managerial Cost Accounting
Budget	Net Present Value
Budget—Performance Report	Operating Margin
Capital Budgeting	Owner's Equity
Cash Sources and Uses Statement	Payback Period
Cost	Profitability
Cost Benefit Analysis	Ratio Analysis
Cost-per-test	Revenues
Cost Volume Profit Analysis (Breakeven)	Return on Investment
Debt Ratios	Semi-variable Costs
Economies Due to Scale	Statement of Cash Flows
Expenses	Time Value of Money
Financial Management	Total Costs
Financial Ratios	Unit Costs
Fixed Costs	Variable Costs
Income Statement	

Case Study: Fundamentals of Financial Management

You are the manager of a "for profit" laboratory attached to a community-based teaching hospital. Your lab is housed in a new building adjacent to the main facility. You have been notified by the hospital administration that reimbursements from both private pay insurance and government sources have been reduced due to the process of capitation. The hospital is negotiating with the insurance companies and agencies to increase reimbursements based on the organization's overall cost structure and related costs for specific services. As laboratory manager, you have been asked to determine the cost of your operations in total and pretest as well as analyze the behavior of the costs incurred.

Issues and Questions to Consider:

1. *How do you determine the total costs of the lab operations?*
2. *How do you determine the costs of individual laboratory tests?*
3. *What is driving the costs of the laboratory tests?*
4. *Discuss the financial tools and ratios that may be used in analyzing the financial performance of the laboratory.*

INTRODUCTION

The healthcare industry accounts for a significant portion of the economy of the United States. The industry has experienced tremendous growth, increasing from 5.5% of the gross domestic product (GDP) in 1965 to 15% in 2003. Healthcare, which significantly affects the financial well-being of the United States, must be carefully managed. Efficient operations provide a basis for the allocation of financial, human, and technologic resources. The first steps in understanding laboratory financial management are rooted in the issues of the macroeconomics associated with the healthcare industry.

Clinical laboratory operations are an important aspect of the healthcare industry, with approximately 70% of patient diagnoses being derived from results of clinical laboratory diagnostic testing. Cost containment has changed the clinical laboratory from the highly profitable enterprise of the 1970s and 1980s into an industry striving for survival under the weight of current and pending government regulations, accreditation standards, and reimbursements. With increased focus and scrutiny on the financial aspects of the healthcare industry, and the laboratory in particular, efficient operations are of paramount importance and must be managed judiciously.

This chapter introduces the reader to the aspects of the fiscal and organizational environment of the healthcare industry as they relate to laboratory managers. This background information provides the framework for a detailed discussion of financial management, an essential portion of a laboratory manager's job. The discussion begins with a review of accounting terminology and reporting. Next, the chapter will cover the concepts of revenue management, budgeting, and ratio analysis to assist managers in financial decision-making. Finally, the chapter will focus on the types of costs and use in determining cost of services and other productivity measures.

FISCAL ENVIRONMENT OF THE HEALTHCARE INDUSTRY

The Social Security Act of 1964 created the single-most significant increase in healthcare industry revenues, whereas the current managed care negotiations have significantly reduced revenues. The laboratory industry's financial philosophy has evolved from one of a revenue center to a cost center over the last 30 years. The challenge to healthcare providers today is to provide low cost medical services while maintaining high standards of quality and easy access. In today's managed care environment and ever-increasing governmental regulations, the laboratory manager must have an understanding of the complex relationships between and among costs, productivity, and revenues. Alternative uses of funds are complex but remain a basic component in the financial decision-making processes of the laboratory manager.

Regardless of whether the clinical laboratory is managed by a hospital or acts as an independent business, the manager must be able to understand the cost structure of the organization. In addition, the manager must view this cost structure in relationship to the complex external healthcare environment of regulations, third party payers, capitation and service reimbursements based on a set fee or rate regardless of the laboratory's formal charges (or costs). To properly manage a laboratory in this environment, the manager first must understand the sources of cost information that are used to analyze the laboratory's cost structure. Next, the manager should use these sources to determine what the lab's base costs of services are and what causes these costs to occur. Next, the manager must understand the tools necessary to analyze the magnitude of the costs (both total and per unit) and compare these with past performance. Finally, the manager should be able use the data to negotiate a better reimbursement rate or use the data to prepare budgets for future operations.

The Healthcare Industry and its Organizational Environment

Healthcare organizations in the United States are categorized either as *for-profit* (taxable entities) or *not-for-profit* (non-taxable entities) organizations. Regardless of the category, the organization's primary goal is to provide services in a cost effective manner to maintain the fiscal viability of the organization. To some extent, the type of organization may affect its business structure and corporate philosophy; however, regardless of the business structures, it is the manager's responsibility to plan, organize, staff, and control the organization. For purposes of illustration, this chapter will assume a for-profit organization, with an emphasis on financial planning and control. A not-for-profit organization plans and controls in a similar fashion without, however, the constraint of answering to owner-investors; although they may have to answer to the board of directors or to legislative oversight.

Review of Financial Accounting Concepts

The primary goal of financial management is to ensure the profitability and the survival of the organization. The manager must have sources of information from which to plan and later evaluate the outcome of operations. The primary source of information is the organization's **financial accounting system** that captures the necessary data on the revenues, expenses, assets, and liabilities and provides reports for the manager to both review and control operations. In contrast to the financial accounting system, **managerial accounting** takes and analyzes the information to make it useful for budgeting, decision-making, and organizational evaluation.

For the profit making company, the statement **Assets = Liabilities + Owners' Equity** provides the framework for financial accounting, and represents the structure of the common Balance Sheet. The nature and definitions related to the Balance Sheet and other financial accounting terms are discussed below.

Balance Sheet (Table 9–1) is a document that represents the financial position of an organization at a particular point in time or at the end of an accounting period. The Balance Sheet reports on the organization's assets, liabilities, and owner's equity . . .

TABLE 9–1. Sample Balance Sheet For Profit Labs Balance Sheet December 31, 2006

Assets		Liabilities	
Cash	15,936	Short-term Debt	1,999
Accounts Receivable	54,962	Accounts Payable	21,874
Restricted Funds	6,467	Accrued Expenses	39,436
Third Party Allowances	7,212	Other Current Liabilities	18,448
Inventory	10,722	Advances from Third party payers	20,397
Prepaid Expenses and		Unearned Revenue	2,642
Other Current assets	4,896		
Total Current Assets	**100,195**	**Total Current Liabilities**	**104,796**
Plant Property			
and Equipment (PP&E)			
Property and Equipment	567,877	Accrued Retirement Costs	783
Less			
Accumulated Depreciation	(160,075)	Long-term Debt	175,309
Net PP&E[1]	**407,802**	**Total Liabilities**	**280,888**
Debt Service	13,946		
Construction	15,188	Equity	
Investments	76,865	Common Stock	100,000
Deferred Financing	4,746	Retained Earnings	242,295
Other Assets	4,441	Total Equity	342,295
Total Other Assets	**115,186**		
Total Assets[2]	**$623,183**	**Totals Liabilities and Equity[3]**	**$623,183**

[1]Depreciation is the systematic allocation of long-term cost to expense over the estimated life of the asset and Net PPE represents the accounting or book value of the fixed assets after depreciation accumulated over a number of years has been recognized.
[2]Total Asset Calculation = Total Current Assets + Net PP&E + Total Other Assets
[3]Total Liabilities and Equity Calculation = Total Liabilities + Total Equity.

Assets represent the resources owned by the organization. These assets can have physical form and a value, such as a building, or may be intangible and be difficult to value, such as a trademark.

Liabilities are the obligations that an organization has to its creditors. These may be short-term or long-term in nature with each type influencing the organization's cash flows in a timely fashion.

Owners' equity represents the "book value" of the organization. In the case of nonprofit organizations, the terminology is simply the excess (or deficit) of assets over liabilities. In a for profit organization, the Owner's Equity is usually made up of Capital (or common) Stock which represents ownership in the company, and Retained Earnings which are all of the company's earnings over time less any dividends that have been distributed. The Retained Earnings is reconciled each year using the Income Statement. In a not-for profit organization, the equity will be represented by either the terms "Net Assets" or the "Excess of Assets over Liabilities" because such an organization cannot use the term "net income" which implies taxability.

Income Statement (Table 9–2) is a document that represents the financial outcome of an organization over a period usually monthly or yearly. In a for profit organization the terminology will be Net Income, however in a not-for-profit organization it will be phraseology such as "excess revenues over expenses" to explain that the organization had a non-taxable "profit."

Revenues are inflows of assets into the organization. They are recognized (or accounted for) when they are earned. For example, when the lab test is completed and reported to the physician. If the revenues have not been collected as of yet, these uncollected revenues are represented on the Balance Sheet by an asset called **Accounts Receivable**.

TABLE 9–2 **Sample Income Statement**

For Profit Labs
Income Statement
For the year ended December 31, 2006

Sales	$240,000	
Cost of goods and services	168,000	
Gross margin (Sales – Cost of Goods Sold)		**72,000**
Operating Expenses		
Wages and salaries	46,000	
Miscellaneous expenses	8,000	
Depreciation	2,000	
Insurance	800	56,800
Total Operating Income		**15,200**
Interest expense		1,220
Net Income[4]		**13,980**

[4]If this were a taxable entity, one more step would be required. The tax liability would be calculated by multiplying a tax rate times this Net Income Before Taxes and that result would be subtracted from Net Income Before Taxes to get after tax net income.

Expenses are outflows of assets and are recognized (or accounted for) when incurred. For example, when a lab test is completed, the labor and materials used can then be recognized as an expense. If the expenses have yet to be paid, the unpaid bills are represented on the Balance Sheet by a liability called **Accounts Payable**.

Costs are assets that have been purchased such as inventories of lab supplies that have yet to be used, or equipment whose cost has not been expensed through depreciation, which is a systematic allocation of long-term costs to current expenses.

EVALUATION OF OPERATIONS—REVENUE AND EXPENSES

Managers of organizations learn about the levels of costs, expenses, and revenues through a system of formal **financial statements**. In addition, there are other internal reports such as budgets and performance reports designed to organize and report the financial information reported to management or other decision makers. The most frequently used statements are the aforementioned balance sheet and income statement. The Income Statement reports and evaluates the Revenues and Expenses of the organization.

Revenue essentially pays the bills for laboratory services and testing, and contributes to profitability. To be an economically successful laboratory, the revenues generated by laboratory operations must cover the cost of medical testing conducted by the laboratory, its administrative costs and generate a commensurate amount of profit. Though a not-for-profit organization by definition does not have a profit motive as the result of its operations, it must still meet or exceed its costs, just like a profit making entity, in order to remain open.

The amount of the revenue or reimbursement for a particular test or service will vary depending on the type of test and the reimbursement policies of the third party payer. If laboratory reimbursements do not cover the costs, there will be insufficient funds to provide the service and the laboratory will begin to operate at a loss. Understanding and managing the costs of the laboratory will be covered in an up-coming section of this chapter, but at this point, it is important for the managers to understand that the expenses of the lab are tied directly to its operations. Because of this, "paying the bills" can come only from the timely collection of the revenue, so efficient billing operations are essential.

The term **operating income (or margin)** refers to the profits that are generated from the excess of revenues received for providing the service. In the highly regulated healthcare industry, however, one laboratory cannot expect to be reimbursed at a higher rate than another for the same services just because it costs more for them to perform that service. Therefore, it is vital that correct information be identified in computing cost per test analysis and that every effort be made to provide services at as low a cost as possible. With increased focus and scrutiny on the finances and reimbursements of the healthcare industry and the laboratory in particular, efficient operations are extremely important and need to be managed judiciously.

The laboratory will receive these actual funds from revenue only after the billing process is completed, and the cash is eventually collected. In the mean time, the laboratory needs money to cover its bills and salaries. This seems simple enough, but it can become a rather complicated issue in this era of managed care. It is important to understand the basic concept of revenues in healthcare in order to further our understanding of the importance of financial management in the clinical laboratory. To analyze the timing of the cash-flows from reimbursements and disbursements comes from the Statement of Cash Sources and Uses.

Statement of Cash Sources and Uses (Table 9–3) is a document that analyzes the sources of cash inflows (collections of revenues or borrowing) and uses of cash (payment of expenses, purchase of equipment, or loan payments) to identify the timing of cash needs. This type of activity can also be incorporated into the budget system by developing a forward-looking cash-

TABLE 9–3. Cash-Sources and Uses Statement

	9/30/06	10/31/06	11/30/06	129/31/06
Beginning cash balance	$10,000	$10,480	$10,860	$10,195
Cash receipts				
Collections	46,000	68,000	68,000	54,000
Total cash available	56,000	78,480	78,860	64,195
Cash disbursements				
Purchases	42,700	48,300	40,600	32,900
Wages and commissions	9,250	12,250	13,000	10,750
Miscellaneous expenses	2,500	4,000	3,000	2,500
Equipment purchases	3,000			
Lease Payments per month	2,000	2,000	2,000	2,000
Total disbursements	59,450	66,550	58,600	48,150
Minimum cash balance desired	10,000	10,000	10,000	10,000
Total cash needed	69,450	76,550	68,600	58,150
Excess (deficit) cash	(13,450)	1,930	10,260	6,045
Financing				
Borrowings (at beginning)	14,000			
Repayments (at end)		1,000	10,000	3,000
Interest (@ 6% annually)[5]	70	70	65	15
Total effect of financing	14,000	1,070	10,065	3,015
Ending cash balance[6]	**$10,480**	**$10,860**	**$10,195**	**$13,030**
Loan Balance	**$14,000**	**$13,000**	**$3,000**	0

[5]Assuming interest is accrued for the entire month, September Interest Calculation = /12 x .06 x $14,000= 70; October Interest Calculation = 1/12 x .06 x $14,000= 70; November Interest Calculation = 1/12 x .06 x 13,000 = 65 December Interest Calculation = 1/12 x .06 x 3,000 = 15
[6]September Ending Balance Calculation = $56,000 – $59,450 + $14,000 - 70 = $10,480; October Ending Balance Calculation = $78,480 – $66,550 - $1,070 = $10,860; November Ending Balance Calculation = $78,860– $58,600 - $10,065 = $10,195; December Ending Balance Calculation = $64,195 – $48,150- $3,015 = $13,030.

budget based on the estimated timing of revenue collections and expense disbursements.

Ratio Analysis A primary responsibility of the laboratory manager is to evaluate the financial operations of the laboratory. The financial statements themselves provide only numbers that are then compared with other data to make them useful and meaningful. The first comparison should always be with prior year's results, so that a trend can be ascertained. In addition, the manager should seek tools for further analysis of understanding and managing operating results.

The most widely used tool to manage finances and analyze the financial statements is the use of **ratio analysis.** Financial ratios can be grouped into the following categories: **liquidity, debt, and profitability.** A liquidity ratio, such as the current ratio or times interest earned ratio, is used to determine the organization's ability to meet short-term debt obligations. Debt ratios, such as the debt to equity ratio are used to determine the organization's ability to meet long-term debt obligations. Finally, the profitability ratios such as the **Return on Investment or ROI ratio** demonstrates the organization's efficiency of operations. The rate of return is used to evaluate the operation of the organization as a whole by comparing Net Income with the organizations Total Equity.[7] In this case, $13,980 ÷ $342,295 = 4.08% return on Investment. A full review of such ratios and the related analysis techniques is out of the scope of this chapter but a review of any financial management or managerial accounting text book (see bibliography at the end of the chapter) will help design a proper analysis regimen.

In addition to the financial ratios that relate to the financial statements, the laboratory manager can also develop internal statistics to control costs and evaluate operations. Cost data to develop these internal ratios can come from the financial accounting system. Certain non-financial data such as testing time can be married to the financial data to make a more robust analysis. Ratios developed from internal operating data can typically pull together individual elements of the laboratory's financial operating statements, and give a clearer picture of both the efficiency of the laboratory and financial viability of the individual tests performed. Examples of ratios important to the laboratory manager are:

- Cost per test (procedure)
- Total cost per billable test
- Direct cost per billable test
- Technical labor cost per billable test
- Billable tests per labor cost
- Billable tests per patient admission
- Revenue per billable test
- Profit margin per billable test

Each of these ratios provides information to the manager, but each must be compared with an industry standard, previous internal laboratory performance, or an alternative performance measure to provide usable information for evaluating the laboratory's operations.

---

[7]Depending on the purpose of the analysis, ROI can also be calculated using an organization's total assets.

A related topic to ratio analysis is investment analysis (**capital budgeting**) where a laboratory manager must make decisions related to the effective use of the long-term funding allotted to support the goals and objectives of the laboratory. With the primary goal of financial management to ensure the profitability and survival of an organization, it is necessary to have techniques to evaluate individual investments. This allows the manager to understand how each alternative investment will meet the organization's goals, and how to choose from among those alternatives. As this is a complicated process, please refer to a managerial accounting book to help to devise evaluation strategies; however, three common ones can be mentioned here.

The first is a variation of the above-mentioned **ROI ratio**. Here individual projects are evaluated by comparing the annual income generated by the project with the original project outlay or investment. For example, if a project, which has a no salvage value after five years, generates $1,000 per year on an outlay of $10,000, then the **project rate of return** over the life of the project is 20%, or about 4.0% per year.[8] Next, the **Payback Period** is a ratio that identifies the time it will take for revenue or other positive cash flows to cover the initial outlay related to an investment project. For example if the Investments is $5,000, and the organization will make $2,500 per year, the payback will occur in two years. Finally, for a more robust evaluation of long-term projects, **Time Value of Money** techniques such a **Net Present Value** (NPV) may be employed. NPV is a calculation that compares the initial outlay of a project with the discounted present value of a stream of cash flows generated by that project. A full discussion of this technique is out of the scope of this chapter. Please refer to a managerial finance book to better understand the techniques of capital budgeting and time value of money analysis. Finally, Chapter 10 covers material related to the subject of **Cost Benefit Analysis**.

In conclusion, using these financial statements and other financial management techniques, the manager can first learn the outcome of operations for the previous accounting period. Next, the manager can determine the current financial position of the organization. Third, the manager can use this information to evaluate the organization's results in light of budgets and other standards. Finally, as will be explained in the next section, the data will be the basis for determining cost of service to help plan for and control operations.

---

[8]The calculation for a project rate of return, (sometimes called the **Accounting Rate of Return**) for this example would use the formula: **Annual Cash Flow/ (Initial Outlay + Salvage Value) ÷ 2.** Using the above data, the calculation would be $1,000 / (($10,000 + 0) ÷ 2) or $1,000/ $5,000= 20%. Over five years this is 4.0% per year. The element of the ROI (Initial Outlay +Salvage Value) ÷ 2 represents the average value in the investment account over time. In this case, the beginning balance in the account would be $10,000 and the ending balance in the account would be zero so the average investment value over time (assuming straight-line depreciation) would be ($10,000 + 0) ÷ 2 or $5,000. Note: the standard depreciation model for straight-line depreciation is (Cost − Salvage value) ÷ depreciable years. If the $10,000 investment is depreciated over five years, the depreciation would be (10,000 − 0)/5 or $2,000 per year in depreciation would be recognized and the account reduce eventually to either zero or the amount of estimated salvage value.

Review of Planning and Management Accounting

Financial management is defined as the process of planning, controlling, and evaluating available monetary resources of an organization. The goal of financial management is the proper and efficient allocation of these resources to the necessary parts of the organization, and the application of continuous quality improvement techniques to ensure quality results flowing from efficient, cost-effective operations. As we have discussed, the laboratory management team must understand basic accounting, economic and financial principles, and their relationship to daily laboratory operations to achieve and maintain success. Equally important is the manager's understanding of the planning process and control of internal operations through planning and budgeting. Figure 9–1 provides and graphic of this process.

The laboratory manager must be aware of the funds needed to perform testing and provide services for patients. (How much does it cost to provide testing?) Understanding revenues and reimbursements is also important to maintain financial efficiency in the department. (How much is the laboratory being paid for the testing?)

The relationship between the costs and revenues determines the operating funds the laboratory has available. If the cost to provide service and testing is greater than the revenue, the laboratory will be operating at a loss. However, if the revenues are greater than the costs to provide the service and testing, the laboratory will generate a profit. With a profit or operating margin, the laboratory manager will have financial resources to expand operations or increase salaries to maintain a qualified work force. To make these decisions, planning for future operations is necessary and often comes in the form of a budget, with formal performance reports acting as the managerial control mechanism.

Budgeting is a system for formalizing in writing a quantitative financial plan, supportive of the institution's financial mission, for a given time period. The

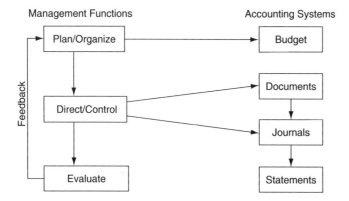

FIGURE 9–1 How does management use budgets?

TABLE 9–4. For Profit Labs Budget and Performance Report Year to Date April 2006

	April Actual	April Budget	April Variance		March Actual	February Actual	January Actual	YTD Actual	YTD Budget	Total YTD Variance		Total YTD Percentage Variance
Wages and Salaries												
Technical Salaries	26,686	25,000	1,686	U	28,333	25,112	26,201	106,332	100,000	6,332	U	6.33%
Non-Technical Wages												
Regular	6,700	6,600	100	U	6,700	7,500	6,300	27,200	26,400	800	U	3.03%
Overtime	2,602	1,700	902	U	2,602	2,200	1,906	9,310	6,800	2,510	U	36.91%
Total Non Technical Wages	9,302	8,300	1,002	U	9,302	9,700	8,206	36,510	33,200	3,310	U	9.97%
Total Salaries & Wages (TS&W)	35,988	33,300	2,688	U	37,635	34,812	34,407	142,842	133,200	9,642	U	7.24%
Benefits												
Retirement (9.6% X TS&W)	3,455	3,197	258	U	3,613	3,342	3,303	13,713	12,787	926	U	7.24%
Health (18.4% X TS&W))	6,622	6,127	495	U	6,925	6,405	6,331	26,283	24,509	1,774	U	7.24%
Total Benefits	10,077	9,324	753	U	10,538	9,747	9,634	39,996	37,296	2,700	U	7.24%
Total Salaries Wages and Benefits	46,065	42,624	3,441	U	48,173	44,559	44,041	182,838	170,496	12,342	U	7.24%
Operating Expenses												
Reagents	20,756	19,900	856	U	20,756	18,780	19,735	80,027	79,600	427	U	.54%
Supplies	16,575	14,900	1,675	U	16,575	15,982	15,631	64,763	59,600	5,163	U	8.66%
Maintenance	725	800	-75	F	725	725	3,200	5,375	5675	-300	F	-5.29%
Repairs	225	200	25	U	225	177	164	791	800	-9	F	-1.13%
Equipment lease	225	225	0		225	226	227	903	900	3	U	0.33%
Utilities	358	400	-42	F	358	321	568	1,605	1,600	5	U	0.31%
Total Operating Expenses	38,864	36,425	2,439	U	38,864	36,211	39,525	153,464	148,175	5,289	U	3.57%
Total Expenses	84,929	79,049	5,880	U	87,037	80,770	83,566	336302	318,671	17,631	U	5.53%

Note 1:—YTD Actual is January through April actual that has been added up; YTD–Budget is given.; YTD–percentage is YTD–Variance ÷ YTD - Budget

Note 2:—Subtract Actual—Budget—If the result is negative there was a Favorable variance and the company saved money compared to budget, if there was a positive result there was an Unfavorable variance and the company spent more compared to budget.

Note 3—Investigation of variances is based on the percentage magnitude (also called materiality) of the variance. The higher the percentage of the variance compared to budget (either favorable or unfavorable, the greater the need for investigation. The internal policy of the lab will dictate materially parameters.

budget is the actual plan for allocating funds to cover the expenditures, for supplies, salaries, equipment, and overhead, involved in the day-to-day operations of the laboratory. The **budget planning process** begins with establishing **goals, objectives,** and prioritizing the use of financial resources. A successful budget blends past expenditure history with projections of expected expenses for a future period. The details of developing a budget are covered in Chapter 11.

Budget—Performance Report (Table 9–4) is a document that takes the forward-looking financial information (the budget) for a given time period and compares these budget expectations with actual performance. The variances (actual performance – budgeted performance) allow the manager to track both the actual and relative magnitude of the laboratory's performance against the budgeted amounts. Comparing the actual expenses with the projected budgeted expenses provide important information to the laboratory manager and help to evaluate the original allocation of funds and available financial resources for a given period. The laboratory manager must pay close attention to and scrutinize the variances between budget and actual expenditures. This variance analysis must provide information in a timely fashion so that the manager can adjust laboratory operations to correct for any inefficiency.

ANALYZING COST OF SERVICE

Cost Behavior

Managerial Cost accounting is a system for providing an analysis of cost information used in financial decision-making. In today's managed care environment and with industry competitiveness, correct cost information ensures participation in those contracts and stabilizes profitability for the laboratory. To accomplish this process, the manager should identify the total costs associated with services, and assign responsibility for those costs. In today's highly regulated environment, the costs of adhering to the accreditation and certification agencies must also be considered a cost of the service, along with traditional costs such as labor, materials, and depreciation. The laboratory manager must also be efficient in defining and itemizing those costs associated with the testing, and the other services provided by the laboratory. **Total costs** for the laboratory consists of two-component cost behaviors (Figure 9–2), fixed and variable. Cost behaviors are defined in relationship to the laboratory's testing volume as follows.

Fixed costs are those that do not change over a given period regardless of testing volume; examples of fixed costs are administrative salaries, rent, and lease commitments (Figure 9–3). The "per unit fixed cost," however, does change in an inverse proportion to laboratories' test volume, and represents a measure for the laboratory's **"economies due to scale."** For example, if the lab has $10,000 in fixed costs and performs 1,000 tests, the fixed

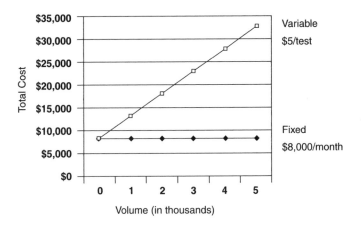

FIGURE 9–2   Example of Total Costs

cost per test is $10.00. If however, the lab completes 10,000 tests, the fixed
cost per test drops dramatically to $1.00 per test.

Variable costs are those that move in relationship to the laboratory's testing volume and change in a direct relationship to that volume (Figure 9–4).
Reagents and supplies required to perform a specific test are variable costs.
Managing variable costs require an understanding of both the type and
cost the inputs used to conduct a test, as well as the "normal" usage of the
materials. For example, if a certain test requires two ounces of liquid
reagent, then normal (or standard) volume of 20,000 ounces is used to complete 10,000 tests. If, however, an inventory reveals that 21,000 ounces were
used, then an unfavorable quantity (or efficiency variance) of 1,000 ounces
has occurred and the manager must investigate this problem. By contrast,
a favorable variance of 1,000 ounces would indicate that less material than
normal actually was used leading the manager to have possible concerns

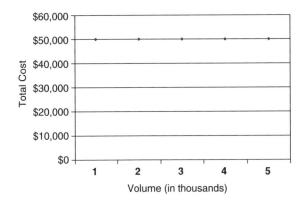

FIGURE 9–3   Example of Fixed Costs.

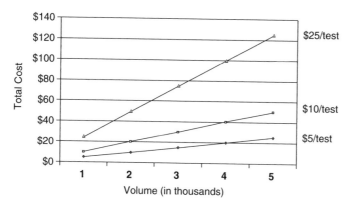

FIGURE 9–4   **Example of Variable Costs.**

about problems related to service quality. The same analysis can be applied to areas such as labor hours and prices of supplies using the following two formulas:

Actual unit quantity purchased × (Actual Price per Unit–Budgeted Price per Units) = Price Variance	Budgeted Price per Unit × (Actual unit quantity used–Budgeted unit quantity used) = Quantity Variance

Note: Some expenses incurred in the laboratory will vary but only incrementally. These costs are termed *semi-variable costs* or *mixed costs* and change in increments based on workload volume change. An example of a semi-variable cost is a part-time technologist's salary. When workload has increased to a certain level, another technologist will be added to the labor force; likewise, if the workload is decreased to a certain level, a technologist will be removed from the workforce.

Understanding the cost behavior of the laboratory allows the manager the opportunity to analyze the position of the lab with respect to profitability and determine what measures are needed to control costs (or increase revenues if that is possible). One of the primary tools for completing this analysis is **Cost Volume Profit Analysis,** (CVP) more commonly called **Breakeven.** To complete a CVP analysis it is important to determine behavior of the lab's costs.

To illustrate CVP, (Table 9–5), assume a lab had fixed costs to cover of $500. The question is simple, if it charges $8.33 per test when the cost is $5.00 per test, how many tests need to be completed to cover the lab's fixed costs? One way of portraying this process is through the following table that shows at 150 tests the lab breaks-even. Any test completed past 150 will yield the lab $3.33 ($8.33-$5.00) contribution towards income per test completed.

For simplicity sake, the lab can determine the amount of tests it needs to perform to breakeven using the following formula

$$\frac{\text{Total Fixed Cost}}{\text{Revenue Per Test–Variable Cost per Test}} = \frac{\$500}{\$8.33-\$5.00} = 150 \text{ tests}$$

TABLE 9–5.   Break-Even Analysis (CVP)

Tests Performed	Revenue $8.33/unit	Variable Cost $5.00/unit	Contribution Margin	Fixed Costs	Operating Income[9]
100	833	500	333	500	-167
110	916	550	366	500	-133
120	1,000	600	400	500	-100
130	1,083	650	433	500	-67
140	1,166	700	466	500	-33
150	1,250	750	500	500	0
160	1,333	800	533	500	33
170	1,416	850	566	500	67
180	1,499	900	599	500	100
190	1,583	950	633	500	133
200	1,666	1,000	666	500	167

[9]Operating Income = Contribution Margin –Fixed Cost. Note All numbers are rounded for illustration purposes.

Finally, the analysis also can be portrayed in graphical format (Figure 9-5).

Cost Volume Profit (Break-Even) Analysis as illustrated in the table above, and the projection of costs and revenues at a given change in volume and pricing, provides the necessary information to make decisions regarding potential service contracts with payers (insurers, managed care, or other third-party organizations). In addition, such analysis allows for planning purchases of materials and staffing as the volume changes.

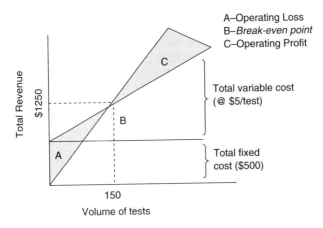

FIGURE 9–5   Example of Break-even Analysis.

In order to complete a CVP analysis, it may be necessary to identify and allocate the various costs to the services being rendered to determine **cost per test.** The process of determining fixed versus variable costs is covered more in more detail in the next section of this chapter.

This cost per test information is extremely useful for decision-making. Examples include pricing decisions for choosing between alternative contracts to offer in response to managed care or group purchasing request for bids, or in choosing between alternative analyzers for the laboratory. In addition, decisions about providing testing in-house or sending it out to a reference laboratory can be made by comparing costs of the alternative service methods. A **cost-benefit analysis** (discussed in Chapter 10) can be performed using the costing information to determine which alternative is the most financially acceptable for the organization.

PRODUCTIVITY MEASURES (COST-PER-TEST)

Cost-per-test analysis is a means of identifying the productivity of a laboratory. Within the obvious guidelines of quality and efficacy, the lower the cost per test, the more efficient the laboratory is in providing its services. A laboratory with high productivity should yield a lower cost per test compared to a less productive counterpart. A cost-per-test analysis begins with the identification and allocation of component costs and their identification and relationship to the service provided. As previously discussed, the laboratory manager must first identify the lab's fixed costs (i.e., those costs that remain constant regardless of volume). Examples of fixed costs are administrative salaries, rent, and lease payments. In addition, the variable costs, those that vary proportionally with volume of testing, must then be identified. Examples are supplies and reagents needed to perform a test. Depending on the manner the medical technologists are paid (hourly versus salaried), labor costs may fall into either and sometimes both categories. All testing services in the laboratory will inevitably consist of both fixed and variable components.

Costs per Test (or more generically - Unit costs) are the sum of both fixed and variable costs divided by the number of unit tests. The unit cost per test is used to measure the laboratory's productivity and demonstrate the laboratory's economies compared with other comparable laboratories.

One of the primary objectives of the process is to identify the costs associated with the testing process, both direct and indirect, and efficiently attach or allocate all of the costs related to the test to determine the cost of that particular unit or test. In the case of indirect costs, they must be allocated using a particular unit of production such as, in this case the glucose assay. Table 9–6 can serve as a template to determine the costs associated with testing.

Test-specific (variable) costs are the simplest to identify and allocate. For example, the cost of both glucose reagents and calibration and/or control materials specific for the glucose assay test are known from previous purchases and usage. Costs of consumable supplies, such as sample cups (cuvettes) and pipette tips

TABLE 9–6.   Cost Analysis Checklist:

Fixed:	**Labor:**
____ Rent	____ Base wage
____ Utilities	____ Taxes
____ Compliance costs	____ Insurance
____ PT Subscriptions	____ Retirement
____ Leases	____ Other benefits
____ Management	

Variable Costs:

Test specific costs:	*Test-system costs:*
____ Reagent	____ Sample cups
____ Calibration	____ Sample tips
____ Control	____ Reagent kit
____ Other	____ Cuvettes
	____ Multianalyte cals/controls
	____ Printing supplies

needed to perform the assay, are also be identified, and allocated appropriately.[10] Finally, fixed costs associated with the laboratory services must be identified and allocated. To illustrate the of cost allocation and the determination of cost per test in more detail, the example of a glucose assay test performed on a random access automated analyzer will be the focus using the following data.

Total tests per month	50,000
Glucose tests per month	3,120
Runs per month	40
Tests per run	78
Test repeats	3
Patient dilutions	6
Controls per run	2
Control repeats	2
Failed runs per month	1
Calibrators (per 6 months)	12
Reagent cost per month	$400
Control cost per month	$60
Calibrator cost per month	$60
Cuvettes per month	3,405
Cost per Cuvettes	$.05
Technologist time per run in minutes	20
Fixed cost per month	$500

[10]Consumable supplies may be shared among other assays being performed on the same analyzer and thus the portion of the purchase cost that can be attributed only to the glucose assays performed must be determined.

Analysis of Cost per Test

Variable Costs:

Cost one cuvette per test	$.0500

Total reagent, control, and calibrator cost per month

(Allocated based on curvette usage)

÷

Cuvettes per month

$520 ($400 +$60 + $60) ÷ 3405[11]	$.1527

---

[11]The total number of patients per run is 78, and 3 patient samples per run require dilution, adding 3 additional . The 2 controls per run are analyzed and there are 6 calibrators run in duplicate, once per each 6 months; therefore 2 are allocated per month. In all 83 (78 + 3 + 2) are needed per run, which equates to 3320 (83 × 40 runs) per month. The one failed run per month and the additional control repeat increases the total to 3405 (3320 + 83 + 2) per month

Labor Costs (Depending on the situation these may
  be variable fixed or semi-variable)

$24.00 X 20minutes/60 minutes = $8.00 per run ÷ 78 tests per run =	$.1026

Fixed Costs (The allocation rate is based on number of tests)

Fixed Costs ÷ Total Annual Test = Fixed Cost per Test

$500 ÷ 50,000 =	$.0100
Total Cost per test	$.3153
Total Glucose tests Performed	3,120
Total Cost for completing glucose assay test is	$983.67

As the analysis indicates, all of the costs need to be considered including the fixed costs. These types of costs are often shared with other tests, thus need to be allocated by some common measure. In this case, the fixed costs are allocated or applied to each test based on the number of tests performed by the lab; whereas, variable costs of reagent, control, and calibrator reagents are allocated based on the usage of cuvettes. This analysis allows for a proper understanding of the lab's costs of operations per unit and total, as well as the charges to the patient necessary to cover the costs. This type of analysis will also help in negotiating reimbursements from third-party payers.

IMPORTANT POINTS TO REMEMBER

1. Knowledge of financial accounting terminology and application is necessary to properly run a medical laboratory and make decisions.
2. Budgets should be prepared annually to chart the future financial course of the laboratory
3. Financial Statements containing current operating results should be obtained and analyzed through ratio analysis or historical comparisons.

4. Current operating results should be compared with budgeted expectations and any variances analyzed and dealt with to enhance the laboratory's efficiency.
5. Determine the cost behaviors associated with the laboratory activities and conduct a breakeven analysis to determine the current profitability position of the laboratory.
6. Determine the "cost per test" of the laboratory.
7. Use the "cost per test" as a standard to compare the laboratory's operating efficiency over time.
8 The "cost per test" can also be used to negotiated reimbursement with third party payers.

SUMMARY

Making decisions that ensure future financial performance is an important aspect of any laboratory manager. Financial management provides a variety of benefits. First, for the patients, it provides for better quality services at a reduced cost. Next for the healthcare administrator, it provides information for strategic planning and the best use of available funds. Finally, for the laboratory manager, it provides financial information for effective cost reductions, appropriate test utilization, equipment utilization, staffing utilization, and material usage.

SUGGESTED PROBLEM-BASED LEARNING ACTIVITIES
Chapter 9: Fundamentals of Financial Management

Instructions: Use Internet resources, books, articles, colleagues, etc., to present solutions to the problems listed below. There is no one correct solution to any problem.

Note to Instructor: Students in class may be divided into groups and given the problem-based learning activity to discuss and solve. Once the group has reached consensus as to a solution, the group may present it to the other students in the class. This activity will provide all students with information regarding solutions to the problem.

Problem #1
Develop a plan to increase your department's financial productivity and illustrate this process using financial productivity means.

Problem #2
Prioritize and discuss the financial issues that will be affected by laboratory consolidation.

Problem #3
Discuss financial information flow and how the laboratory manager uses financial and statements reports.

<u>*Problem #4*</u>
Develop a plan to evaluate your lab's productivity and cost structure using managerial accounting measures.

BIBLIOGRAPHY

Baker J. J., Baker R. W.: *Health Care Finance, Basic Tools for Nonfinancial Managers.* Aspen Publications, Gaithersburg, MD., 2000.

Brigham E. F. and Houston S. C.: *Fundamentals of Financial Management,* 10th ed. South-Western College Publications, Cincinnati, OH., 2004.

Fields, E.: *Essentials of Finance and Accounting for Non-Financial Managers.* AMACOM, New York, 2002.

Horngren, C. T., Sundum, G. L. and Elliot, J. A.: *Introduction to Financial Accounting 9th edition. Pearson Prentice Hall and Company.* Upper Saddle River, 2006.

Horngren, C. T., Sundum, G. L. and Stratton W.O.: *Introduction to Management Accounting 13th edition. Pearson Prentice Hall and Company.* Upper Saddle River, NJ., 2005.

Ives, M., Razak, J. A., Hosch, G.A.: *Introduction to Governmental and Not-for-Profit Accounting. Pearson Prentice Hall and Company.* Upper Saddle River, NJ, 2004.

Snyder J. R., Wilkinson D.: *Management in Laboratory Medicine,* 3rd ed. Lippincott , Philadelphia, PA., 1998.

Internet Resources

AACC—(American Association for Clinical Chemistry)
www.AACC.org
ASCP—(American Society of Clinical Pathology)
www.ASCP.org
CLMA—(Clinical Laboratory Management Association)
www.CLMA.org
CDC—(Center for Disease Control)
http://www.cdc.gov/nchs/fastats/hexpense.htm
OECD—(Organization for Economic Cooperation and Development)
http://www.oecd.org/dataoecd/44/18/35044277.xls

10

Cost/Benefit Analysis

JANET S. HALL, MS, CC(NRCC)

Chapter Outline

Objectives

After successful completion of this chapter, the learner will be able to:

1. Define and manipulate the key elements of managerial cost accounting.
2. Identify and discuss the five types of expenses (costs).
3. Identify and describe the information required to calculate expected revenue.
4. List potential intangible factors that should be assessed when performing a make versus buy analysis.
5. Perform a break-even analysis for a proposed new test.
6. Price a new test.

7. Evaluate the special considerations for capital equipment acquisition.
8. Summarize the relationship between micro, departmental, and institutional financial analysis and planning.

Key Terms

Billable Procedure
Cost
Depreciation
Direct Expense (Cost)
Expense

Indirect Expense (Cost)
Microcosting
Overhead
Payback Period
Return on Investment

Case Study: Cost/Benefit Analysis

You are a manager in a clinical laboratory in a small community hospital. You currently refer specimens for free PSA (prostrate specific antigen) to a large commercial laboratory. A prominent physician on your staff has requested that you start doing the test in-house to improve turnaround time. To do this, you would need to offer a total PSA and a free PSA together. You currently perform the total PSA. The physician states that if he can have timely results for the paired test, he estimates that it will eliminate the need to perform approximately 60 prostate biopsies a year.

Free PSA is available on equipment that you currently use under a reagent rental agreement (you pay only for reagents, as the cost of the equipment is rolled into the cost of the reagents). The vendor has quoted a price of $8.00 per test (not $8.00 per billable test) for free PSA reagents.

How would you go about evaluating whether the test is profitable to bring in-house?

Issues and Questions to Consider

1. *How will your direct costs be affected?*
2. *Will there be an increase in your indirect costs?*
3. *Will you need to evaluate equipment costs (capital)?*
4. *Will the test be reimbursed and at what rate?*
5. *What intangibles should you factor into the decision?*
6. *How will you price the test?*
7. *Is it worth bringing in?*

INTRODUCTION

One of the most important tasks of a laboratory manager is assessing and comparing expense (cost) with associated revenue (benefit), a process known as a cost/benefit analysis. This chapter provides the reader with a global perspective on using financial information followed by details on the nuts and bolts of cost/benefit analysis including evaluation of expenses, evaluation of revenues, and pricing formulas. Two related topics—making business decisions and capital purchases—are also discussed. Finally, the chapter includes suggested resources to assist laboratory managers in evaluating the financial position of their institutions, as well as to compare their findings to financial situations of other comparable institutions.

USING FINANCIAL INFORMATION: THE BIG PICTURE

Healthcare is a huge business in the United States that is composed of a complex system of providers and payers. The providers perform healthcare services and attempt to maximize the reimbursement received. The payers, on the other hand, pay out only what they deem necessary. It was not always that way.

The healthcare market before 1982 was based on fee-for-service reimbursement. A healthcare provider performed a service (e.g., a laboratory test) and a payer paid for that service. Cost was not an issue. When the cost of performing a test increased, the provider increased the price to the payer, and the payer paid the increased rate. This system eventually began to burden payers. In 1982 laboratories came to realize that they needed to act like businesses when the federal government instituted a payment system for Medicare patients that was based on DRGs (diagnostic-related groups). Under that system, all services provided for hospital inpatients were grouped together, and a single payment amount was made based on the DRG assigned to the case. Whether the laboratory charged $5.00 or $50.00 for a test, the amount received to cover the test plus all other services performed, was the same. It suddenly became important for laboratories to contain costs. In the year 2000, the same system was applied to hospital outpatients.

In 1983 TEFRA (Tax Equity and Fiscal Responsibility Act) was passed. TEFRA set limits of reimbursement and established a system to monitor and adjust reimbursement to providers. Most recently the Balanced Budget Amendment of 1997 set more limitations on Medicare payment schedules and defined a systematic scheme for decreasing payments over time. Healthcare providers, including laboratory technologists, have been forced to take a hard look at expenses and revenues and to modify operations to control expense.

Entities providing healthcare in the United States are divided into two categories: for-profit and not-for-profit. A **for-profit entity** is privately held (e.g., a corporation). Its profits are distributed to the owners (individuals or shareholders) and its primary purpose is to generate revenue. Any profits it is able to generate are taxed. Examples of for-profit healthcare entities include the large commercial laboratories and some large hospital systems such as Columbia HCA. A **not-for-profit entity** (e.g., most community based hospitals) is one whose profits are held by the entity to further its cause. These entities usually exist to provide a service, such as healthcare. In these entities the "profits" are not taxed and are retained by the entity and used for purchase of capital equipment or other goods and services required to keep the entity in business. The objectives of for-profit and not-for–profit businesses are different, but the bottom line is that both must balance expense and revenue to remain solvent.

TABLE 10–1. Accounting Relationships

Public Accounting	Governments Outside Accountants (Auditors) Stockholders Regulatory Agencies Income Tax Services	
Private Accounting	Strategic Planning Forecasting Department Audits	<—— *Financial Accounting*
	Budgets Line Item Analysis Microcosting	<—— *Management Accounting*

Further, in the business world there are two levels of oversight of the financial side of a business. The first, **management accounting**, is the analysis of cost and revenue data that provides information on operations and budgeting for managers. Managerial accounting is also called **cost accounting.** In the laboratory, managerial accounting includes activities such as *microcosting* (the process of determining the actual cost of performing a billable procedure), performing analyses of services and equipment in order to evaluate their profitability, and budgeting (the compilation of expected expenses and revenue into a financial plan).

Information generated through management accounting in all departments of a hospital is then collated and evaluated by the Department of Finance, which generates financial records and forecasts and performs strategic planning for the entire entity. These activities are called **financial accounting.**

The activities performed in the laboratory and other departments which are evaluated and reported by the Department of Finance are facets of **private accounting** (i.e., they are performed by an entity for its own managerial activities). Once done, however, they are made available to regulatory, government, and private accounting firms for both informational purposes and to meet regulatory requirements. This activity is called **public accounting.** Table 10–1 shows the relationships between private and public accounting and between management and financial accounting.

All entities, whether for-profit or not-for-profit, go through the same general accounting processes, although the information may be distributed differently outside the entity based on applicable regulations.

EVALUATING EXPENSES

It is important for managers to know what it costs to operate a laboratory section or department. It is the only side of the cost/revenue equation over which they have direct control. For this discussion, *expense* is defined as the *cost* of providing a billable procedure. In the laboratory, a ***billable procedure*** is a test that is billed to a payer. The payer may be an individual or a private or government insurance. The charge for a billable procedure includes all the expenses (costs) incurred in generating the test result, including the cost of collecting and processing the specimen, performing the test (reagents, consumables, laboratory and equipment costs), and numerous other costs plus some measure of profit. A **nonbillable procedure** contributes to the generation of a billable test result, but which is not directly reimburseable. Examples of nonbillable procedures include standards, quality control specimens, and repeats. Some nonreimbursable procedures are occasionally performed in the laboratory, but should not be billed because payment is unlikely. These include tests considered to be experimental and tests for which appropriate medical necessity or diagnosis information has not been gathered. Obviously the volume of such tests should be kept to a minimum, if allowed at all.

The most effective method for determining the actual cost to perform a billable procedure is to perform a microcost analysis. Microcosting (also known as cost per test) accounts for all expenses associated with performing a given test including reagents, consumables, laboratory costs, and reporting costs and includes preanalytical, analytical, and postanalytical expenses. It is a structured approach that, when built into a template, can be used to price any new test being considered or to be an ongoing evaluation tool for tests currently being performed.

There are two types of expenses to consider when performing a microcosting evaluation. ***Direct expense (cost)*** includes all costs directly related to performing a test. It includes the reagents, consumables, labor and benefits, etc. Examples of direct costs are shown in Table 10–2.

Indirect expense (cost) includes expenses that are part of doing business, but that are not directly related to the cost of the test being evaluated. Indirect costs are also called ***overhead.*** Examples of indirect costs are shown in Table 10–3.

Direct costs are relatively easy to determine and should be calculated using a line-by-line approach. For example, the cost of consumables needed to collect a blood specimen is straightforward:

Alcohol swab	$ 0.10
Needle	0.25
Vacutainer tube(s)	0.37
Adapter	0.12
Gauze pad	0.02
Band-Aid	0.05
Total cost	$ 0.91

If more than one test is performed per collection, the cost of the collection expendables can be spread over multiple tests, thereby decreasing the cost per test. The same can be done for processing costs. Pricing information for the consumables used is available from the purchasing department and from utilization reports generated monthly by the finance department.

TABLE 10–2. Examples of Direct Costs

Specimen collection consumables (preps, Vacutainers, needles, etc.)
Processing consumables (tubes, caps, transfer pipets, labels, etc.)
Reagents
    Calibrators
    Controls
    Reagents, stains, etc.
Analytical consumables (sample cups, tips, media plates, etc.)
Proficiency testing materials
Labor
    Collections
    Accessioning
    Analysis
    QC
    Reporting
    Other
Equipment costs
    Monthly lease/rental cost
    Depreciation (purchases only)
    Maintenance
        Ongoing/inhouse/daily/weekly/monthly
        Contracted
Office supplies
Reporting costs (fax, paper, printheads, etc.)

TABLE 10–3. Examples of Indirect Costs

Licenses
Marketing
    Labor
    Materials
Information Systems Requirements
    Programming (ongoing)
    Maintenance fees
    Training
        Initial
        Ongoing
Supervisory and Administrative salaries
Secretarial support
Other facility overhead (as determined by facility)
Intangibles
    Signatures—ABN (Advanced Beneficiary Notice) risk,
      F/U (Failure/Unable) to obtain
    Liability costs (insurance)
    Public Relations
    Involvement in product line
        Physician relations
        Markets
        Network requirements
        Long-term survival
    Medical Involvement

When calculating reagent costs, the cost of the reagent actually used to run a single test is easy to calculate based on the known volume of reagent used and the cost per volume. These numbers are readily available from contracting information generated by vendors or from records in the purchasing department. The cost of calibrators and controls is also available, but the actual cost of these per test can be determined by dividing the total amount used by the total number of tests performed using a particular calibration and/or control schedule. For example, if three levels of control are run once per shift and the instrument uses 0.2 ml of control, the cost of 0.2 ml of control can be divided by the total number of reportable tests run on that shift to determine the actual cost of the control per reportable result. Sometimes, when these numbers are very small, they can be included as a factor and not evaluated directly.

Laboratory labor cost calculations are generally done using the number of minutes required to perform the test multiplied by an average hourly rate plus 25% of the rate to cover benefits. For example, if a test takes 3 minutes of a medical technologist's/clinical laboratory scientist's time to perform and report a laboratory test and the hourly rate of the medical technologist is $16.00 + 25% for benefits (total $20.00 per hour):

$$\frac{\$20.00}{60 \text{ minutes}} = \$0.33 \,/\, \text{minute} \times 3 \text{ minutes} = \$0.99$$

then the cost of technologist labor to perform this test is $0.99. The cost of labor for collections, accessioning/processing, etc. can be calculated in the same way using the hourly rates of the personnel who perform these tasks.

Equipment costs per test can be determined in a similar fashion. Reports of monthly rental costs for rented or leased equipment and any additional ongoing maintenance costs are available from the purchasing department. Generally, calculating the part of those costs that apply to a single analysis of a single analyte can be performed by dividing the total cost over a given period by the total number of tests performed on the equipment during the same time period. Depreciation cost for owned capital equipment should be calculated as a direct cost, but it will not vary with the number of tests performed. Each analyzer should be evaluated independently based on how it is used.

Indirect costs may be calculated in two ways. The first is to do a line-by-line analysis of all indirect costs. This method can be time consuming, and sometimes the information is not readily available. The second method is to multiply the direct cost by a factor that is a reasonable assumption of the total indirect cost. Many not-for-profit laboratories use a factor of 1.3, but the factor for any given entity may vary greatly, depending on the type of entity and the overall overhead costs. The finance department is the best source for determining the factor for your institution.

When costing out a test that will be added to the menu of a current piece of equipment, it is sometimes valuable to consider only the direct variable costs involved, as the indirect costs will not change. In that case, the true indirect cost per analysis is not performed, but only the additional direct cost is of significance.

Costs may also be fixed, variable, or semivariable. A fixed cost remains constant despite any change in the volume of tests performed. Examples of fixed costs include salaries and benefits for supervisors and administrators, the cost of a courier, and depreciation on a piece of equipment. Variable costs, however, vary proportionately to the change in test volume. Examples of variable costs include reagent costs and consumables (e.g., pipette tips, cups). Semivariable costs vary with the volume, but not in direct proportion. Technologist labor is a good example. If a 5% increase in test volume occurs, and the work can be covered by current staffing, the total labor cost does not increase and the labor cost per billable actually decreases. If a 30% increase occurs, additional technical staff is required and the total cost will increase. The cost per labatory may remain the same or increase.

Knowing the cost of what the laboratory does is an important first step in determining profitability. Unfortunately, not enough laboratories have done a microcosting analysis of much of what they do, but rely instead on historical data generated during the budget process. Unfortunately, many actually have little or no idea of their true costs.

EVALUATING REVENUE

Revenue is defined as the price of services rendered. It is the amount charged for a test or service. Do not confuse revenue with reimbursement, which will be discussed later (in Chapter 12).

In medical laboratories, the charges billed for a test are attached to a specific CPT (current procedural terminology) code. The CPT coding system is maintained by the American Medical Association (AMA) and is considered the standard for healthcare billing practices in the United States. Codes are assigned for all healthcare procedures, including operating room, imaging, respiratory therapy and others, and are updated annually. Codes for laboratory tests are in the range of 80000 to 89999. Examples of current laboratory CPT codes are:

80162	Digoxin
82465	Total cholesterol
80048	Basic metabolic panel
85025	Hemogram and platelet count, automated, with automated complete differential white blood cell (WBC) count (CBC)
87060	Throat culture
86900	Blood type ABO

CPT codes may refer to a single test (total cholesterol) or to specific panels of tests that are constructed by the AMA and approved for reimbursement by Medicare. Only tests that have CPT codes are reimbursed.

Generally the hospital has a list of all billable services, their associated CPT code, and the price charged to the patient or insurance carrier. This list is called a **chargemaster**. As a manager, you should be closely involved in updating and validating the information in the chargemaster that applies to your area of responsibility in order to maximize revenue and avoid Medicare fraud and abuse issues. The chargemaster is used to price inpatient and on-campus outpatient or regulated visits. A separate chargemaster may be in place for unregulated (non-inpatient) visits, which include laboratory outreach programs. This chargemaster is used for outreach business, which may be brought in to expand the hospital laboratory's revenue base. Although the CPTs are the same for the tests rendered, the charges usually differ. Both taxable and nontaxable entities may have one chargemaster, but may offer discounted pricing to other entities to which they provide services. This is possible because they are not billing the patient directly (or Medicare), but are billing the institution who is purchasing the tests. The institution, in turn, bills the patient or other payer.

Revenue projections for the laboratory are compiled using a number of means including the following:

1. Historical data
2. Patient day forecasts
3. Regulatory changes
4. Growth projections based on new markets and changing technologies

Historical data are gathered from the budgeting process of the previous fiscal (financial) year and modified based on expected or actual regulatory changes and growth projections related to strategic planning initiatives. Revenue based on patient day forecasts is based on the expected DRG reimbursement rate multiplied by the number of patient days expected to fall into each DRG. Most of these calculations are performed by the finance department, but input by laboratory management, especially that related to outreach initiatives, is important.

In theory all billed charges are reimbursed. However, there are several caveats that can affect whether a billed charge is actually paid. Most of these apply to Medicare and Medicaid (state run programs), and many of the commercial insurances are following Medicare's lead and not reimbursing without having secured the appropriate information.

First, all work reimbursed by Medicare must be authenticated as "medically necessary" by the person ordering the test. To do that, there must be a physician signature with the order (many Medicare programs accept other providers) or an indication in the patient's chart that a physician ordered the test. Second, there must be a valid ICD-9CM code, which is a numerical code indicating a specific diagnosis for which the test is ordered. A narrative description of symptoms or diagnosis is generally not acceptable. If the ICD-9CM code does not match criteria developed by Medicare for tests it considers to be medically necessary for that ICD-9CM code, the test will not be reimbursed. Laboratories have the option of having a Medicare patient sign an ABN (advanced beneficiary notice), which certifies that the patient accepts financial responsibility for tests not covered by Medicare. Accomplishing this task on inpatients can be difficult; even on outpatients and outreach patients, it is a complex and tedious procedure. Medicare holds laboratories responsible for obtaining ABN signatures and also for educating their users about the necessity of providing this information. It is a difficult task for laboratories and a cause of ongoing concern.

The type of insurance held by the patient is also a factor in determining what is paid. Medical assistance programs (Medicaid), which are run by states but partially funded by the federal government, have many of the same rules as Medicare. In addition, many patients are enrolled in managed care insurance plans that do not pay fee-for-service, but instead pay the institution a flat per-member-per-month rate. These contracts are becoming more common and involve the shared risk by healthcare providers and insurance companies to keep utilization low. If the laboratory bills most HMOs (Health Maintenance Organizations) for fee-for-service, it will not be reimbursed. The laboratory "piece" is all included in the flat rate.

Although budgeted revenue is carefully calculated and based on inpatient rates, actual revenues collected may differ. Actual reimbursement, however, is constantly monitored, and changes noted are included in the next year's revenue projections.

Pricing Formulas

Pricing for inpatient and outpatient work may be done using several methods (Table 10–4).

Using the **surcharge/cost plus method,** the actual cost of performing the test is determined using the microcosting method. The total cost is then multiplied by a factor (e.g., 1.5 times cost) or a dollar amount is added to the cost (surcharge) to arrive at the final price.

Pricing based on weighted value/RVUs (relative value units) is performed by assigning an RVU to the test. RVUs are generally based on the complexity and time required to perform the test, although other factors such as reagent cost for more esoteric tests may be included. The RVU so determined is then multiplied by a fixed dollar amount to determine the pricing for the test. For example, if cholesterol is weighted at 4 RVUs and the fixed dollar amount per RVU is $1.50, the price for a cholesterol test would be $4 \times \$1.50$ or $6.00.

Pricing may also be determined based on historical data, which may be modified to reflect current market trends and expected adjustments.

Reimbursement issues (see chapter 12 for more details) are key in evaluating real revenue, as where a test is priced and what the expected reimbursement is determine how much revenue is actually generated. More important on the inpatient side is the need to control utilization so that unnecessary tests are not performed for which the laboratory incurs expense, but not reimbursement.

TABLE 10–4. Pricing Formulas

Surcharge/Cost Plus
Weighted Value/RVU
Historical Data

MAKING BUSINESS DECISIONS

The evaluation process for bringing in a new test or deciding to continue to perform a test should include a break-even analysis. The **break-even point** is the point at which there is no profit or loss from performing a test, but that the total of all fixed and variable costs equals the amount of revenue generated by the test. The reasons for performing a break-even analysis are (1) to determine where to price the test and (2) to determine the volume of tests required to meet the break-even point.

The break-even point is determined by dividing the fixed costs plus the dollar amount of the profit expected per test by the revenues generated minus the total variable expense. Figure 10–1 shows the relationships among the factors used to calculate the break-even point.

The break-even point may be expressed by the following:

Where V = the volume of tests needed to break even, R = the expected revenue generated by the test, VC = the total variable cost per test, FC= the fixed cost per test, and I = the net income.

$$V = (FC + I) / (R - VC)$$

Comparing the expected number of tests to the number of tests required to balance the equation will indicate whether the test will be profitable. Adjusting the price of the test will also change the volume required to break even.

The break-even analysis formula is based on several assumptions.

1. When costs increase, profits decrease.
2. When costs decrease, profits increase.
3. When volumes increase, costs and profits increase.
4. When volumes decrease, costs and profits decrease.

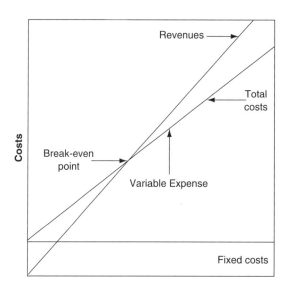

FIGURE 10–1 Break-Even Point
Source: Donna Falcone, *Medical Laboratory Observer*

Although the increases and decreases may not be linear, it is prudent to keep in mind that these relationships do exist. Quantifying their relationships is generally possible, given the availability of appropriate information.

The astute manager also needs to remember that many things other than volumes can affect costs. Those include, but are not limited to, changes in method, changes in equipment, changes from manual to automated methods or vice versa, changes in test mix, changes in unit prices for laboratory, consumables or purchased services, and changes in regulations. The best defense in monitoring these potential changes is to become fast friends with the purchasing department, the human resources department, and the group purchasing organization, if you belong to one, and to keep abreast of regulatory issues and information via Internet access, publications, and professional associations.

The degree of profitability should also be evaluated in light of a number of "intangibles." These may include the following:

1. Will this give us a foothold in a not-yet-developed market?
2. Is this necessary for a new service or program being developed by ours or another department?
3. Is this required to keep us competitive in the outreach market?
4. Is there a particular high profile physician who requires this test?
5. Will providing this test shorten the length of stay?
6. Will providing this test decrease downstream costs by not having to perform expensive interventional procedures that might otherwise be ordered?

In some cases it is better to break even while managing to accommodate an intangible than to make a large profit for profit's sake alone. Particularly in the community-based hospital, not all testing will be profitable. These hospitals do not have the luxury enjoyed by the commercial laboratories of accepting only "good" business. Instead, they provide the continuum of care and the support services required in the community setting, while having to work harder on at least breaking even on their overall business volume.

Taking all of these factors into account, the make-versus-buy decision can be made with some certainty. If it is determined that it is more profitable to perform the test than to send it elsewhere and incur the additional cost, the test should be brought in. In not-for-profit institutions, it may even be logical to bring in a test if doing so saves expense downstream, even if the expense to the laboratory is slightly higher. If, on the other hand, there are either financial or intangible reasons not to perform the test, it should continue to be referred out.

CAPITAL PURCHASES

Capital purchases have their own set of unique requirements and considerations. When selecting a new piece of equipment, the cost of renting or leasing that equipment should be compared with the cost of interest and depreciation expense of purchase. Most equipment companies will perform these analyses for the laboratory, but the finance department will likely want to perform the same analyses themselves. The issue of capital equipment lies in the **current value of money.** The outlay of a sum of money that has a current value, but that will increase in value over time and that if not spent today will be more valuable in purchasing goods or services at a future date, is the center of discussion. Once spent, that money is no longer available and must be written off over the life of the equipment. If that money is spent in increments over a period of time, it has a greater total value over that time.

The evaluation of *depreciation* of capital equipment is key. The amount of depreciation is determined by the number of years over which the equipment is accounted for on the general ledger. Most hospitals use a straight-line depreciation formula, where the dollar value of the equipment is "written off" at the same rate over the useful lifetime of the instrument. That period of time is determined by the hospital's general accounting practices.

The calculation of the *return on investment* is another common practice when evaluating the cost-versus-rent or lease option. The return on investment (ROI) can be expressed in many ways, but generally ROI = profit margin × asset turnover. Profit margin and asset turnover, therefore, work in opposite directions. For the profit margin to increase, the turnover in assets (money) must decrease. Several factors increase profit margins, including automation, decreasing discretionary costs, eliminating obsolete and redundant services or testing, increasing collections of billed revenue, and decreasing direct costs. If a direct cost of a piece of equipment increases, the profitability of the testing scenario decreases. The goal is to at least break even on the return.

A *payback period* calculation should also be made. The payback period indicates the time it will take to generate the incoming revenue that compensates for the money paid out for the equipment (outgoing assets). For example, if an instrument costs $100,000 and it generates $25,000 annually in incremental cash, the payback period would be $100,000 divided by $25,000 or 4 years. The goal is to keep the payback period as short as possible, so that funds are not tied up. This is critically important when cash flow is tight and capital funds are at a premium.

These are only a few of the different types of justifications that can be performed on capital equipment. By starting with these and working with the finance department, you will ensure that appropriate capital decisions are made.

RESOURCES

Many resources are available to assist laboratory managers in evaluating their own profitability and in comparing that to the profitability and practices of other institutions. Information on cost accounting is available both in hard copy and on line and is provided not only by financial institutions, but by government agencies and professional associations affiliated with the healthcare field. The College of American Pathologists, the Clinical Laboratory Management Association, and the Centers for Medicare and Medicaid Services (formerly the Health Care Financing Administration) are but a few. The attached bibliography is only a starting point for locating additional information.

SUMMARY

This chapter has presented a basic overview of the interrelationships of financial and managerial accounting, methods to evaluate expenses and revenues, issues surrounding reimbursement, methods for pricing tests, factors related to capital purchases, and a short list of resources available to laboratory managers. In an industry where competition is brutal and change is rapid and extensive, it becomes critical for the manager to understand and constantly evaluate the financial status of the laboratory. A strong knowledge of financial methods and practices will allow the manager to do that and to remain financially strong and competitive.

SUGGESTED PROBLEM-BASED LEARNING ACTIVITIES
Chapter 10: Cost Benefit Analysis

Instructions: Use Internet resources, books, articles, colleagues, etc., to present solutions to the problems listed below. There is no one correct solution to any problem.

Note to Instructor: Students in class may be divided into groups and given the problem-based learning activity to discuss and solve. Once the group has reached consensus as to a solution, the group may present it to the other students in the class. This activity will provide all students with information regarding solutions to the problem.

Problem #1
Suppose you have just been given a project to provide new laboratory services. Project revenue and costs for this new service.

Problem #2
You have just purchased a piece of new equipment and must determine what testing to perform in-house and what testing to send to a reference laboratory.

Problem #3
Suppose your institution just received notification that the reimbursement for your in-patient laboratory testing will be reduced by 6%. What alternative do you have to maintain your current profit level?

BIBLIOGRAPHY

Bozzo P (ed): *Cost-Effective Laboratory Management.* Lippincott, Williams & Wilkins Publishers, Philadelphia, 1998.

Brock HR, Herrington LA: *Cost Accounting: Principles and Applications.* McGraw Hill, Glencoe, 1998.

Cooper R, Kaplan RS: *Design of Cost Management Systems.* Prentice Hall, Upper Saddle River, 1998.

Horngren CT, Foster G, Datar SM: *Cost Accounting: A Managerial Emphasis.* Prentice Hall, Upper Saddle River, 1999.

Kimmel, P., Weygandt, J., Kieso, D.: Financial Accounting: Tools for Business Decision Making. John Wiley & Sons, Inc., Danvers, 2005.

Kirschner CG et al: *Current Procedural Terminology 2000.* American Medical Association, Chicago, 1999.

Schultz D: *ICD-9CM Code Book for Hospitals.* St. Anthony Publishing, Inc., Reston, VA, 2000.

Travers EM: *Clinical Laboratory Management.* Williams & Wilkins, Philadelphia, 1997.

Wallace MA, Kosinski DD: *Clinical Laboratory Science Education and Management.* WB Saunders, Philadelphia, 1998.

Williams, J., Haka, S., Bettner, M.: Financial and Mangerial Accounting: The Basis of Business Decisions. McGraw-Hill/Irwin, New York, 2004.

Internet Resources

The American Association for Clinical Chemistry
www.aacc.org

The American Medical Association
www.ama-assn.org/

Centers for Medicare and Medicaid Services (formerly The HealthCare Finance Administration)
www.cms.hhs.gov

The Clinical Laboratory Management Association
www.clma.org

The Maryland Hospital Association
www.mdhospitals.org, www.mhaoline.org

11

Effective Budgeting in the Laboratory: Practical Tips

IRINA LUTINGER, MPH, H(ASCP)DLM

Chapter Outline

Objectives

Following successful completion of this chapter, the learner will be able to:

1. Describe the operating budget types.
2. Explain the steps for preparation of a successful budget process.
3. Identify common budgetary problems and recommend possible solutions.
4. Describe how to write proper budget justifications.

Key Terms

Appropriation budget
Budget Justification
Fixed Budget
Flexible Budget
Operating Budget
Program Budget

Resource Allocation
Resource Management
Rolling Budget
Variance Analysis
Zero-Based Budget

Case Study: Planning to Open a New Satellite Laboratory

You are a supervisor of the clinical laboratory in the hospital. The hospital administration wants to penetrate the market and expand the business by opening a Breast Center outpatient facility. It will be dedicated to the detection, treatment, and prevention of breast cancer. Hospital administration graciously appointed space allocated for the laboratory services. The center will provide services in an elegant, "boutique" environment where all patients receive expedited care.

Issues and Questions to Consider

1. *What type of budget should be used for this satellite laboratory?*
2. *What other departments need to be involved in developing this laboratory?*
3. *What assumptions should be made developing this operating budget?*
4. *How many laboratory personnel will be required for this appointed facility?*
5. *Which are the major aspects of concern in proposing the new facility?*

INTRODUCTION

In the healthcare industry, the demand for services inevitably exceeds the availability of resources. It is necessary to optimize the use of resources available and make decisions amidst competing demands. In attempting to respond to the challenge, most hospital managers are confronted with a lack of information about the expected resource requirements, the actual resources used, and the subsequent results.

The budget process becomes demanding and unpredictable as a result of various changes in government regulations and cuts; laboratory professionals become much more accountable. The laboratory manager/supervisor should be able to respond to the following questions:

- How much did the laboratory spend on various subscriptions (such as proficiency testing) last year?
- How much is it expected to spend on developing new in-house assays?
- Did increased expenditures for the send-out tests to the reference laboratory result in more cost-effective patient care?

The current healthcare environment of limited resources forces laboratorians back to the basics of good management. As a result, budgeting has taken on greater importance. An understanding of the planning, budgeting, and managing process is vital in allocation of available resources not only to meet anticipated needs but also to control actual use. The laboratory must be viewed as a business. Once this fact is recognized, considerations of long-term and short-term planning should be included, with emphasis on operating requirements; clear goals and objectives must be identified; and monitoring and control of ongoing operations must be implemented. Budget is a business tool to be used for effective resource management.

Resource management is different from *resource allocation* because it includes accountability for results. Managers are asked to justify resources needed in terms of expected results; therefore cost accounting is an important tool to accomplish this objective on an on-going basis. Cost accounting identifies, defines, measures, reports, and analyzes the elements of costs associated with providing a unit of output (test) and appropriately assigns and allocate costs to that test. For example, operating costs requires daily review including but not limited to payroll, reagents, and consumable utilization. Constant justification for variances is required to explain why the better/less expensive results can't be obtained by using fewer resources. Payers, patients, and the community ask questions about prices and charges, which increases pressure on the budgeting process and hospital resources. In this climate of high demands and low resources, sufficient information provided during the year from the hospital to the laboratory manager is imperative for a successful budgetary planning. The challenge of the budgeting and resource management is to improve existing resources, to identify realistic expectations, and to communicate it to all appropriate parties.

The *operating budget* is a tool for laboratory managers throughout the year. It is the overall plan for coordination of resources, a plan for identification of resources and expenditures, and a plan for projections. Today's budget must evaluate appropriate use of resources in relation to results, instead of being used as a projection and monitoring tool. Furthermore, the operating budget is a communication tool to be used with internal and external customers, but it is not a crystal ball.

When reviewing a budget, it is important not to focus on numbers only, but to understand the objectives of the **department** and organization behind it to be able to objectively assess the resources and appropriate allocations. The budgetary package should explain the objectives regarding future growth, and then the manager will be able to objectively estimate and identify the realistic expectations. The budget should be used not only to comply with the annual process but also to improve the financial aspects of one's job and the department to solve problems as they arise. This chapter defines the types of operating budgets, offers guidelines for the budgetary process, identifies the most common budget problems, and provides tips on surviving budget justification.

TYPES OF OPERATING BUDGETS

The laboratory's operating plan or budget cycle covers a 1-year period, and is goal oriented with specific levels of attainment. Accountability during the cycle is maintained so that objectives are reached. The hospital information system can provide the laboratory with report(s) identifying how well the department is achieving its identified goals and objectives.

The type and format of the operating budget selected depend on the organization's requirements. Among budget types are the following: fixed, flexible, program, appropriation, rolling, and zero-based budgets.

A *fixed budget* assumes a single level of activity, and the entire budget is built around that level. If the laboratory is confident that its expenditures won't change during the budget cycle, there will be no new tests brought in and no new equipment purchased, then this type of budget can be used. A fixed budget is not a tool to monitor and control resources during changes. A *flexible budget* reflects expected laboratory revenue and expenses and it anticipates changes. In this budget some expenses are fixed and some are variable. The flexible budget recognizes the difficulty of establishing a single level of achievement and provides a tool for controlling costs. It can also point out the priority expenses and its variances. The flexible budget provides the information on specific objectives, such as appropriate resource usage, and adjusts budgeted expenses to the actual activity on the basis of specific activity indicators.

A *program budget* is created based on a specific program matrix. Included in this matrix are all proposed services and the resources required. A proposed program can include a set of activities, services, staffing, and equipment related to the program. This type of budget can be used for short-term planning.

An *appropriation budget* is usually found in governmental organizations that depend on an outside source of funds. During the review process the outside agency reviews the budget in detail and authorizes specific dollar amounts. If expenses exceed the appropriated amount, the responsible party must obtain the supplemental appropriation from the granting agency.

A *rolling budget* is a continuous budget that is updated periodically in preparation for the next budget cycle. A rolling budget for a 12-month period is reviewed and revised every quarter. The past quarter becomes history and the new quarter is added to the projection to move ahead. This type of budget is used for cash projections and therefore frequently updated. Incremental Budget addresses only changes like new equipment, new positions, and new programs. It assumes that all current operations are essential to the process and working at its peak performance. The advantage is the minimal time commitment for incremental budget preparation and the disadvantage is assumption that all existing operations are essential for business.

In a *zero-based budget,* management annually reevaluates all activities to decide whether they should be eliminated or funded. Projects are approved based on funds availability and funding levels are determined by priorities. A zero-based budget helps to determine levels of resource requirements within a service or program and the possible expenditure level within each responsibility center. Each department manager is required to justify the entire unit budget annually as if all of its activities were totally new.

Based on the preceding discussion in our case study, the new satellite laboratory that we're planning to open, what budget should we use? We don't know the exact expenditures, but based on assumptions, we can develop an estimated

TABLE 11–1. Example of Variable Costs for Reagents and Supplies

Number of tests	Costs of Reagents and Supplies	Total Variable Costs
1	$.25	$.25
10	$.25	$2.50
100	$.25	$25.00

budget, anticipating possible adjustments during the year. To be successful, we need to carefully account for all the services required in this venture.

The budget will be based on various components of costs such as direct, indirect, variable, and fixed. The direct costs can be easily tied to a laboratory test, but the indirect costs are not involved in the production of the test. For example, direct costs include consumables and supplies, labor, and equipment to do the test. In contrast, the major component of indirect costs is the cost of time in which personnel are doing things other than producing reportable laboratory results. Supervisory personnel not doing testing, secretarial support, phlebotomist time, photocopying, utilities, employee benefits, computing services, and space are examples of indirect costs. Costs can behave as fixed or as variable. Fixed expenses do not vary with the test volume for a given period when variable expenses change proportionately with changes in volume of tests performed. Variable costs increase or decrease proportionally as activity changes. Table 11–1 provides an example of variable costs for reagents and supplies.

Total costs = Fixed costs + Variable costs.
Average cost per test=Total costs/# tests
The average cost per test decreases as volume increases.

Labor expenses are important to accurately estimate the budgetary needs. An example of direct variable costs is presented in Table 11–2.

Because the laboratory in our example will be a satellite laboratory in the Breast Center, we need to make sure that all the regulatory requirements are met appropriately, the equipment is selected and validated, the staff training is completed, and the critical telecommunication and informational services are not only in place but completely functional. Telecommunication services will ensure functionality of the telephone lines and cabling for computer-related equipment. The information services staff will be responsible for connecting laboratory

TABLE 11–2. Example of Direct Variable Costs

- Labor: Tech time $14/hr/60 min = $0.233/min
- Time to perform test 13 minutes 13 minutes × $0.233/min = $3.03
- Benefits @35% of time to perform test = $1.06
- Consumables expense is $1.05
- Therefore our cost is $5.14

TABLE 11–3.   Example of a Projected Payback Period for Capital Equipment

- Instrument costs = $150,000
- Estimated annual cash flow =$30,000/year
- Payback period for the instrument =5 years ($150,000/$30,000)

---

information, clinical information, and registration systems operations. Failure of any of these systems could lead, for example, to the inability of the laboratory information system to retrieve, transmit, or compile results for clients or their patients leading to a loss of both revenue and future business. Furthermore, it is important to start immediately to negotiate with vendors regarding the equipment for the new facility. Based on available resources, it must be determined whether analyzers should be purchased, leased, or reagent rented. When lump sum capital dollars are not available, a hospital can choose to **lease** an instrument. In a lease agreement, monthly payments are spread over a specified period of time (60 months) and are based on the purchase price plus interest and taxes, insurance, and maintenance. Because lease expenses can be depreciated, leasing can represent an advantage over purchase when cash availability is an issue for the institution. Leasing also offers 100% financing at fixed rates, no money down, and protection for the laboratory against inflation. The disadvantages of leasing include locking the laboratory into a long-term relationship with one vendor and higher reagent and consumables prices, in most cases.

In a **reagent rental** agreement, the cost of the instrument is included in the reagent cost charged by the vendor. The laboratory signs an agreement, which usually commits it to a minimum volume of reagent, purchased over a specified period at a set price. Again, the advantage is that there are no capital costs for the laboratory. Whereas direct purchase requires a large amount of money up front, and leasing requires capital money spread over time, reagent rental requires no capital money. If the allocated resources do not allow for lease or purchase, reagent rental can be used for the first year and the equipment leased or purchased later working with the financial services of the institution and appropriate vendor(s). If the choice is for a capital purchase of an instrument, it is important to realize the concept of the payback period. The payback is the number of years it will take to pay back the original instrument purchase cost. A projected payback period for capital equipment is presented in Table 11–3. The financial services department can help with various financial calculations presented by vendors.

The Successful Budget Process

The success of the budget process depends on the following elements:

1. Clear goals and objectives that can guide the resource allocation.
2. Project volumes.
3. Convert volumes into revenue.

4. Convert volumes into expense requirements.
5. Detailed statistical data, economic trends, and accurate information about existing and potential clients.
6. A defined budget period and procedures for development of the budget.
7. Reports to identify actual financial and statistical information for comparison with the budget and for variance analysis.

There are three important segments for the complete budget: **income forecasting, expense budget,** and **cash flow projections.** Income forecasting estimates future revenues and should be used to set goals. In our example, what is the projected volume of testing planned for the Breast Center? Because it is a new facility, the operating budget will need to be constructed based on the forecasted volume. If one knows the number of physicians re-locating to the Breast Center from the main campus, the history of utilization can be reviewed and used as a base line for the operating expenses. Once the above is determined, convert volumes into revenue. What number should the price per test be? One needs to calculate the variable and the fixed costs for a particular test and then it can be multiplied by a specific number of tests projected. Then you will be able to convert volumes into expense requirements: Labor expense with benefits, non-labor expense, and overhead expense.

In order to control the labor expenses one can hire part-time and/or temporary employees instead of only full-time employees, if possible. Part-time employees receive benefits in proportion to the number of hours worked. The temporary workers receive only benefits required by law. Expense budget should also include upcoming cost-of-living raises, if any.

The non-labor expense will be based on projected volume of testing. But managers can reduce these expenses by using generic supplies wherever possible in the laboratory. In reality, it is almost impossible to use generic materials because the main bulk of its reagents and consumables must come from a specific vendor to be used on their analyzers. The non-labor expenses also should include an estimate of anticipated increases in supplies and service contracts. Overhead expenses such as depreciation, heating, cooling, insurance premiums, etc. are assigned to each department as a specific percent.

A realistic estimate of future growth can demonstrate to management the need for additional staff to meet future revenue standards. The expense budget can also forecast expense categories. For example, a growth in an outreach services area will require a greater commitment to travel, administrative support, and telephone and other expenses. The cash flow projections are just as important for future planning and are based on the accuracy of projected volumes and expenses. Several factors can adversely affect cash flow, including excessive investments or a too high level of debt. All of these components must be interrelated and coordinated for successful budget planning.

For our satellite laboratory budget we need to perform a careful analysis based not only on the cost of opening this laboratory site but also on the expectation of profit. We need to assess the potential volume of specimens and tests based on clinicians' projected patient population, evaluation of existing services, and the forecast of clients relocating to this new facility. We will need a full-time laboratory technologist to process specimens efficiently and timely. A full-time phlebotomist will collect, label, and send specimens to the technologist in the laboratory. Physicians and clients in this high quality oncology operation are expecting rapid and accurate results. In addition, by meeting with various services that will be involved in the Breast Center operation, one can realistically project assumptions of future growth. Once operations begin, monthly operating reports will compare actual to budget expenses, outlining variances. The **variance analysis** will capture changes and trends in the market place that affect the operation.

Analyzing variances will improve the quality of the original forecasts, point out changes in operation, and offer a means of asking why goals were not met. Proper budgeting and forecasting cannot entirely eliminate problems. We can't predict the future accurately, but we can make proper distinctions.

COMMON BUDGET PROBLEMS AND POSSIBLE SOLUTIONS

Losing sight of real objectives occurs when too much emphasis is placed on completing a complex procedure in a short time, involving endless revisions and paperwork. People are so pleased that this process is over; they often forget that it is only actually beginning. Control reactions that go into effect during the year can be practical when they result from discovered variances (i.e., when something is wrong with the budget or the actual results such as expenses overbudget or revenue below projected levels). The budget requires a monthly review to use all the necessary control opportunities and put them into the effect.

To avoid losing sight of the reason for budgeting, it is important to remember the following:

- Focus decisions toward clear objectives.
- Think of the budget as a standard and focus performance against it.
- Analyze monthly variances by comparing actual expenses to budget expenses and examining causes.
- Look in the budget for specific keys to higher profits and identify ways to either reduce expenses or improve income.
- Make a list of suggestions included in the budget, monthly recommendations, and approvals by management.

Budgeting above 100% of the previous year is known as **historical-based budgeting** and is the easiest way to budget without major effort. To budget in this way, the total spent in the previous year is divided by 12. The number obtained plus a percentage for inflation is used to budget for the upcoming year. Accepting this approach builds lack of control into the process and encourages further spending. Other factors, when used as the only criterium, may result in a poorly developed budget and include:

- Using historical information as the only assumption source.
- Only examining the accounts that show unfavorable variances.

- Looking for solutions not to increase the budget but to enforce realistic spending limits.
- Making budget increases automatically.

Another important aspect of a budgetary process is to not accept arbitrary changes, but in practice logical philosophy isn't always possible. Individuals who prepare budgets and develop assumptions rarely have the final word. No matter how careful the budget is assessed, it is not possible to prevent someone higher up from changing the budget. To help ensure approval of a budget, the following points may be helpful to consider:

- Present a strong case based on sound assumptions.
- Do not defend a budget that has been changed randomly.
- Use discretion when arguing with a superior. Avoid ego confrontations.

Realistic expectations help explain the inevitable variances (the difference between budgeted and actual dollar amounts) that may arise. A variance is a sign that control over expenses is needed. A problem can be solved only if it is identified. Budgets should be a tool not for blame but for improvement. Follow the steps below when explaining variances:

- Always go back to the assumption when writing a variance explanation, and base it on a comparison.
- Identify real problems and recommend solutions.
- Recognize the budgeting process as one that monitors process.
- Acknowledge that budget is only a guideline and no one can do better than estimate.

Furthermore, the explanations that don't identify causes but rather attempt to indicate a trend are not a positive development.

- Don't try to excuse the previous year's excessive variances by referring to a previous period. Confront the problems that exist each year.
- Don't ask for a budget increase this year based on not being able to meet last year's budget.
- Try not to use weak assumptions. It leads to an inability to identify or explain problems.

Table 11–4 lists the major areas of concern for planning the satellite Breast Center laboratory. One problem with budgeting is that problems are often left unresolved and allowed to continue. Changes must be suggested immediately to respond to major budget errors. Management must understand that problems will not go away and must be solved. If the manager does not have a voice in the decision-making process, it is important to point out the problem to those in a position to make changes. Try to meet a challenge by asking for authority. Keep all lines of communication open with internal and external customers to ascertain the necessary information. Always attempt to develop joint solutions rather than being an adversary.

TABLE 11–4. Major Aspects to Consider in Planning a Satellite Breast Center Laboratory

Equipment Selection	Cost/Impact
Computer system	Compatibility with other systems
Space	Adequacy
Specimen processing	Location/convenience
Manpower	Number of employees
Cost justification	Expense/Savings/Growth
Implementation	Schedule/Training

SURVIVING BUDGET JUSTIFICATION

The real test of a budget's value is how it compares to actual expenses. This will determine the accuracy of the forecast and whether problems can be identified and solved during the year. Most organizations prepare a monthly report that lists both actual and budgeted costs, highlighting the variances. A good *budget justification* report can propose concrete solutions rather than just describe the variance. An explanation of variances can be devised to satisfy administration or to provide an opportunity to propose corrective actions for the existing problems.

The following budgeting standards can present justifications as opportunities:

- Review and prepare justifications monthly.
- Present recommendations for corrective action.
- Make sure that actual results are not manipulated.
- Make all staff aware of budgetary limits and goals.

Justification should present information as clearly as possible. The reader should be able to answer these questions: Why did variances occur? What's being done to correct the problem?

The best way to structure monthly justifications is to compare the year-to-date (YTD) results. Remember, variances are not always problems. On the contrary, they present opportunities to correct problems.

> Variance = actual-budgeted
> Revenue variance = actual revenue-budgeted revenue
> Expense revenue variance = actual expense-budgeted expense

TABLE 11–5. Example of Comparison of a Monthly Budget Justification to Year-to-Date (YTD) Results

- Reagents budgeted YTD expenses $100,000
- Actual expenses $120,000.
- The variance percentage is:
$120,000 – $100,000 = $20,000
$20,000/$100,000 = (20%)

Table 11–5 compares a monthly budget justification to year-to-date results. Justifications should include favorable as well as unfavorable variances. Justifications can fall into one of these areas:

1. The variance is a timing difference that will disappear in coming months. No action is needed.
2. The assumption in the budget was wrong, as proven by negative variance. The budget should be revised.
3. Expenses are not being controlled. Corrective action is needed to eliminate the unfavorable trend.

Consider another <u>example</u>: The 10% unfavorable variance is an improvement over the last year, when the same items were 20% over budget. This explanation tells nothing about the underlying cause of this problem. A possible explanation could be: The 10% variance is due to two major causes. The new proficiency subscriptions were not included in the budget and the inspection fees have increased since last year. Specific reasons are given for the unfavorable variance and the corrective action that can be taken.

An additional example of variance justification is provided in Table 11–6.

TABLE 11–6.   **Example of Variance Justification**

Salaries for 9 months:	
YTD (Year to date)	$207,130
Forecast	$172,400
Variance	$(34,730)
Percent Variance	$(34,730)/$172,400 = (20.1%)

Explanation

The original budget for salaries was based on the assumption that current staff levels were adequate for workload projected into this year, but the volume increased by 40%. The unfavorable variance was caused by overtime.

Analysis

The negative trend will continue given the present staff levels. The present budget level is unrealistic, and the level of growth was not anticipated when the budget was prepared.

Recommendations

• Revise the department's salaries in line with current information about volume.

- Authorize the hiring of two additional staff members.
- Review procedures and determine whether a more efficient system would improve the operation.

It's important to be mindful of various causes of variances before opening and during the operation of the center. Some common causes of variance are listed in Table 11–7. By generating effective and realistic justifications, you can make constructive recommendations for trend corrections to management. An effective justification should contain the following elements: comparison between actual and forecast, an explanation of causes, analysis of factors affecting its performance, and recommendations.

TABLE 11–7. Common Causes of Variance

Causes of Variances	Example	Action Needed
Periodic large expenditures	Equipment maintenance	No action needed
Increased usage due to special circumstances	Increase in volume of tests	Document
Incorrect budgeting	Decreased reagents usage	Document
Changes in method of testing not known at the time of budgeting process	Modification of existing assay testing due to changes in the analyzer	Rebudget appropriately and inform administration

Summary

Budgeting is a process that every laboratory manager has to face. It is a way to take control of the laboratory environment, master the financial aspects of a department, and solve problems before they become critical. The budget is a tool to reassure, to clarify, to lower the risk, to keep on track, and to help obtain goals. The budget defines the steps taken in the annual cycle to keep the plan on target. It is a management resource that defines the plan for the department and informs management of progress in achieving targets.

If properly prepared, a budget can increase revenues, decrease spending, and identify ways to make improvements. For the significant amount of effort that is invested into the budgetary process, it should generate recognizable results. Out-of-control situations should be avoided and actions should be taken immediately by planning and monitoring trends.

The goal of the budget is to set standards. An expense report reflects the accuracy of assumptions. It also demands that problems must be identified and explained, and solutions recommended. By knowing the common budgetary problems, one can develop a sense of what to avoid and how to make the budget succeed. Table 11–8 is an example of a budget for a clinical laboratory.

TABLE 11-8. Example of a Detailed Budget

Clinical Laboratory

Salary	Description	FTE Expense Proposed	FTE Expense Target	FTEs
1	S-Level Management Reg.	228,384	218,384	3.00
2	M-Level Management Reg.	232,791	222,791	3.00
3	Lab/Tech Staff Union Reg.	1,910,629	1,900,629	34.00
4	Lab/Tech Staff Union OT	98,000	88,000	1.51
5	Lab/Tech Staff Non Union	55,159	45,159	1.10
6	Lab/Tech Staff Non Union OT	18,480	8,480	0.22
7	Clerical Employees Reg.	113,355	103,355	3.00
8	Clerical Employees OT	1,620	1,620	0.03
9	Service Employees 1199 Reg.	118,439	108,439	4.00
10	Service Employees 1199 OT	1,650	1,650	0.04
11	Casual A-Level Management	1,620	1,620	0.03
12	Casual Office/Clerical Emp.	1,620	1,620	0.03
Salary–Total:		**2,781,747**	**2,701,747**	**49.96**

Non Salary	Description	Budget Proposed	Budget Target
1	Medical/Surgical Supplies	84,400	80,400
4	Reagents	1,588,699	1,584,699
6	Food and Dietary Supplies	500	500
7	Non-Medical/Non-Surgical	1,600	1,600
8	Office Supplies	6,995	2,995
9	Purchased Services	1,200,000	1,196,000
10	Conference Registration and	3,000	3,000
11	Travel	2,000	2,000
12	Other Direct Expenses	20,000	16,000
13	Repairs and Maintenance	1000	1000
14	Painting & Decorating	2,500	2,500
15	Rpr/Maint Eqpt P&M Cost Id	1,500	1,500
16	LockSmith Shop	500	500
17	Telephone	1,000	1,000
18	Telephone Usage from	2,500	2,500
19	Rentals and Leases	19,476	15,476
Non Salary—Total:		**2,679,129**	**2,675,129**
TOTAL EXPENSE		**5,460,876**	**5,376,876**	84,000

SUGGESTED PROBLEM-BASED LEARNING ACTIVITIES

Chapter 11: Effective Budgeting in the Laboratory: Practical Tips

Instructions: Use Internet resources, books, articles, colleagues, etc., to present solutions to the problems listed below. There is no one correct solution to any problem.

Note to Instructor: Students in class may be divided into groups and given the problem-based learning activity to discuss and solve. Once the group has reached consensus as to a solution, the group may present it to the other students in the class. This activity will provide all students with information regarding solutions to the problem.

Problem #1
Suppose your laboratory budget is cut. Indicate how you as the laboratory manager would maintain your current level of quality laboratory testing.

Problem #2
Prepare a laboratory budget forecasting an 8.5% increase in patient admissions.

Problem #3
Suppose that administration informed you that you must reduce your operating/personnel budget by 10%. As laboratory manager, you have been asked to design a plan indicating how you will handle and survive this cut.

BIBLIOGRAPHY

Esmond TH Jr: *Budgeting for Effective Hospital Resource.* American Hospital Publishing Inc, Chicago, IL., 1990.

Helman EZ: *Cost Containment in the Clinical Laboratory.* Berkeley Scientific Publication, Denver, CO., 1995.

Nigrom D: Clinical Laboratory Management. McGraw-Hill Companies, Inc., New York, 2000.

Snyder J: *Administration and Supervision in Laboratory Medicine,* 3rd ed. JB Lippincott, Philadelphia, PA., 1998.

Thomsett M: *The Little Black Book of Budgets and Forecasts.* AMACOM, New York, NY., 1988.

Travers E: *Managing Costs in Clinical Laboratories.* McGraw-Hill Information Services Company, New York, NY., 1989.

Travers E, Wilkinson D: Developing a budget for the laboratory. *Clin. Lab. Manager Review* 1997, Jan-Feb; 11(1):56-66.

Travers E, Krochmal C: *A new way to determine test cost per instrument.* Part I. MLO Med Lab Obs. 1988, Oct;20(10):24-9.

Travers E, Krochmal C: A new way to determine test cost per instrument. Part II. *MLO Med Lab Obs.* 1988 Nov;20(11):59-62.

Internet Resources

http://www.ed.gov
http://www.napavalley.edu/Projects/51/Effective-Budgeting.pdf
http://www.pitt.edu/~offres/proposal/budget.html
*http://www.widelearning.com/website/02_e-library/fi_accountancy-training
   _effective-budgeting.html*
http://www.secaf.org/Effective_Budgeting.pdf
http://www.afe.org/vip/portal/media/topics/Planning/murphy994.pdf

12

Healthcare Reimbursement

JEANNE M. DONNELLY, MBA, RHIA
THOMAS H. PETERS, JR., MT(ASCP)

Chapter Outline

Objectives

Following successful completion of this chapter, the learner will be able to:

1. Identify and discuss the following reimbursement methodologies used by the Center for Medicare and Medicaid Services (CMS) for Medicare patients:
   a. Diagnostic Related Groups (DRGs)
   b. Resource Based Relative Value Scale (RBRVS)
   c. Ambulatory Payment Categories (APCs)

2. Calculate the payment rate for each methodology based on CMS formulas.
3. Discuss other payment methodologies such as:
   a. Fee-for-service
   b. Capitation
   c. Per diem
   d. Per case
   e. Carve out
4. Calculate payment based on a capitated rate.
5. Identify reasons why healthcare costs have escalated and discuss how the healthcare industry has responded.

Key Terms

Ambulatory Payment
  Categories (APCs)
Capitation
Carve Out (Carved Out)
Diagnostic Related Groups (DRGs)

Fee-for-service
Per Case
Per Diem
Resource Based Relative Value
  Scale (RBRVS)

Case Study: Healthcare Reimbursement

As the manager of a clinical laboratory, you have been asked to calculate the reimbursement rates for certain laboratory tests with Ambulatory Payment Categories (APCs) under the new Outpatient Prospective Payment System. You must estimate what your laboratory will receive for Medicare patients under this system to assist you in the budget process.

Issues and Questions to Consider

1. *What coding system is used to assign APCs?*
2. *What allied health professional is preferred for assigning code numbers?*
3. *What is the formula for calculating the payment rate?*
4. *Where can you find the most current information regarding the APC rates and the conversion factor used in determining the payment rate?*
5. *How can this information be used in planning for the budget?*
6. *What is another way that laboratory tests are billed for non-Medicare patients?*

INTRODUCTION

This chapter provides the reader with a basic understanding of healthcare reimbursement. A brief history of healthcare costs shows why costs have escalated and how payers have responded. The different types of reimbursement mechanisms are discussed. These are broken down into governmental and private sectors. It is important to note that more than one of these mechanisms may be used by the payers.

Certain terms related to reimbursement are used throughout the chapter. A **provider** refers to the hospital, the outpatient department, the physician or other healthcare professional who furnishes care to the patient. A **payer** refers to the **governmental payers** (such as Medicare, Medicaid, and other public sources of funds), **private payers** (such as Blue Cross and other commercial insurers) or **self-payers** who do not have any other type of insurance.

HISTORICAL PERSPECTIVE

In 2002, healthcare represented 14.9% of the Gross Domestic Product (GDP) or the equivalent of $1.5 trillion. Clinical laboratory costs account for approximately $30 to $40 billion of that amount. It is estimated that total healthcare costs will increase to 16.2% of the GDP or $2.2 trillion by the year 2008. Yet, in 1965, healthcare accounted for only 5.5% of the GDP. How did healthcare come to consume such a large portion of our national expenditure? Several elements have contributed to the increase in healthcare costs.

1. *Increase in technology:* Technology advances in testing, surgical procedures, and diagnostic procedures required new, cost intensive equipment. Not only did equipment need to be purchased, but in some cases, new facilities needed to be built to house the equipment.
2. *Increase in skilled personnel:* These new technologies required staff with different skill sets to operate the equipment. This resulted in new categories of allied health personnel that needed to be educated, trained, and hired.
3. *Aging population:* As we age, we access healthcare services more frequently. Also, the improved technology resulted in a longer life span and increased the need for skilled nursing care to accommodate an elderly population.
4. *Consumer awareness and expectations:* The consumer expected and demanded the high-priced technology. Where an x-ray study would have sufficed in the past, now a magnetic resonance imaging (MRI) or positron emission tomography (PET) scan is the expectation.
5. *The uninsured/underinsured:* Individuals who do not have access to insurance use emergency room services to receive routine care, or wait until they are very ill before accessing the healthcare system.

As the cost of healthcare continued to rise, the cost of health insurance increased as well. Government and private insurance plans had to increase their premiums to keep pace with the rising costs. Employers sponsoring the health insurance benefits for employees initially bore the cost increase; however, as time went on, the employee had to share in the increased cost of insurance through higher premiums, deductibles, and co-payments, or face a decrease in benefits. *Premiums* are the amount charged by the insurer to insure against specific risks. *Deductibles* represents the amount the insured must first pay (usually annually) before benefits are payable. *Co-payments* are the proportion of total medical costs that the insured must pay out of pocket each time health services are received after the deductible has been paid. As the employer and consumer become responsible for more of the cost of healthcare, they became more cost conscious regarding the use of healthcare dollars.

The healthcare industry has responded in several ways to try to manage such a large segment of spending. There is an increased emphasis on preventive medicine and alternative care options. Employers have initiated programs to decrease occupational health hazards. Spending limitations and benefit exclusions have been added to insurance plans to try to slow the growth of spending.

The main sources of healthcare funding are federal government programs and private insurance. Both have sought new ways to curb costs. The private sector has incorporated parts of the federal programs and the federal programs have seen value in the private arena. But the goal is the same in both cases: obtain the best quality care at the correct level of service for the least cost.

FEDERAL REIMBURSEMENT SYSTEMS

As seen in Figure 12–1, the federal government pays for approximately 45% of healthcare expenditures through Medicare, Medicaid, and other public programs. Medicare came into being as an amendment to the Social Security Act (SSA) in 1965. It is funded by the federal government through a payroll tax and is administrated by the Center for Medicare and Medicaid Services (CMS). Medicare pays for healthcare for persons 65 and over, disabled individuals entitled to Social Security benefits, and patients with end stage renal disease. The Medicare Program benefits were originally separated into two parts. Part A covers certain hospital and outpatient costs; Part B covers certain individual physician costs. In recent years, "Part C" managed care plans were added as options for many beneficiaries, modeled after private sector managed care plans (discussed later in this chapter).

Medicaid, also created by the SSA of 1965, is a state-run healthcare plan for the poor. It is funded jointly by state and federal funds based on income levels for each state. Each state has a different methodology for reimbursement, but all must meet the funding limitations set by the federal government. Each state must also provide certain basic health services as mandated by the federal government. Most states reimburse under a fee-for-service basis; however one third of the states use a managed care program. Under the Balanced Budget Act (BBA) of 1997, states were given the authority to mandate managed care enrollment.

Other types of public health aid funded by the federal government are programs for veterans health care, Indian health care, school health programs, and maternal and child health services.

Because the government subsidized such a large portion of healthcare expenditures, it became evident that the rapid growth in healthcare costs needed to be controlled. The first area to be addressed, hospital costs, accounted for one third of the healthcare dollar.

"My costs are higher because I have sicker patients" was the rallying cry for hospitals in the 1970s to explain away their higher costs, but there was no

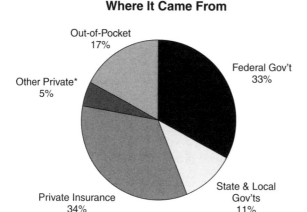

**The Nation's Health Dollar: 2001
Where It Came From**

Out-of-Pocket
17%

Federal Gov't
33%

Other Private*
5%

Private Insurance
34%

State & Local
Gov'ts
11%

FIGURE 12–I   The Nation's Healthcare Dollar: 2001.

mechanism to justify this claim. Data were collected on patients' diagnoses and procedures, but there was not a way to relate the diagnosis and treatment to costs.

Prior to the early 1980s, hospitals were reimbursed on a *fee-for-service* basis. This meant that the provider was paid by either the government, the commercial insurance company, or patients themselves, for all services the physicians ordered. Each test, shot, examination, and procedure generated a separate charge. There were no controls or incentives to order only those tests that were necessary to treat the patient, because the physician and hospital would get paid whether or not the test was necessary. Tests were also ordered to prevent litigation and to provide teaching opportunities. Medicare spending was increasing at a rate that outpaced inflation. Between 1980 and 1990, healthcare spending increased from approximately $247 billion to $699 billion—a 183% increase. The government needed a mechanism to control the increase in spending. The CMS looked to research being done on a patient classification system to assist in the endeavor.

Diagnostic Related Groups (DRGs)

Diagnostic Related Groups (DRGs) are a patient classification system initially developed to evaluate quality and resource consumption in a hospital setting. Patient data were collected and categorized into groups that consumed similar resources. In 1982, the Tax Equity and Fiscal Responsibility Act (TEFRA) stated that Medicare reimbursement would be based on DRGs, and in 1983, the Social Security Act was amended to include a DRG-based reimbursement system for all Medicare patients. This system is referred to as the **Prospective Payment System (PPS).** Under the PPS, hospitals would receive a set amount of reimbursement per patient discharge.

DRGs are used to reimburse hospital costs for Medicare inpatients only (Part A services). They are not used for physician services. As patients are discharged, the hospital provider assigns code numbers for the diagnoses and procedures relevant to that hospital admission using the International Classification of Diseases, 9th Revision, Clinical Modification (ICD-9-CM) classification system. These code numbers, along with certain patient demographic information are "grouped" via decision trees into a DRG specific to the patient's episode of care. There are currently more than 500 DRGs. The CMS assigns a weight to each DRG based on the severity of the diagnoses, type of procedure, number of laboratory and diagnostic tests, number and type of drugs prescribed, and presence of complications or co-morbid conditions.

Each hospital is assigned a specific rate by the CMS that has been calculated based on several factors: type of hospital (community versus teaching) setting (urban versus rural) and location (western United States versus northeast). These factors determine the **case mix** of the facility. The CMS weight multiplied by the hospital rate determines how much the hospital will be reimbursed for the care of patients who have been grouped to the DRG. See example (Table 12–1).

The hospital's rate does not vary greatly from year to year unless there has been a dramatic change in the case mix. The CMS weights are evaluated annually and modified based on changes in treatment. Additional DRGs have been added over the years to account for new diseases and updated treatment methodologies.

Using PPS, hospitals are now able to determine how much reimbursement they will receive for Medicare patients. If a hospital can treat a patient for less than the reimbursed amount, it will make a profit. If it costs more to treat the patient than the amount it receives, the hospital must absorb the cost. The patient cannot be billed for the excess cost.

Assume that we are evaluating two patients who have been categorized to DRG 126 from the preceding example (see Table 12–1). The reimbursement rate for a patient in this DRG at Community Hospital is $3,873. To determine if the hospital will make a profit or loss we compare the cost with the reimbursement rate.

Patient A
Cost: $3,500   3,873 – 3,500 = $373   *Profit*

Patient B
Cost: $4,000   3,873 – 4,000 = (-) $127   *Loss*

TABLE 12–1. Example of Using DRGs to Calculate a Hospital's Reimbursement

Community Hospital has a rate of $1500

DRG	Definition	CMS weight	Hospital's Reimbursement
126	Acute endocarditis	2.5820	$3,873
235	Fracture of femur	.7260	$1,089

It is now possible for hospitals to estimate the amount of reimbursement they would receive from Medicare. Historically, if they discharged 150 patients annually in DRG 126, they could estimate $580,950 worth of reimbursement. With this kind of information, hospitals can begin to evaluate all aspects of care to ensure all tests and drugs ordered were necessary, and to increase efficiencies in providing those services. Any nonessential services, or extended length of stay due to inefficiency, will cost the hospital money.

Resource Based Relative Value Scale (RBRVS)

While hospitals were dealing with DRGs and their impact, physician's finances were not affected directly because they were still reimbursed by payers on a fee-for-service basis. Physicians were responsible for ordering the laboratory tests and diagnostic procedures reimbursed to hospitals under PPS, but their services were reimbursed under a separate payment system. Once the DRG system was in place and operational, CMS turned its attention to physician services.

In 1985, the Consolidated Omnibus Budget Reconciliation Act (COBRA) mandated that Congress explore a new payment system for physician reimbursement and in 1992, CMS began implementation of a physician payment schedule using the *Resource Based Relative Value Scale (RBRVS)*. The program was fully operational by January 1996.

The RBRVS is used to reimburse physicians for their services under Part B of Medicare. Each patient visit receives a code number using the Current Procedural Terminology (CPT-4) or CMS Common Procedure Coding System (CCPCS). The code numbers are usually assigned by either a Health Information Management professional or a staff member trained in coding. Each code has three relative value units (RVUs) associated with it: work, practice expense or overhead, and malpractice expense. In addition, a geographic index is applied to each of these RVUs to account for cost differences based on locality (Table 12–2 and 12–3).

Each RVU is multiplied by the geographical practice cost index (GPCI) for each RVU to calculate an unconverted number. This unconverted total is then multiplied by a national conversion factor, determined annually by CMS, to establish the amount of reimbursement for the physician. The conversion factor, RVUs and geographical index are published in the *Federal Register* that can be located at *www.cms.gov*. The conversion factor for the year 2005 is $37.8975.

TABLE 12–2.   **Relative Value Units (RVUS) for Three Selected CPT Codes**

Relative Value Units

CPT Code	Description	Work RVU	Practice RVU	Malpractice RVU
88104	Cytopathology, fluids	0.56	0.68	0.03
88305	Tissue examination by pathologist	0.75	1.28	0.05
88319	Enzyme histochemistry	0.53	2.16	0.03

TABLE 12–3. Geographic Index by Relative Value Units (RVU) for Three Selected Localities

Geographic Index by RVU

Locality	Work GI	Practice GI	Malpractice GI
St. Louis	1.000	0.938	0.893
Los Angeles	1.056	1.139	0.955
Manhattan	1.094	1.351	1.586

GI, Geographical index.

The formula for calculating payment for a given CPT code is:

Payment = [(RVU work × GPCI work)
+(RVU practice expense × GPCI practice expense)
+(RVU malpractice × GPCI malpractice)] × CF.

Table 12–4 illustrates what the different payment rates would be for different localities.

As with the DRG system, physicians could look at historical data and determine what impact the RBRVS would have on their practice.

TABLE 12–4. Calculation of RBRVS Payment for Cytopathology, Fluid in Two Localities

Locality	CPT Code	RBRVS Calculation	Payment
St. Louis	88104	[(0.56*1.000) + (0.68*0.938) + (0.03*0.893)] * $37.8975	$46.24
Manhattan	88104	[(0.56*1.094) + (0.68*1.351) + (0.03*1.586)] * $37.8975	$59.88

Ambulatory Payment Categories (APCs)

As hospitals absorbed the impact of DRG-based reimbursement, certain procedures that had been done on an **inpatient** basis were moved to the **outpatient** setting. Improved technology and changes in practice protocols allowed this to happen without compromising the quality of care. Hospital-based outpatient care (including emergency room) was still being reimbursed on a fee-for-service basis and resulted in higher revenue for the facility. This was the next arena that CMS was to target to control expenditures. The Omnibus Budget Reconciliation Act (OBRA) of 1986 mandated that Congress investigate an outpatient prospective payment system, but it wasn't until the Balanced Budget Act of 1997 that CMS was mandated to implement an Outpatient Prospective Payment System (OPPS) using *Ambulatory Payment Categories (APCs).*

APCs are based on a combination of the CCPCS and the ICD-9-CM coding systems. Services performed during an outpatient or emergency room visit are

TABLE 12–5.   Calculation of APC Payment for Two Procedures

CPT/CCPCS	Description	APC	Weight	Payment Rate
88305	Tissue examination by pathologist	0343	0.43	$24.55
88319	Enzyme histochemistry	0342	0.21	$11.99

APC, Ambulatory Payment Category; *CPT,* Current Procedural Terminology; CCPCS, CMS Common Procedure Coding System

coded using the CCPCS/CPT-4 coding system. In addition, diagnoses are coded using the ICD-9-CM classification system to justify medical necessity for the treatments and laboratory tests ordered. Services that are similar clinically and in terms of resource consumption are then grouped into APCs. Laboratory tests have been grouped into certain levels based on time and supplies needed to run the tests. Unlike the inpatient DRG system, it is possible for one patient encounter to generate more than one APC. As with DRGs, CMS has assigned weights to each APC. This weight is then multiplied by a national conversion factor determined annually by CMS to calculate reimbursement for the hospital. The conversion factor for the calendar year 2005 is $57.10. (See Table 12–5)

Summary of Medicare Payment Systems

The federal government has adopted three payment methodologies (DRGs, RBRVS, APCs) to help control the rate of growth in healthcare expenditures. *DRGs* are used to pay hospitals for inpatient services. *RBRVS* is used to calculate payments to physicians for inpatient and outpatient visits or services. *APCs* are used to pay hospitals for outpatient services and emergency room care. CMS evaluates and adjusts the programs on a continual basis to ensure that they remain viable mechanisms for healthcare payment. Some private insurers have adapted these or similar payment systems for their beneficiaries.

PRIVATE INSURERS/MANAGED CARE REIMBURSMENT

Increasing healthcare costs were also affecting the private sector of health insurance. As seen in Figure 12–1, private insurance accounted for one third of the total healthcare dollar. The increase in healthcare costs and consumer demand for higher technology in treatment forced the private sector to evaluate their reimbursement methodologies. Increased premiums affected employers who were providing health insurance for employees. Employees were now expected to pay for an increased portion of the premium, a deductible, and a co-payment for healthcare. Individuals without employer-sponsored insurance found it very difficult and expensive to obtain health insurance. Private insurers began to take a greater interest in the type, amount, and cost of healthcare services being provided to their beneficiaries.

Managed care is a "means of providing health care services within a network of health care providers. The responsibility to manage and provide high quality and cost effective health care is delegated to this defined network of providers" (Samuels, 1996). Although there are different types of managed care plans, the common denominator is that the insured individual must see a physician who particpates in the managed care plan, or else they must pay a higher co-payment to obtain services outside the network. A health maintenance organization (HMO) is the most common type of managed care organization.

Types of Reimbursement

Managed care plans are reimbursed in several ways. The more common methodologies are described here. A managed care plan will typically use a combination of these methodologies.

Capitation   *Capitation* is a prospective payment agreement between an insurance plan and a provider. Under capitation, a physician is paid x dollars per member per month (PMPM). From this amount, the physician agrees to provide services to all of their patients covered by the plan. For example, assume Dr. Williams has 200 active patients who belong to Community HMO. She has agreed to a reimbursement rate of $20.00 PMPM. That means she will receive $4,000 per month or $48,000 per year to treat those 200 patients. Dr. Williams' contract may state that this amount includes outpatient care and any necessary diagnostic or therapeutic tests. Any office visit, laboratory test, or radiology study ordered for any of the 200 patients during the year will come from the $48,000. If Dr. Williams can see her patients and treat them for less than $48,000, then she makes a profit; but if she orders too many tests, or sees the patient too frequently, she may experience a loss of income by the end of the year.

Capitation can also be established for individual treatment areas. Insurance plans may contract separately with a laboratory to provide outpatient testing for plan members served by the laboratory. The laboratory supervisor may be called on to determine the PMPM payment rate the laboratory is willing to accept. Assume that a laboratory provides only three levels of tests. Based on the data in Table 12–6, the annual cost to the laboratory for these tests would be $105,900 as

TABLE 12–6. Sample Average Cost and Volume Data for Three Different Levels of Laboratory Testing

Level of Testing	Average Cost	Average Number of Tests Performed
Level I	$11 per test	3,000
Level II	$19 per test	2,100
Level III	$33 per test	1,000

TABLE 12–7. Example Calculation of Annual Cost and Per Member Per Month Cost

Level of Testing	Average Cost	Average Number of Tests Performed
Level I	$11.00 per test	3,000
Level II	$19.00 per test	2,100
Level III	$33.00 per test	1,000

Annual Cost per patient: $105,900 ÷ 2,000 = $52.95
Per Member Per Month: $52.95 ÷ 12 = $4.41

depicted in Table 12–7. If there were 2000 patients in the Community HMO, the laboratory would need to receive from the HMO a fee of at least $4.41 per member per month to cover their costs. If the laboratory performs less than the estimated number of tests, or can lower their unit cost, they can realize a profit on testing. If testing orders exceed estimation, the lab would be responsible to absorb the additonal costs.

Per Diem Inpatient care may be reimbursed on a *per diem* or per day basis. The hospital may negotiate, with the managed care program or other insurers, a set amount of reimbursement per day that the patient is in the hospital. Assume a hospital had 39,652 patient days during the year. The cost for treating these patients, including meals, laboratory tests, and ancillary services, was $5.7 million. The average cost per patient day is $144. The hospital will use the cost per day to negotiate the per diem rate. If the hospital can decrease the services provided without compromising the quality of care, or lower the unit cost of providing the care, it will have an increased profit.

Per Case Reimbursement on a *per case* basis is similar to the federal prospective payment systems. The cost for certain diagnoses or procedures that have a relatively similar treatment protocol can be determined. The provider and themanaged care plan or private insurer can then agree on a per case reimbursement rate for those specific diagnoses or procedures. This method may be used for physician reimbursement as well as hospital reimbursement.

Carve Out ("Carved Out") There may be some instances where certain types of care will be *"carved out"* of the set reimbursement amount. In the discussion under per diem, the contract may state $144 per diem *except* special care unit days (ICU, CCU, NICU, etc.). Those "carved out" days may have a separate per diem rate, or they may be reimbursed on a fee-for-service basis.

For laboratories, it may be critical to "carve out" certain tests from a prospective payment arrangement. Cytogenetic testing, molecular diagnostic assays, and esoteric testing sent to a reference laboratory all have significantly higher unit costs that cannot be covered by the usual PMPM negotiated rate.

SUMMARY

The federal government, managed care plans, and private insurers may use all of the reimbursement plans described in this chapter to provide healthcare coverage for their plan members. Hospitals, physicians, laboratories, and other ancillary departments must understand what their services actually cost to perform in order to negotiate appropriately with the insurers. These areas must also know the level of activity at which they are operating. Hospitals must know the number of patients, patient days, diagnoses, and procedures. Physicians must know the number of visits.

Laboratories must know how many and what types of tests they perform. They need to know how many and why duplicate tests are done. The reimbursement area of healthcare is complex and data driven. If the manager of a department cannot supply the information needed to adequately estimate costs, then that department is at risk of negotiating an arrangement that will not provide adequate reimbursement for their services.

SUGGESTED PROBLEM-BASED LEARNING ACTIVITIES
Chapter 12: Healthcare Reimbursement

Instructions: Use Internet resources, books, articles, colleagues, etc., to present solutions to the problems listed below. There is no one correct solution to any problem.

Note to Instructor: Students in class may be divided into groups and given the problem-based learning activity to discuss and solve. Once the group has reached a consensus as to a solution, the group may present it to the other students in the class. This activity will provide all students with information regarding solutions to the problem.

Problem #1
Research the history of laboratory reimbursement from Medicare and Medicaid services. Itemize and discuss relevant issues.

Problem #2
What problems are generated with DRG reimbursement?

Problem #3
Suppose your institution is providing glucose and occult blood point-of-care testing. Explain how you will charge for this service and why.

BIBLIOGRAPHY

Bersch C. Med tech of all trades; master of many. Medical Laboratory Observer. 2005, June. 24(4).

Burns L: *The Business of Healthcare Innovation.* Cambridge University Press, New York, NY., 2005.

Casto A, Layman E: *Principles of Healthcare Reimbursement.* AHIMA. Chicago, IL., 2006.

DRG Diagnosis Related Groups-Definitions Manual. 3-M Health Information Systems, 1999, p 1.

Elevitch F: Impact of managed care on laboratory economics. *Lab Medicine* 1998; 29:747–52.

Gallagher P (ed): *Medicare RBRVS: The Physician's Guide.* American Medical Association, Chicago, IL., 2000, pp 4–10.

Gapenski L: *Cases in Healthcare Finance,* 3rd ed. Health Administration Press. 2005.

Levit KR et.al: National health expenditures, 1994. *Health Care Financing Review* 1996; 19:220.

Nowinski M: *The Financial Management of Hospitals and Healthcare Organizations.* American College of Healthcare Executives. Chicago, IL., 2004.

Rowell J, Green M: *Understanding Health Insurance: A Guide to Professional Billing.* Delmar Learning. Clifton Park, NY. 2004.

Samuels DI: *Capitation: New Opportunities in Healthcare Delivery,* McGraw Hill Companies, Boston, MA., 1996, pp 20–1.

Shi L, Singh D: *Delivering Health Care in America: A Systems Approach,* 3rd ed. Jones and Barlett Publishers. Sudbury, MA., 2003.

Shi L, Singh DA: *Delivering Health Care in America,* Aspen Publication, Gaithersburg, MD., 1998, pp 178-9; 185–7.

Sultz H A, Young KM: *Health Care USA-Understanding its Organization and Delivery,* 2nd ed. Aspen Publication, Gaithersburg, MD., 1999, pp 209-11.

INTERNET RESOURCES

National Health Care By Type Of Expenditure, 2001
www.cms.hhs.gov/researchers/ pubs/datacompendium/2003/03pg12.pdf

National Health Care Source Of Funds, Selected Calendar Years 1965- 2001.
www.cms.hhs.gov/researchers/pubs/datacompendium/2003/03pg15.pdf

RBRVS Conversion Factor and Payment Schedule, 2005.
www.ama-assn.org/ama/pub/category/3232.html

Personal Health Care Payment Source, Selected Calendar Years 1965-2001.
www.cms.hhs.gov/researchers/pubs/datacompendium/2003/03pg16.pdf

RBRVS Geographic Indexes
www.mgma.com/research/gpci.cfm

Hospital Outpatient Prospective Payment System, 2005
www.cms.hhs.gov/providers/hopps/2005fc/1427fc.asp

OECD – (Organization for Economic Cooperation and Development)
http://www.oecd.org/dataoecd/44/18/35044277.xls

Today's healthcare environment demands attention to operation details by laboratory managers. The reasons for this are many and include the following:

- There are more compliance and regulatory issues.
- Creative workflow and staffing have resulted from an administrative mindset that laboratories must work more and better with less (the current staffing shortage affects these issues even more).
- Information technology is the wave of today as well as of the future.
- Laboratories must now market themselves to customers (such as private physician practices and clinics) that once barely existed.

Section IV of this text covers four important aspects of laboratory operations: compliance issues, process design, computer-based laboratory information systems, and marketing concepts. An introduction to the concepts as well as tips on ways to address the various issues are included. These chapters are designed to equip learners with a knowledge base, tools, and tips necessary to tackle managerial operations situations.

Section IV Contents:

Compliance Issues— The Regulations

SHARON S. EHRMEYER, PhD, MT(ASCP)
RONALD H. LAESSIG, PhD

Chapter Outline

OBJECTIVES

Following successful completion of this chapter, the learner will be able to:

1. In the framework of CLIA'88, discuss the concepts of:
   a. site neutrality
   b. certification
   c. test complexity categories
   d. proficiency testing
   e. quality systems for nonwaived testing
2. Compare and contrast CLIA, COLA, JCAHO, and CAP testing requirements for waived and nonwaived testing.
3. Formulate strategies for meeting the regulations that are applicable to his or her healthcare organization.
4. Describe the OSHA requirements in terms of laboratory testing.
5. Discuss the laboratory requirements for meeting the HIPAA legislation.

Key terms

Centers for Medicare
 and Medicaid Services (CMS)
Clinical Laboratory Improvement
 Amendments of 1988 (CLIA'88)
OSHA's Standard Precautions
Patient Test Management (PTM)

Proficiency Testing (PT)
Provider-Performed Microscopy
 (PPM) Certificate
Compliance Registration Certificate
Waiver Certificate

Case Study: Compliance Issues—The Regulations

You are a supervisory level, clinical laboratory scientist (10 years of experience) in a 300+ bed, Joint Commission on Accreditation of Healthcare Organizations (JCAHO) accredited hospital. The laboratory director informs you that the organization's administrator has asked the laboratory to assess the institution's overall approach to meeting its regulatory responsibilities including point-of-care testing (POCT). In addition to the main laboratory testing, POCT is performed on inpatients, outpatients, at off-site clinics, and through outreach (e.g., visiting nurses). The laboratory director asks you to assume the overall responsibility for this reevaluation.

Issues and Questions to Consider

1. *What regulations govern point-of-care testing?*
2. *What type of quality control for point-of-care testing must be implemented?*
3. *What kind of complexity testing does point-of-care fall under?*
4. *What kind of tests does point-of-care testing offer?*

5. *What is the benefit of point-of-care testing?*
6. *Who is allowed to perform point-of-care testing? What type of training is required?*

INTRODUCTION

This chapter explores the regulations by which laboratory testing including point-of-care testing (POCT) is performed. Central to this discussion is the Clinical Laboratory Improvement Amendments of 1988, referred to as CLIA'88 or just CLIA. CLIA is a federal mandate that identifies laboratory testing standards and supersedes the requirements outlined in the Clinical Laboratory Improvement Act of 1967. This chapter describes this CLIA mandate, discusses the CLIA certificates, and provides an overview of the actual regulations to provide the learner with information that will be of great benefit in the clinical laboratory and POCT setting. Voluntary accreditation, through professional organizations is a means by which laboratories prove that *the entire* CLIA laboratory standards are being met, is also described. Three well-known and respected accrediting organizations are profiled. The regulations related to safety, that is, the Occupation Safety and Health Administration (OSHA) requirements also are discussed along with the protection of patient medical information by the Health Insurance Portability and Accountability Act (HIPAA).

Due to the nature of this chapter, numerous terms that have abbreviations are used. To assist the learner in familiarizing him or herself with these terms, in addition to serving as an easy reference, an alphabetized listing of these abbreviations and their meanings is located in Appendix A at the end of the chapter.

THE CLINICAL LABORATORY IMPROVEMENT AMENDMENTS OF 1988 (CLIA'88)

Definition

All laboratory testing is regulated by the *Clinical Laboratory Improvement Amendments of 1988 (CLIA)* (Public Law, 1988). Because of real and perceived problems in test quality, primarily with cholesterol testing and Pap smear evaluation, Congress passed CLIA to establish quality standards for all laboratory testing to ensure accuracy, reliability, and timeliness of patient test results. CLIA is "test site neutral," meaning that the same regulations apply regardless of the location of testing. Every site examining "materials derived from the human body for the purpose of providing information for the diagnosis, prevention, or treatment of any disease. . ." is subject to CLIA (USDHHS, 1992).

CLIA was signed into law in 1988 by President Reagan and supercedes all former laboratory regulations (Public Law, 1988). The initial testing requirements to meet the intent of the law were published on February 28, 1992 in the *Federal Register* (USDHHS, 1992). The testing requirements are based on the complexity or difficulty to perform a test method. The three categories of tests methods are waived; moderate complexity, which includes the subcategory of provider performed microscopy (PPM) for clinicians and midlevel practitioners only; and high complexity. The most stringent requirements are for methods in the high complexity category. Although the 1992 CLIA regulations were called "final," the requirements have been modified and clarified; these modifications were published in a series of *Federal Registers*. The most up-to-date (codified) version of the CLIA requirements including all of the changes can be downloaded from the *Centers for Medicare and Medicaid Services (CMS)* website (see Internet resource list).

CMS with the Centers for Disease Control and Prevention (CDC) were charged originally with developing and promulgating the CLIA regulations. CMS continues to be responsible for registering laboratories for CLIA certificates, fee collection, on-site and self-inspection surveys, surveyor guidelines and training, for enforcement actions when needed, and approving proficiency testing providers, accrediting professional organizations, and exempting states. The Food and Drug Administration (FDA) categorizes test methods for complexity.

CLIA Certificates

All laboratory testing must be done under an appropriate CLIA certificate. Each certificate has a fee schedule, which is test complexity level and test volume dependent. As mentioned previously, CLIA regulations divide test methods into three categories: waived, moderate complexity, and high complexity. However, if a site develops its own test procedure or chooses to modify an existing FDA-approved procedure, which includes not following the manufacturer's directions, the test automatically falls into the high complexity category and is subject to CLIA's most stringent requirements.

Depending on the test complexity, laboratories will receive one of the following CLIA certificates: (1) *waiver,* which permits a site to perform only those tests methods identified as waived; (2) *provider-performed microscopy (PPM)* a certificate issued to a laboratory for physicians, midlevel practitioners, or dentists to perform PPM procedures or those tests on specimens collected during a physical examination and waived tests; or (3) *registration,* a certificate issued to enable laboratories to conduct waived, moderate, and/or high complexity laboratory testing. Once the laboratory is judged to be in compliance with the requirements through inspection, a permanent certificate of **compliance** is issued to those laboratories inspected by an agent of CMS or a certificate of **accreditation** is issued to laboratories seeking accreditation by a CMS-deemed professional organization. As of April 2005, approximately 190,000 CLIA certificates had been issued. Information on applying for a CLIA certificate (the CMS 116 form) along with associated certificate fees is available on CMS's web site (see Internet resource list).

Overview of **CLIA** Regulations

Waived Testing

The CLIA Law (Public Law, 1988) specifies that laboratory requirements are to be based on complexity of the test method performed and established provisions for categorizing a test as waived, which are test methods waived from regulatory oversight provided they meet certain requirements established by the statute. CLIA defines waived as "tests cleared by the FDA for home use" (patients can purchase the product over the counter) and "tests using such simple and accurate methodologies that the likelihood of erroneous results is negligible." In 1992 when the requirements for meeting CLIA were first published in the *Federal Register*, only simple and foolproof methods for eight analytes were waived: dipstick/tablet reagent urinalysis (visually read), fecal occult blood, visual urine pregnancy and ovulation tests, nonautomated erythrocyte sedimentation rate, blood glucose by monitoring devices cleared by FDA for home use, hemoglobin by copper sulfate, and spun hematocrit (USDHHS, 1992). In November 1997, Congress revised the CLIA waiver provisions (see FDA website in reference list). Under the current process, waiver may be granted to (1) any test listed in the regulation, (2) any test system that the manufacturer or producer applies for waiver in which the test meets the statutory criteria and the manufacturer provides scientifically valid data verifying that the waiver criteria have been met, and (3) test systems cleared by the FDA for home use. Further revisions to the CLIA waiver provisions are anticipated. Currently, the number of analytes on the waived list has expanded by 10-fold and includes hundreds of methodologies to test these analytes. The categories for all test methods are available on CMS's web site (see CMS website). Reagent and instrument manufacturers also have current information on the classification of their products.

For sites using test methods classified as waived, CLIA has no specific personnel or quality control requirements other than to follow the manufacturers' directions. CMS inspectors responsible for determining adherence to CLIA regulations will not inspect waived testing unless a specific complaint has been lodged or fraudulent activities are suspected.

Moderate and High Complexity Testing

Each specific laboratory test system or methodology is graded for level of complexity by assigning scores of 1, 2, or 3 to each of seven criteria shown in Table 13–1. These criteria are considered key elements important in performing a test correctly (FDA website). A score of 1 indicates the lowest level of complexity (waived testing), and a score of 3 is the highest level **(high complexity testing).** For the seven criteria, test systems receiving a total score of 12 or less are categorized as **moderate complexity.** Methods receiving scores above 12 are categorized as high complexity. Of the test systems currently being marketed, more than one-half are classified as moderate complexity and the remaining, excluding

TABLE 13–1.   Seven criteria used to evaluate test method complexity

1.	Knowledge
2.	Training and experience
3.	Reagent and material preparation
4.	Characteristics of operational steps
5.	Calibration, quality control, and proficiency testing materials
6.	Test system troubleshooting
7.	Interpretation and judgment

those in the waived category, are highly complex. CLIA requirements, as well as those of accrediting agencies, vary with test complexity.

Personnel   For sites performing moderate complexity testing, individuals with the proper qualifications must be identified for the positions of director, technical consultant, clinical consultant, and testing personnel. The director, as listed on the CLIA certificate, can range from a physician to an individual with a bachelor's degree in medical technology/clinical laboratory science or a degree in chemical, physical or biological science and having two years of laboratory training/experience and two years of laboratory supervisory experience. The director is responsible for all aspects of laboratory operation and administration. Although the director may delegate the duties to qualified individuals, the director is ultimately responsible for ensuring that all duties are properly performed. When the director is a physician, she or he typically also serves as the clinical consultant or as the liaison between the patient and clinician. The laboratory must employ one or more individuals who are qualified by education and either training or experience to provide technical consultation for each of the specialties and subspecialties of service in which the laboratory performs moderate complexity tests or procedures. The technical consultant establishes the quality standards of the laboratory through selecting and monitoring the laboratory's methods/instrumentation and evaluating and documenting the competency of the personnel. Qualifications for the technical consultant range from a clinician to an individual possessing a bachelor's degree in chemical, physical, biological, or medical technology/clinical laboratory science and one year of laboratory training or experience in the designated specialty of responsibility. The clinical consultant must be a clinician or have a doctorate in chemical, physical, biological, or medical technology/clinical laboratory science and serve as the liaison between the laboratory and its customers. This individual must be qualified to consult with clinicians and patients and give opinions concerning the diagnosis, treatment, and management of patient care. Testing personnel are responsible for specimen processing, test performance, and reporting test results. Minimum requirements for testing personnel include a high school education or equivalent plus appropriate, director-approved training and continued (at least yearly) competency assessment.

For sites performing high complexity testing, individuals with the proper qualifications must be identified for five positions: director, technical supervisor, clinical consultant, general supervisor, and testing personnel. As with moderate complexity testing, the director is responsible for the overall operation and administration of the laboratory. In addition to laboratory training or experience, to qualify as a director, an individual must be a licensed doctor of medicine, osteopathy, or podiatry; have a doctorate in chemical, physical, biological, or medical technology/clinical laboratory science and for those hired after February 24, 2003 be certified by a board approved by Health and Human Services (HHS); or have qualified as a director on or before February 28, 1992. The technical supervisor establishes the quality standards of the laboratory by selecting and monitoring methods and instrumentation and evaluating and documenting the competency of its personnel at least once per year after the first year of employment. The qualifications for this position range from a clinician to an individual possessing a bachelor's degree in medical technology/clinical laboratory science or chemical, physical, or biological science plus specified training and/or experience. The role and qualifications of the clinical consultant are the same as that for moderate complexity testing. The general supervisor provides day-to-day supervision of testing personnel and reporting of results. Requirements range from individuals who qualify as a clinician to persons possessing an associate degree in a laboratory science or medical laboratory technology and two years of laboratory training and experience. Also personnel who have served or would be qualified to serve as a general supervisor on or before February 28, 1992 can fill this position. Testing personnel performing high complexity testing must have an associate degree in laboratory science or medical laboratory technology or education and training equivalent to an associate degree (USDHHS, 2003).

Proficiency Testing   Under CLIA, regulatory *proficiency testing (PT)* plays a key role in assessing the internal quality for CLIA-regulated analytes in test sites performing moderate and/or high complexity testing. Successful participation in PT is a requirement for maintaining the CLIA certificate of compliance. All laboratories must be enrolled in a CMS-approved PT program for at least the CLIA-specified regulated analytes tested (see CMS website). CLIA requirements identify the minimum performance limits for passing each analyte in the three PT events that occur yearly and mandates that PT samples be treated, as much as possible, like patient specimens. Testing sites failing the same analyte in two of three consecutive PT events can be subject to sanctions ranging from being required to submit a plan of correction to mandatory suspension of testing for the failed analyte. However, CMS now views PT less punitive and more educational and has indicated that its intent is not to revoke CLIA certificates, except in cases of clear danger to patients.

Quality Systems for Nonwaived Testing   On January 24, 2003, CMS published the latest "final" rule to CLIA (USDHHS, 2003), which includes a revised Subpart K, Quality Systems for Nonwaived testing. The specified requirements are for all nonwaived testing, meaning that it is applicable to both the moderate and high complexity test categories. This revised section consolidates quality requirements found in multiple sections of the February 28, 1992 version of the CLIA regulations. It is organized to follow the path of patient specimens through the testing process: preanalytical, analytical, and postanalytical. The preanalytical requirements specify the information needed on each test request and the policies and procedures that must be in place for specimen submission, handling and referral. CLIA is concerned with maintaining sample integrity and positive patient identification throughout the testing process. The analytical requirements address the procedure manual, all components associated with a particular test system/instrument, verification of methods performance specifications before routine implementation, maintenance and function checks, calibration and calibration verification, and quality control procedures. This section also includes additional requirements for specialty testing such as bacteriology and immunohematology. Postanalytical requirements include the systems that need to be in place to ensure accurate, reliable and timely reported patient data along with the needed information on the test report.

The requirements for each of the three phases of testing have identical quality assessment and continuous quality improvement mandates. Section '493.1200 states: *establish and maintain written policies and procedures that implement and monitor quality systems for all phases of the total testing process meaning the preanalytical, analytical, and postanalytical phases of the testing process* [and, as part of this ('493.1200(b)] *each of the laboratory's quality systems must include an assessment component that ensures continuous improvement of the laboratory's performance and services through ongoing monitoring that identifies, evaluates and resolves problems.* (USDHHS, 2003).

Procedure Manual   Failure to follow manufacturers' directions (procedures) is the number one deficiency identified by inspectors for CLIA compliance. As a consequence, high quality "standard operating procedures" or SOPs are essential. Procedures, in written or in electronic form, must be available to all testing personnel for all tests performed. The necessary elements of the manual that need to be included are detailed in section §493.1251 of the January 24, 2003 *Federal Register* (USDHHS, 2003). All procedures for nonwaived testing must at least include written policies and procedures for patient preparation, specimen collection, labeling, preservation, transportation, referral, specimen acceptability and rejection; step-by-step performance of the procedure; instrument calibration and calibration verification; reportable range; quality control and corrective actions; limitations to the methodology; reference intervals; panic values; literature references; reporting of patient results; and course of action when a test system becomes inoperable.

Manufacturers' product inserts or operator manuals may be used to partially meet this requirement, however, additional information specific to the laboratory must be included. Initially, the procedures must be approved, signed, and dated by the laboratory director. Any changes to the procedures or changes in directorship require reapproval by the current director.

Method Verification of Performance Specifications   Method verification for nonwaived test methods means collecting data that document the method's performance in the test site and enable the site to make decisions on how to manage the method. The performance characteristics that need to be evaluated include accuracy, precision, reportable range, and verification that the manufacturer's reference intervals are appropriate for the test site's clientele. Sites can use the manufacturer's reference ranges as long as the director determines that these are suitable for the testing site's clientele. Test sites developing their own methods or modifying FDA-approved test systems must also determine, in addition to the above, analytical sensitivity and specificity, appropriate reference ranges, and any other performance characteristics required for test performance.

Quality Control   Section §493.1256 (USDHHS, 2003) specifically describes a series of quality control procedures for nonwaived testing. The section begins with the following statement: *"For each test system, the laboratory is responsible for having control procedures that monitor the accuracy and precision of the complete analytical process."* This section describes what the control procedures must do—detect immediate errors that occur due to test system failure, adverse environmental conditions, and operator performance; and (2) monitor over time the accuracy and precision of test performance that may be influenced by changes in test system performance and environmental conditions, and variance in operator performance. Section §493.1256(d) goes on to break new ground by stating: Unless the Centers for Medicare and Medicaid Services approves a procedure, specified in Appendix C of the 2004 State Operations Manual (see CMS website), that provides "equivalent quality" testing, the test site must perform the control procedures identified. However, as laboratory professionals gained a better understanding of equivalent quality testing or control (EQC), the concept has become controversial. CMS currently (2005) is rethinking the concept and will not cite laboratories in noncompliance with this requirement.

Inspection   CLIA requires those sites performing nonwaived testing (moderate and high complexity tests) to be inspected every two years for compliance to the regulations. CMS assesses a fee for this process. (USDHHS, 2003). While these inspections now are announced, they may become unannounced in the future.

VOLUNTARY ACCREDITATION

CLIA regulations allow CMS to approve nonprofit, professional organizations having laboratory testing and inspection standards that are essentially equivalent to, or more stringent than, those of CLIA (USDHHS, 1992). Testing sites may voluntarily choose to be accredited by such a deemed organization and pay the required fees, which are in addition to the ongoing CLIA fees. In 2005, approximately 190,000 testing sites received CLIA certificates (CMS website); 8% of these are accredited and inspected by deemed organizations. The three principal organizations are the JCAHO, the Laboratory Accreditation Program of the College of American Pathologists (LAP-CAP), and COLA (formerly the Commission on Office Laboratory Accreditation). When these sites meet the accrediting agency's requirements, as assessed through inspection every two years, the test site is, in essence, meeting CLIA requirements. CMS, however, has the right to reinspect up to 5% of testing sites accredited by deemed organizations.

While each aforementioned deemed organization has a slightly different focus to laboratory inspection, each of the accreditation practices must be fully compliant with the CLIA regulations. The choice of accrediting organization is left entirely to the laboratory.

Joint Commission on Accreditation of Healthcare Organizations (JCAHO)

The Joint Commission on Accreditation of Healthcare Organizations (JCAHO) is a voluntary organization that accredits more than 80% of US healthcare organizations (see JCAHO website). Test sites in a JCAHO accredited institution need to adhere, at a minimum, to current standards identified in the JCAHO Comprehensive Accreditation Manual for Laboratory and Point-of-Care Testing (CAMLAB, 2005–2006). These testing standards focus on quality improvement and are designed to promote quality outcomes. Inspection for *compliance* is conducted every two years by inspectors hired and trained by JCAHO. JCAHO charges additional fees for this process.

JCAHO recognizes the test categories including waived test (WT) methods as defined by CLIA, but unlike CLIA, JCAHO has specific requirements, including personnel training criteria, and inspects waived testing. The six WT standards are shown in Table 13–2.

Before a waived test methodology is placed into routine use, JCAHO requires documented evidence (accuracy and precision data, reportable range, and appropriate reference range) that the method is adequately meeting the needs of the site's clientele. If a test (same method, model) is initiated in a new location, the method's performance history is sufficient evidence. JCAHO does not require participation in a CMS-approved PT program for waived testing. More quality testing requirements are identified in Table 13–3.

TABLE 13–2. JCAHO Waived Testing (WT) Standard Requirements

WT Standard	Testing Requirement
1.10	The organization establishes policies and procedures that define the context in which waived test results are used in patient care, treatment, and services
1.20	The organization identifies the staff responsible for performing and supervising waived testing
1.30	Staff performing tests have adequate, specific training and orientation to perform the tests, and demonstrate satisfactory levels of competence
1.40	Approved policies and procedures governing specific testing-related processes are current and readily available
1.50	QC checks, as defined by the organization, are conducted on each procedure
1.60	Appropriate quality control and test records are maintained

Laboratory Accreditation Program of the College of American Pathologists (LAP-CAP)

The Laboratory Accreditation Program of the College of American Pathologists (LAP-CAP) accredits only laboratory testing sites and not the entire healthcare organization (see CAP website). LAP-CAP does not base its requirements on the different CLIA complexity levels of testing; instead its philosophy is "that all clinical laboratory testing needs to adhere to the same requirements" and all testing is inspected. LAP-CAP spells out it its requirements in a series of specialty-related checklists. All test sites must follow the Laboratory General Checklist (GEN) and then the specific checklists appropriate to the specialty of testing (Checklists, 2004–2005).

For high complexity testing, CAP accredited test sites must identify a director, clinical consultant, technical supervisor, general supervisor, and testing personnel. The qualifications are identified in CLIA, section §493.1441–1495, for high complexity testing. The director, as listed on the CLIA certificate, needs to be a physician (preferably a pathologist) or a doctoral scientist with appropriate experience. When test sites cannot find qualified testing personnel, LAP-CAP will allow less qualified personnel to perform tests as long as they meet the CLIA personnel requirements identified for the specific complexity classification of testing and have appropriate "general" supervision (Checklists, 2004). For example, there are no specific educational requirements for personnel performing waived tests under CLIA.

Proficiency testing has long been an important component of LAP-CAP inspection philosophy. CAP-accredited sites must participate in PT (when available) through CAP surveys or other CAP-approved PT surveys for each analyte tested. This includes POCT sites.

LAP-CAP, like JCAHO, emphasizes an overall total quality management approach and continuous quality improvement for the entire analytical process, including management of pre-analytical, analytical and postanalytical errors.

CAP inspections are intended to be educational and are unique in that they are conducted by a trained team of "peer" laboratory professionals. More quality testing requirements are identified in Table 13–3.

TABLE 13–3. Comparison of Testing Requirements (CLIA, JCAHO, LAP-CAP, COLA)

Requirement	CLIA (CMS) Compliance	COLA Accreditation	JCAHO Accreditation	LAP-CAP Accreditation
Waived Testing (WT)	Follow all manufacturers' directions; no inspection unless complaint is issued	Same as for CLIA	Follow WT standards in JCAHO CAMLAB Manual; waived testing is inspected	Considers only one level of testing. Follow standards in Checklists, e.g., POC and GEN; all testing is inspected
QC for waived testing	Follow all manufacturers' directions	Same as for CLIA	Follow manufacturers' directions; if none, develop own system. At least 2 levels/day/procedures	Yes, follow requirements in CAP checklists appropriate for test performed
PT for waived testing	no	no	no	yes
Personnel requirements for waived testing	no	no	Testing personnel identified, orientation to testing performed and on-going competency assessment	Testing personnel identified, orientation to testing performed and on-going competency assessment
Quality Control for Nonwaived (moderate and high complexity) testing	Follow section §493.1256 in codified Federal Register for most analytes and §493.1261,.1267, .1269 and .1254 for some analytes in microbiology, chemistry, hematology/ and coagulation	Same as for CLIA	Follow appropriate QC standards in JCAHO CAMLAB Manual	Follow appropriate QC standards in CAP checklists

Accepts manufacturer's internal/ procedural controls to fulfill QC requirements Nonwaived testing	Yes, 2-year educational survey to meet new QC requirements will be extended indefinitely until concerns with "equivalency" qualifying options have been resolved	yes	Yes, with verification of manufacturer's claims and periodic method assessment with liquid controls	Yes, with verification of manufacturer's claims and periodic method assessment with liquid controls
Regulatory PT for nonwaived testing	Regulatory PT for CLIA regulated analytes only (for each CLIA certificate). Follow §493.901-941 in codified Federal Register	Same as for CLIA	Same as for CLIA	For all analytes tested, if PT program is available
Testing personnel— moderate complexity testing	Follow §493.1425 in codified Federal Register, including training/ competency assessments. Staffing of four positions— director, technical and clinical consultants and testing personnel are required.	Same as for CLIA	Same as for CLIA	Same as CLIA, however, a pathologist is preferred as the director. At a minimum, follow CAP Checklist GEN .54750 for testing personnel.

(continued)

TABLE 13–3. Comparison of Testing Requirements (CLIA, JCAHO, LAP-CAP, COLA) (Continued)

Requirement	CLIA (CMS) Compliance	COLA Accreditation	JCAHO Accreditation	LAP-CAP Accreditation
Testing personnel—high complexity testing	Follow §493.1487 in codified Federal Register, including training/competency assessments. Staffing of five positions—director, technical and general supervisor, clinical consultant and testing personnel are required.	Same as for CLIA	Same as for CLIA	Same as CLIA, however, a pathologist is preferred as the director.
Ongoing assessment of reportable range (every 6 months) for Nonwaived testing	yes, in codified Federal Register §493.1255(b)(3) (accomplished through calibration if use ≥ 3 calibrators or the calibration verification process)	Same as for CLIA	Same as for CLIA	Same as for CLIA. Clinical reportable range is a one time activity performed with the initial performance verification
Method correlations (at least every 6 months)	Between all methods, instruments, sites under same CLIA certificate	Same as for CLIA	Same as for CLIA except across entire healthcare organization (testing may be done under more than one CLIA certificate)	Same as for CLIA
Accuracy assessment (at least every 6 months)	Yes, all analytes. Proficiency testing is one means to accomplish this assessment	Same as for CLIA	Same as for CLIA	Same as for CLIA

COLA

COLA, formerly the Commission of Office Laboratory Accreditation, initially focused on accrediting physician office laboratories (COLA website; Laboratory Accreditation Manual, 2005). Today COLA accredits many other types of test sites including those in small hospitals. COLA's philosophy is one of education and problem solving. Inspectors usually are medical technologists/clinical laboratory scientists who are prepared to assist test sites in meeting the regulations and generating quality test results. To prepare for the accreditation process, COLA provides sites with an initial, preinspection (self-inspection) checklist. The COLA inspector then uses this same checklist during the on-site inspection. COLA's requirements essentially follow the CLIA regulations. COLA does not inspect sites performing only waived testing. More quality testing requirements are identified in Table 13–1.

OCCUPATIONAL SAFETY AND HEALTH ADMINISTRATION (OSHA) REQUIREMENTS

In addition to the CLIA regulations and requirements from the various organizations (JCAHO, LAP-CAP, and COLA), the U.S. Department of Labor, under the **Occupational Safety and Health Administration (OSHA),** is responsible for regulations relating to general workplace safety and protecting the health of US workers. These regulations are most commonly known as the "OSHA Bloodborne Pathogens Standard 1910.1030." In general the handling of biological specimens, fall under the part of the OSHA regulations addressing "Universal Precautions." They require that all blood, body fluids, tissue and other potentially infectious materials be treated as equally hazardous. OSHA regulations require facilities to devise an exposure control plan for blood-borne pathogens that is updated annually. Facilities must have in place a classification system for each job based on the level of exposure to blood-borne pathogens. In addition, the facility must develop and implement procedures that are in compliance with OSHA regulations to protect workers and that minimize the risk of exposure. Employees must be informed of the occupational hazards, provided with personal protective equipment (such as goggles, masks, gloves, gowns, and laboratory coats), and monitored to ensure compliance with safety procedures. Employees at risk for exposure must receive employer-financed hepatitis B vaccinations unless they sign an affidavit stating that they refused the vaccine. Upon employment, employees must participate in an on-the-job training program that minimally covers the facility's exposure control plan, use of personal protective equipment, procedures to be followed in the event of exposure to a blood-borne pathogen, and the labeling system for biohazardous materials. The training program is repeated annually for all employees or more frequently whenever changes occur. OSHA inspectors may choose to make an unannounced inspection; they cannot (legally) be refused admittance to the workplace. An extended discussion of workplace safety requirements is beyond the scope of this chapter. The reader, unfamiliar with OSHA requirements, is referred to the agency's website *http://www.osha.gov/*.

HEALTH INSURANCE PORTABILITY AND ACCOUNTABILITY ACT [HIPAA]

The Health Insurance Portability and Accountability Act of 1996 (HIPAA), was the result of efforts by the Clinton Administration and healthcare reform proponents. The primary goal of this "health insurance focused" legislation was to make it easier to detect and prosecute fraud and abuse and enable workers of all professions, even those with pre-existing medical conditions, to change jobs without loss or interruption of health insurance protection. Safeguarding patient privacy, with respect to health related information was a paramount concern. As part of this legislation, HIPAA established new privacy rules for "covered entities" including laboratories, which took effect April 14, 2003. While not all information needs to be protected under HIPAA, most patient information is considered protected and is subject to HIPAA requirements For example laboratories must ensure confidentiality when transmitting health information electronically. This rule requires healthcare organizations (laboratory test sites are part of this), insurers and payers using any electronic means of storing patient data and performing claims submission to comply with the Final Rule for National Standards for Electronic Transactions.

The full scope of HIPAA related requirements is beyond this text. However, larger institutions are required to have a "HIPAA Privacy Officer" to provide information. The extensive **Standards for Privacy of Individually Identifiable Health Information** are designed to help guarantee privacy and confidentiality of patient medical records. Healthcare providers must be in HIPAA compliance, which means that staff need to be educated and trained and documentation for these activities available to demonstrate compliance with the HIPAA requirements. Staff also are subject to ongoing compliance monitoring and application of appropriate sanctions when necessary. For more details on HIPAA, the government has prepared a website: *http://www.cms.hhs.gov/hipaa/*

SUMMARY

Today's laboratories must meet multiple regulations, CLIA, HIPAA, OSHA and others. With CLIA, all laboratories are required to implement minimum standards to ensure quality laboratory test results that are available in a reasonable timeframe. Proof of meeting these standards, which may be achieved through a CLIA-deemed professional organization, is critical in providing high quality laboratory services to the healthcare community. Laboratory managers must be familiar with *all* regulations and constantly work toward ensuring that they are met at minimum and preferably at an exceeded level.

SUGGESTED PROBLEM-BASED LEARNING ACTIVITIES
Chapter 13: Compliance Issues—The Regulations

Instructions: Use Internet resources, books, articles, colleagues, etc., to present solutions to the problems listed below. There is no one correct solution to any problem.

Note to Instructor: Students in class may be divided into groups and given the problem-based learning activity to discuss and solve. Once the group has reached consensus as to a solution, the group may present it to the other students in the class. This activity will provide all students with information regarding solutions to the problem.

Problem #1

Suppose you are told that your laboratory will soon have a CAP/AABB/JCAHO inspection. As the laboratory supervisor, you must develop a plan to prepare for and initiate this process.

Note: AABB stands for the American Association of Blood Banks, an organization that issues standards for and blood bank practices, conducts inspections, and accredits blood bank laboratories.

Problem #2

Correlate your laboratory practices to the CLIA regulations for your type of operations.

Problem #3

Identify and explain the OSHA regulations that apply to your laboratory operations.

BIBLIOGRAPHY

Checklists. Laboratory Accreditation Program-College of American Pathologists (CAP) 2005, Northfield IL.

Comprehensive Accreditation Manual for Laboratory and Point of Care Testing. 2005–2006 Joint Commission on Accreditation of Healthcare Organizations (JCAHO), Oakbrook Terrace, IL.

Laboratory Accreditation Manual. COLA, Columbia, MD, 2005.

Public Law 100-578, Section 353 Publish Health Service Act (42 U.S.C. 263a) October 31, 1988.

U.S. Department of Health and Human Services: Medicare, Medicaid and CLIA programs: regulations implementing the Clinical Laboratory Improvement Amendments of 1988 (CLIA). Final rule. *Fed Reg* 1992; 57:7002–186.

APPENDIX A

List of Abbreviations and Their Meanings Pertinent to Compliance Issues— the Regulations

Abbreviation	Meaning
CAP	College of American Pathologists
CDC	Centers for Disease Control and Prevention
CLIA'88 (CLIA)	Clinical Laboratory Improvement Act of 1988
CMS	Centers for Medicare and Medicaid Services (formerly HCFA, the Health Care Finance Administration)
COLA	Formerly the Commission of Office Laboratory Accreditation
FDA	Food and Drug Administration
JCAHO	Joint Commission on Accreditation of Healthcare Organizations
LAP-CAP	The Laboratory Accreditation Program of the College of American Pathologists
OSHA	Occupational Safety and Health Administration
POCT	Point-Of-Care Testing
PPM	Provider-Performed Microscopy
PT	Proficiency Testing
PTM	Patient Test Management
QA	Quality Assurance
QC	Quality Control
WT	Waived Test

U.S. Department of Health and Human Services: Medicare, Medicaid and CLIA programs: Laboratory Requirements Relating to Quality Systems and Certain Personnel.

Qualifications; Final Rule. *Fed Reg* 2003; 68:3640–3714. Available at *http://www.phppo.cdc.gov/clia/docs/CMS-2226-F.htm*

U.S. Department of Health and Human Services: Medicare, Medicaid and CLIA programs: regulations implementing the Clinical Laboratory Improvement Amendments of 1988 (CLIA). Final rule. (codified 10–1–03 edition including all changes from 1992) Available at *http://www.phppo.cdc.gov/clia/pdf/42cfr493_2003.pdf*

Appendix C, Survey Procedures and Interpretive Guidelines for Laboratories and Laboratory Services. Available at *http://www.cms.gov/clia/appendc.asp*

Internet Resources

http://www.hcfa.gov/medicaid/clia/cliahome.htm
http://www.fda.gov/cdrh/clia/cliawaived.html
http://www.jcaho.org
http://www.cap.org

http://www.cola.org
http://www.osha.gov/
http://www.cms.hhs.gov
http://www.phppo.cdc.gov/clia/pdf/42cfr493_2003.pdf
http://www.cms.hhs.gov/hipaa/

Process Design— Workflow and Staffing

SANDRA S. BROWN, MBA, MT(ASCP)
KELLY L. MCLEAY, RN, MSN
DALE C. SCUTRO, BS, MT(AMT)

Chapter Outline

Objectives

Following successful completion of this chapter, the learner will be able to:

1. Explain the relationship between process design, workflow, and staffing.
2. Identify the factors that must be considered when developing a process design.
3. Construct a table that contains the three phases of workflow and discuss the components of each.

4. Define Process Management and identify various process improvement methodologies.
5. Compare and contrast the written application with the oral interview.
6. Develop a generic schedule using:
   a. 8/80 work rule
   b. 40 hour workweek rule
   c. Self-scheduling guidelines
7. Discuss the importance of retention in the workplace.

Key Terms

40-Hour Work Week Rule
8/80 Work Rule
Analytical Phase
Flowchart
FOCUS-PDSA
Postanalytical Phase
Preanalytical Phase

Process Management
Process Management Tools
Process Design
Self-scheduling
Six Sigma
Staffing
Workflow

Case Study: Process Design—Workflow and Staffing

You are the manager of a small to medium-sized city hospital laboratory. A small rural hospital within an hour's drive has decided to close its microbiology department and has asked if your facility can do the work for them. This would mean a 50% increase in the workload of your department. To determine if this is feasible a process design must be developed, and the workflow analyzed. Staffing must be reviewed and if needed additional employees hired, trained, and scheduled to work.

Issues and Questions to Consider

1. *What factors should be considered when developing a process design?*
2. *How does process design differ from and relate to workflow?*
3. *What are the three phases of workflow?*
4. *What is the purpose of the application and the interview in the hiring process?*
5. *What is the 8/80 work rule? The 40 hour workweek work rule?*
6. *How do the two work rules differ?*
7. *How is a generic schedule developed and what purpose does it serve?*

INTRODUCTION

Process Designs are broad overall plans used to develop and design a process or way of completing work or doing a task. Once the process design is developed **Workflow** can be analyzed. Workflow is the pathway the work follows from the beginning to the end of the task. **Staffing** is the hiring, training, scheduling, and retaining of the employee who will be doing the work or task. Each of these is interrelated and must be developed and studied if the work or task is to be successfully completed. Process designs can be complex or simple depending on the size of the task or the amount of work that needs to be done. In our case study, the addition of a 50% workload is large so it will be fairly elaborate; but it will cover all the thoughts, designs, and processes necessary for this to be a successful endeavor.

Process Management is a systematic data based approach to improving the performance of business. It is a method of continuously seeking improvement opportunities without sacrificing quality. And it is necessary to be successful in the dynamic environment of health care.

This chapter explores in detail how to develop a process design. Then using the process design it explores in-depth workflow, staffing, and the interrelationships of each. Process Management is introduced along with a variety of tools that can be used to improve processes.

To best illustrate the concepts in this chapter, the chapter case study is referred to and discussed throughout. Learners are thus encouraged to revisit the case along with the issues and questions to consider during study of this chapter.

PROCESS DESIGNS

Process designs are the broad plans or overall designs that are developed to provide a blueprint for completing work or a task. They are not unlike an outline in a textbook. To design a process you must know what work or task needs to be completed.

Many factors, which are discussed in the following paragraphs, influence every process design. Each must be identified, understood, and applied if the process design is to be successful. Moreover each factor is related to the other in such a manner that one by itself is not complete. In the laboratory the reliability (i.e., the accuracy and timeliness of test results), is only as good as the process design that produces that result. A process design may be large or small depending on the task, but all must (1) be cost effective; (2) be within organizational needs and budgets; (3) be customer friendly; and (4) produce quality results.

Sometimes to make the process easier to understand, it is helpful to draw a *flowchart* (Figure 14–1), which is a picture or diagram of a process. Flowcharts can be simple or complicated depending on the work or task that needs to be completed. The flowchart has been developed to present all possible factors that can influence a process design. It is global in nature, and not all factors on the chart are relevant to our case study but they may be applicable in other situations. Managers will choose those that work best in their setting. Eight global factors influence the process design, which are numbered 1 though 8 (see Figure 14–1). Each of these are "possibility lines," which in turn influence each of the factors. Process designs are influenced by the following factors:

1. *Size and setting of the laboratory or department:* Is it large or small? Is it in a hospital or is it off site? Is it a commercial or specialty laboratory? In our case study it is a small to medium-sized hospital department.

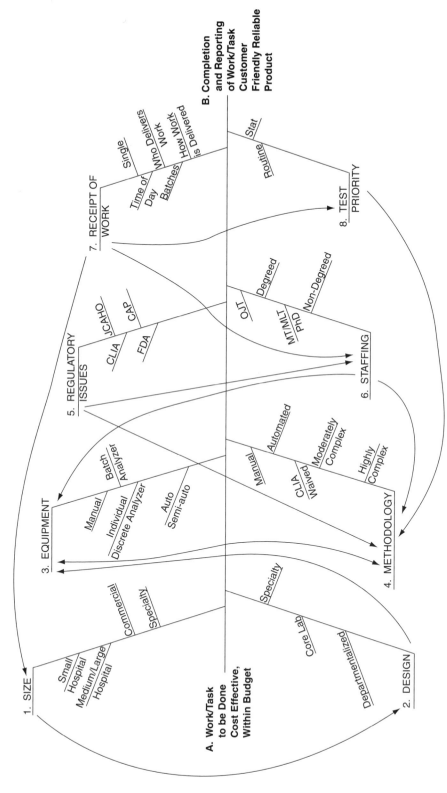

FIGURE 14–1 Flowchart of Process Design.

KEY: OJT, On job-trained; CLIA, Clinical Laboratory Improvement Act; FDA, Food and Drug Administration; JCAHO, Joint Commission on Accreditation of Hospital Organizations; CAP, College of American Pathologists; Auto, Automated; Semi-auto, Semi-automated.

2. *Design of the laboratory:* Is it centralized (all of it is located in one area of a building) or decentralized (parts are located throughout the building or even in different buildings)? Is it a core laboratory design (the routine or most commonly performed tests in the areas of hematology, chemistry, coagulation and urinalysis are grouped together in one area of the laboratory), or is it departmentalized (all tests in one discipline such as hematology are grouped into one area or department)? If it is a core laboratory design, nonsimilar tests, tasks, or instruments are grouped in such a way that one person can do many things. If it is departmentalized people will need to be assigned to each department. In the case study, microbiology is the department that will be affected. Microbiology is a specialized area of a laboratory and is usually separate because regulatory issues require that some of the work processes must be isolated from other work areas.

3. *Equipment:* What type of equipment is being used? Is it fully automated (it does most of the work with very little interaction from the employee), or is it semiautomated (it does some of the work and the employee does the rest manually)? Is it a batch analyzer (it does only one type of test at a time), or is it a discrete analyzer (it can process many different tests at the same time or in any order)? In our case study the microbiology department has a semiautomated piece of equipment that assists with culture processing.

4. *Test methodology:* Is the test performed manually or is it automated? Is it (Clinical Laboratory Improvement Act-CLIA waived or moderate/highly complex testing, see Chapter 13)? Most of the work in microbiology is considered highly complex under CLIA.

5. *Regulations:* Regulatory issues are complex and a laboratory must answer to many. CLIA, Joint Commission on Accreditation Healthcare Organizations (JCAHO), College of American Pathologists (CAP), Food and Drug Administration (FDA), state and local authorities may all apply depending on the process or testing method used. In our case study, the microbiology department has interactions with each of the organizations listed.

6. *Staffing.* How many and what type of employees are needed to do the work? Do they need to have a degree (PhD, MT, MLT), or no degree (technical assistant, phlebotomist or on-the-job trained)? What is the availability of each type? In our case study most of the work in microbiology must be done by someone with a degree in laboratory sciences.

7. *When/how will the work be received?* Will the work come one or two times during the day? Will it be received in off hours? Will it come in batches or one test at a time? Who delivers the specimens (i.e., laboratory or nonlaboratory personnel)? In our case study we will look at this issue under workflow and staffing.

8. *Test priority:* Is the test to be performed routinely or is it stat? If it is stat, can it be done immediately as that term implies? Most microbiology work can be collected stat but not performed immediately.

Developing a process design can be complex as seen by the flowchart. It may look confusing, but all the factors must be considered and they are interdependent. Work experience, and in some cases, additional education may be necessary to complete all the parts of a process design; therefore this chapter is limited to introducing the learner to basic concepts.

To return to the case study, you as the manager need to develop a process design for the 50% increase in work. To do this you must ask many questions and then try to answer them.

- What needs to be done?
- What costs are associated with increasing the workload, and is there a benefit to the organization if this work is done?
- How will the work get done, and will it affect the current workload?
- Will new equipment be needed?
- Will more staff be needed and at what level?
- Will the department need remodeling?
- When and how will the work get to the laboratory and then to the microbiology department?

After further examining Flowchart 1, *Process Designs*, it can be seen that each of these questions falls under one or more of the design influences (#1 – 8 on flowchart) as illustrated on the chart.

1. *What needs to be done?*

The answer may seem obvious—it must be the work. On the flowchart the A – B line represents this question. The question must consider not only the work but the kind of work. In the microbiology department cultures such as wounds are much more complex to process than a voided urine culture. In our case study the work that will need to be done is similar to that already being done in the department. There will just be more of it.

2. *What costs are associated with increasing the workload, and is there a benefit to the organization if this work is done?*

Remember that the work needs to be cost effective (best product for the lowest cost), within the budget (historical data usually provides this information such as cost/test and projected costs), timely (increased workload does not mean it takes longer to complete the work), customer friendly, and reliable (easily available and understood) (see Chapter 10).

3. *How will the work get done and will it affect the current workload?*

Adding a 50% increase to the current workload sounds like a lot of work, and it may be a burden to the existing processes. A burden on the department would exist if the staff is unable to perform the tests within acceptable time frames or incurs overtime in completing the work. On the flowchart, #3, #4, #5, and #6 represent this question. In our case study, the department has a semiautomated instrument that assists with culture processing. Everything else is done manually. All processes except culture setups are considered highly complex by CLIA. It must be determined if there is room for expansion i.e., will the department be able to do more work as it now stands. Also when referring to a 50% increase do not forget to express this as a number. Fifty percent may be only 2 cultures, or it may be 150 cultures per week. In the case study, the increase represents 75 cultures per week. The department with a current workload of 150 cultures per week is close to capacity with the existing processes. To handle the increased work, the processes will need to be changed. This may mean adding staff, getting new equipment, or remodeling the department to be more efficient. A combination of all three considerations will probably be needed, but until everything is studied the answer is uncertain.

4. *Will new equipment be needed?*

On the flowchart #3 represents this question. The department has a semiautomated piece of equipment that assists with processing cultures. It will be able to do the type of work projected in the increase because it is doing similar work now. It can also handle the extra capacity. It is not interfaced with the laboratory computer and can not be interfaced. Every result produced must be manually entered. With the workload nearly at capacity an automated piece of equipment should be considered. When considering new equipment, determine the age and value of the current instrument, the cost of purchasing the new instrument, the cost of operating both, and how much more work can the new piece do than the old. Also when choosing an instrument do not get the biggest and most expensive one on the market. Instead choose a reliable instrument with a throughput (number of tests completed in one hour) matched to the needs of the work. Another consideration is the ability of the new instrument to interface with the computer. This ability reduces the need for manual entry, which is often time consuming and fraught with clerical errors. This could also influence a staffing decision.

5. *Will more staff be needed and at what level?*

On the flowchart (Figure 14–1) #5 and #6 presents this question. In the case study it has been determined that with the current workload and present staff, the department is working at nearly full capacity. The type of work in microbiology requires it to be done or supervised by a person with a laboratory science degree. Some of the work could be done by an assistant such as setups, Gram staining, and ordering supplies. Would an employee at this level allow the technical staff more time to perform the rest of the work? An assistant's salary expense is less than that for technical staff, but there is less flexibility because the employee can not do all tasks within the department. A technical employee's salary expense is higher but this person can perform all tasks. The equipment decision will influence the type of employee needed. If a new instrument is obtained, the technical staff may be able to handle all the technical work quite well if the nontechnical work is not a responsibility. The availability of staff at the level needed must also be considered. A nontechnical employee will probably be easier to hire than a technical person because they are more easily obtainable. In the case study, it has been determined that the automated piece of equipment will be purchased and nontechnical staff will be added to the department. This decision was made after all costs and benefits were studied.

6. *Will the department need remodeling?*

On the flowchart, #2 (Figure 14–1) refers to this question. The physical layout should be efficient. Instruments or tasks should be grouped so that people can operate without either tripping over each other or having to do a lot of walking from one work station to another. They should also be grouped so that one employee may be able to do multiple tasks. In the case study, remodeling is also dependent on two other considerations, the new equipment's size and shape and/or whether a new work station will be created.

7. *When and how will the work get to the laboratory and then to microbiology?*
On the flowchart, #7 refers to this question. Will the work be received once a day or throughout the day, in batches or as single specimens? Will the work be brought to the hospital by a courier from the other hospital, or will our hospital send a courier to pick it up? There is a cost associated with the delivery whether their courier, ours or someone from the outside does the work. In addition to the cost of delivery, turnaround should be considered in this step. If the specimens are delivered only once a day this can add up to 24 hours to the turnaround time. This means if it would normally take 48 hours to report a result, it will now take 72 hours for a culture that is collected right after the courier has left. On the other hand, if every specimen is delivered as it is collected, this will add a significant cost to the process. A good compromise would be two deliveries a day, one in the morning and one late afternoon or early evening. Once the specimens are received who will deliver them to the department? Currently this is being done by nontechnical staff in a receiving area. Two deliveries a day will not add burden to the current workload, so this process will not change.

The preceding discussion shows that designing a process can be complicated. To make sure that everything is considered, it is helpful to produce a paper product similar to the flowchart in our illustration with everything being specific to the process that is being developed. It is a good guide for getting from point A to point B.

Workflow

Once the broad questions are identified and solutions are proposed, then setting up how the work transitions through the department—workflow—is the next step. The process design development is the overall plan or outline from which to work while workflow, although a part of the process design, is more detailed. Workflow (Figure 14–2) is the pathway the work follows from its beginning to its completion. Policies and procedures are developed at this stage.

Workflow can be divided into three phases: *preanalytical,* the *analytical* and *postanalytical* (Table 14–1). The preanalytical phase consists of everything that occurs before actual testing. It is collecting the right specimen at the right time and under the right set of circumstances. The analytical phase is the actual testing of the sample. The postanalytical phase consists of everything that needs to be done, including reporting the results, after all testing is complete. It ties everything together and finishes the whole process. Of the three phases the preanalytical is the hardest to control. The greatest number of errors occur in this phase because many more people are involved with it than in the other two. The people involved are more likely not to be laboratory employees. Communication and training are important if the right specimen is to be collected and delivered to the department at the right time. The analytical and postanalytical phases are much easier to control because they are performed by laboratory employees who are under the management of a laboratory supervisor or manager. Each of these workflow phases is further described in the following sections.

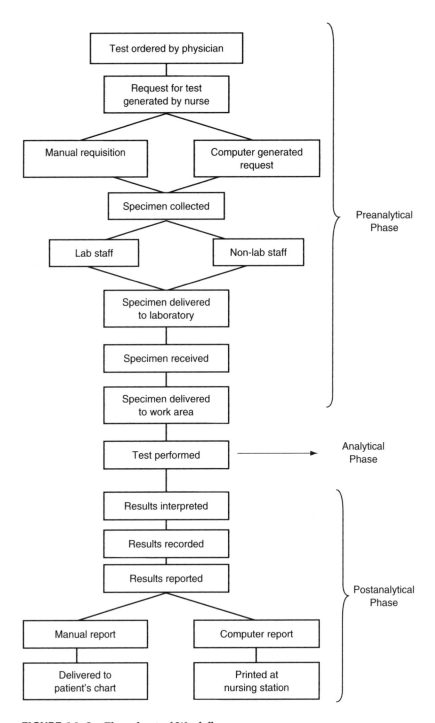

FIGURE 14–2 Flowchart of Workflow.

TABLE 14–1.   Workflow Phases

Preanalytical	Analytical	Postanalytical
Ordering	Testing	Interpreting
Collecting		Recording
Transporting		Reporting
Processing		

Preanalytical phase   In the preanalytical phase, uniformity of procedures is important. If everyone is taught to do things the same way, errors can be reduced. The procedures should not be so complicated or cumbersome that no one wants to follow them; this causes an increase in errors. This especially applies to the collection process. If a specimen is improperly collected, it can affect the test results, which ultimately affects patient outcome. In any setting, well-written manuals with thorough training is vital.

The ordering process should use a standard language. Everyone should call the test by the same name and should use the same abbreviations. Deviations cause confusion and can lead to misinterpretations. The wrong specimen could be collected or the wrong test performed.

After the specimen is collected, it must be transported to the laboratory. In a hospital this may be as simple as walking down the hall. When specimens are delivered from an off site location, the transportation process becomes more complicated. In the case study, the specimens are coming from a small hospital located an hour's drive away. Courier schedules will need to be established. Also before delivery, specimens must be stored so that specimen integrity is not compromised. The specimens need to be protected from such things as exposure to heat or cold. The specimens should not be too old to produce reliable results; hence time frames must be established for "from time of collection to time of delivery." This will affect the courier schedule.

Once the specimen is ordered, collected, and transported, it must be received in the laboratory. This refers to the acceptance of the specimen, whether logging it manually or in the computer. The receiving procedure should include what to do if the specimen is not acceptable, the wrong test has been ordered, or patient information is not complete. Then the specimen must be delivered to the work area. It does no good if it sits in the receiving area.

Analytical phase   When the specimen arrives in the work area the testing is done. The physical layout of the area and how the test will be performed are important for efficiency. Will it be done by a manual method or will it be automated? What equipment should be used? These types of decisions are made during the process design development.

Postanalytical phase   After the test is performed the results must be interpreted (i.e., put into a format for reporting). Then it must be recorded and the results manually written on a log or placed in a computer log. The log is usually available only to laboratory staff. From the log the results are then reported; that is, they are made available to the person(s) that ordered the test or needs them to care for the patient. Until the final product is available to the people that need to know, the task or work is not complete. Many media, depending on the circumstances, are used to report tests such as the computer, paper, phone, mail, or fax. Remember, reports are not useful if they are hard to read and understand or if they are not easily accessible.

Workflow can be a complicated process. To help identify all the steps it is beneficial to draw a flowchart that is specific to the workflow being analyzed (Figure 14–2). Each step should be specific to the work and department. It then serves as a guide for getting from the beginning to the end of a task.

PROCESS MANAGEMENT

The business of the laboratory is to provide information to the clinician to assist in patient care decisions. The clinical – or hospital-based – laboratory is integral to patient care and as such, integrated with the healthcare delivery system in which it resides. A reference or freestanding laboratory provides service in a different manner, yet is still a crucial part of patient care. In either case, the goals of the laboratory must be aligned with the overall goals of the healthcare system. It is then possible to analyze and define the current state, and all inherent processes, to determine if purposeful change can bring about measurable improvements that fit with the stated goals.

Process Management is defined as a systematic data based approach to monitoring and improving the performance of business. It is a management strategy that identifies opportunities for improvement using proven problem-solving methods. Process improvement has been around informally for thousands of years – theoretically ever since the caveman made the 2nd wheel. Formal programs began in the 1940's and 50's when Japanese businessmen discovered the methods taught by Drs. Deming, Juran, and Shewhart. The roots of process management have evolved from the basic Shewart Cycle (see Chapter 4) popular in the 1950's to the more complex Six Sigma Methodology applied by modern businesses. Although a variety of names such as Total Quality Management and Continuous Quality Improvement have been used to individualize these methods, they all have a common goal: an efficient, effective process that produces highly satisfied customers. They also involve a number of quality – or process management – tools including PDSA (*Plan, Do, Study, Act*) (a.k.a. PDCA, Deming's Cycle, or Shewhart's Cycle.) Many modern businesses have segued into the more complex Six Sigma methodology. Numerous models of process management, process improvement methods, and quality tools exist. Regardless of which quality management system is utilized, the expected results are the continuous monitoring of processes, looking for ways to make improvement without sacrificing quality.

Every organization can potentially improve its processes and the systems in which they operate. By mapping current processes, and defining a more efficient and smoother functioning future state, we can achieve measurable improvement in multiple areas: care delivery, cost effectiveness, and the work environment. The team members actually performing the work become better informed about how their individual tasks contribute to the success of the entire organization.

How then can we, as laboratory managers, best serve the customer and ultimately achieve the best outcomes for the patient? How can we monitor and improve the performance of the laboratory to more resourcefully provide the delivery of services? How can we manage the process?

PROCESS MANAGEMENT TOOLS

Many businesses including health care organizations develop a Quality Philosophy or Quality Model based on a variety of process improvement methodologies. Time and money is invested in teaching the chosen methodology and some are groomed to be expert facilitators. If your organization does not offer this, you can still take advantage of these proven problem-solving methods. An example of a Process Management Tool called FOCUS-PDSA is shown here (See Figure 14–3). Each letter of the FOCUS-PDSA acronym stands for a phrase that describes a step in the order it needs to be taken to enact a process improvement. A Quality Improvement (QI) Review Form can be used to keep the team on track. (See Table 14–2) Skipping steps can be tempting, but is discouraged as it usually calls for rework further along in the project.

The acronym FOCUS-PDSA stands for:

F – Find an Opportunity   P – Plan your Actions
O – Organize a Team   D – Do the Actions
C – Clarify Current Process   S – Study the Results
U – Understand Variation   A – Act on your Conclusions.
S – Select Improvements

The first step is often easy as the *Opportunity* finds you, perhaps as a recurrent customer complaint or a directive from administration. If the opportunity is not so clear, try surveying your customers and team members. You will find ideas that you may not have considered independently. *Organizing a Team* is not to be taken lightly. You must identify key players who are familiar with the process, have the ability to affect the process, are customers–internal or external, and have a stake in the outcome in order to select a lasting, meaningful change.

The next step–*Clarify the Current Process*–is done by gathering information from the users of the process so that a true picture of current operations can be mapped out. This stage consists of direct observation, measurement, and numeration. A process flow chart is often utilized at this point. If the climate of the organization is non-threatening and conducive to change, the team member whose tasks are being studied will welcome the analysis and participate by collecting data and providing frontline insight to the team. The accuracy and appropriateness of the information collected at this stage is important and every effort should be made to collect unbiased data. The participation of the individuals most affected by the proposed improvement should be emphasized and is crucial to its

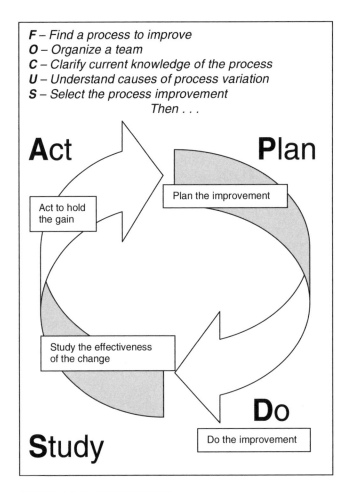

F – *Find a process to improve*
O – *Organize a team*
C – *Clarify current knowledge of the process*
U – *Understand causes of process variation*
S – *Select the process improvement*
                    Then . . .

Act

Plan

Act to hold
the gain

Plan the improvement

Study the effectiveness
of the change

Do

Study

Do the improvement

FIGURE 14–3 FOCUS-PDSA

success. The team member needs to understand that process improvement is a tool for positive change and will result in innovation that better aligns the actions of an individual worker with objectives and visions of the organization.

Understanding Variation is next. This step is key to every Quality Management theory. It consists of determining which specific steps in the overall process need improvement. Quality is inversely proportional to variability. Questions to ask at this stage include "How does this process vary from what the customer wants? What are the common causes of variation in the process? What are the special causes? What can be done to reduce variation?"

The options for improvement are then outlined and *Selected*. At this stage the creative floodgates are opened and various ideas are entertained and analyzed for feasibility, practicality, cost, and effect on outcome. Once an idea is chosen, usually through a variety of quality tools (i.e., Brainstorming, Benchmarking,

TABLE 14.2 QI Review Form

Find an Opportunity
- Describe the data that quantifies the need: _____
- How can you narrow the scope? _____
- Opportunity Statement: *We have the opportunity to improve the* _____*process.*
  This process begins with _____ *& ends with* _____.
  If we meet our goal of _____, *our key customers,* _____*will benefit.*
- Describe the set of numbers that would tell you if the above process has changed:_____

Organize a Team
- Name key players & customers. (Which team members and customers are most familiar with the process?)_____
- Establish team ground rules: i.e. Meeting dates, team etiquette, etc. _____
- Review Opportunity Statement for clarity _____
- Establish timeline–write in projected completion date of each step:

F	O	C	U	S	P	D	C	A

Clarify Current Process
- Using input from the people listed above, make a flowchart of the current process.
- What are easy problems that could be solved immediately? _____
- Describe the data that quantifies the customer's expectations? _____

Understand Variation
- How does this process vary from what the customer wants? _____
- Why do special cause and common cause variations occur? _____

Select Improvements
- What are the root causes of the problem? _____
- List several ways that the process can be improved: _____
- What criteria will you use to evaluate the list of improvements? _____

Plan your Actions
- Describe only one process improvement that will be piloted: _____
- Does your action plan describe who, what, when, and where? _____
- How long will you try the process before studying the data collected? _____

Do the Actions
- Are you following an Action Plan? _____
- Are you collecting data during this trial period? _____

Study the Results
- Did you make progress toward your goals? Why or why not? _____

Act on your Conclusions
- Should the change be made permanent? _____
- Is another improvement needed? _____

Multi-voting, or a Selection Matrix) the change is introduced into the process flowchart and effects of the change on the future state are explored. If the change is doable, and not contraindicated by the outcome analysis, the change is *Planned* or incorporated into the future state map.

The *Doing* stage translates to controlled implementation of the process change. Controlled in the foregoing sentence means that the effects of the change are observed, monitored, and measured. It is important that a measurable variable be defined prior to the implementation so that an objective assessment of the benefits of change can be made. Without empirical measurements of outcomes, we have no reliable way of *Studying the Results* – or in other words – of knowing if the change has brought about improvement.

The final step of the FOCUS-PDSA method is to review the change by monitoring the effect it had on a measurable outcome. You will *Act on Your Conclusions* by determining if the change should be made permanent or if another improvement is needed. It is not unusual to have multiple cycles (often referred to as Rapid Cycle Changes) of the PDSA part of the formula. By introducing one small change at a time, studying what works and what does not, you can refine the process to relative perfection.

In recent years, efforts have been made to incorporate more sophisticated process management tools into the health care environment and specifically into the clinical laboratory. This is the methodology mentioned earlier and developed in manufacturing industries of *Lean Thinking, Lean Tooling*, and *Six Sigma*.

What are Six Sigma and the Lean Philosophy? The term Sigma comes to us from the world of mathematics and is the statistical measure of variability within a selected process. In the manufacturing environment, it has been used to measure the number of products produced that do not meet quality control standards or that simply do not function as intended. In service industries, it may be a measure of the number of transaction failures or an inordinate delay in the delivery of a service.

The underlying assumption of the Sigma methodology is that the cause of a defect or failure is variation. If something works most of the time, then one can eliminate the reasons that create differences in the outcome of the process with the goal of eliminating failure. The number preceding Sigma, in this case Six, refers to the order of magnitude of the reduction in variation: Thus the higher the number, the fewer the failures. Six Sigma improvements mean that a process has been refined to reduce errors to 3.4 per one million opportunities. For practical purposes, an error rate at this level is virtually perfect.

The fundamental concepts of the Lean Philosophy are to define value by challenging traditional definitions, discovering what is of value to the customer, and then determining the value of each step leading to the delivery of the goods or service to the customer. This leads to mapping the "Value Stream" (the flow or movement (physical or informational) between processes) and redesigning the structure to respond to the needs of the customer. By adding value, and eliminating what does not add value, or even takes value away, the waste generated in the system is reduced or eliminated. Six Sigma uses a DMAIC (Define, Measure,

Analyze, Improve, Control) tool similar to the FOCUS-PDSA tool for improving existing processes.

The full application of the Six Sigma methodology and Lean Tooling require extensive training and experience. A person achieving mastery of these system design methodologies are awarded certifications as "Black Belts," "Green Belts," and "Lean Tool Masters." As these technologies are applied even more broadly in the health care environment, improvements and efficiencies can be realized making the health care environment safer for everyone.

Teaching Quality Improvement programs is an industry in itself. Much more information is available about the quality process, quality tools and how to use them via literature and the Internet. Several websites to begin with include: *http://curiouscat.com/guides/* and *http://www.isixsigma.com/sixsigma/six_sigma.asp.*

Staffing the Laboratory: Hiring, training, scheduling and retaining

Staffing is defined as finding the right person to do the job at the time needed, that is, matching that person to the needs of the job. Staffing includes hiring, training, scheduling, and retaining, each of which is further discussed in the sections that follow. When a decision is made to hire a new employee, the level of staff needed must be determined. Will a degreed person be needed or a non-degreed person? This is usually decided by the type of work to be done and regulatory issues associated with that work. Will the person need to be a specialist or a generalist? A specialist is someone with extensive knowledge in one area while a generalist has knowledge of many. Will the person work full time, part time, or as needed (per diem)? Will there be shift work, weekend work, or holiday work? After deciding what is needed, the hiring process can start.

Hiring The hiring process consists of two components, the application and the interview. The **application** is a written document that lists the prospective employee's education, qualifications, and work experience. It can be used as an initial screening because if these do not meet the needs of the open position, no further action should be taken. If the applicant appears to meet your needs, then an **interview** should be scheduled. The interview is the oral process used to confirm the information in the application and to fill in any gaps. This is also an opportunity to explain to the applicant the job responsibilities, the hours/days/shifts that need to be worked, the benefits package that will be available, and the wages. If everything appears compatible for both parties, a job offer can be made and accepted.

Training Once hired, the employee needs to be taught the procedures in the work area. If you expect an employee to do well in the position then that person must be thoroughly trained (see Chapter 8 for additional information regarding training). The initial training period is referred to as orientation. Having a complete, well-defined orientation helps everyone—the new hire and the trainer—because it defines the expectations and responsibilities of the position. It also helps the new employee to become productive and able to operate independently.

Scheduling   When the training or orientation is complete, the employee must be scheduled to work. Scheduling is assigning the employee to work-specific hours, to a specific department, or to a specific task. The manager has the responsibility for scheduling to meet the needs of the department in the safest and most cost effective way possible. The number of hours that an employee is scheduled depends on their classification, full time, part time, or per diem. A full-time employee works 40 hours a week or 80 hours in two weeks depending on the work rule used. A part-time employee is regularly scheduled and works a defined number of hours that are less than the full-time employee's hours. This could be as little as 8 hours in a week or two week period to as much as 32 hours in a week or 72 hours in two weeks. The number of hours authorized often determines if the employee is qualified for benefits. In our case study, an employee must work at least 40 hours per 2-week pay period to be benefit eligible. The employee can choose to work less than 40 hours but must be informed that they will not be able to receive benefits. This will not affect those who have benefits elsewhere, but often benefits play a large part in the job search. A per diem employee (also known as PRN – as needed – or pool) is not regularly scheduled and has no set number of hours. This employee works when needed such as filling in for someone on vacation, someone absent due to illness, or during heavy workload periods. They can fill out the schedule when the core staff members are done – or be called to work at the time they are needed.

Two major scheduling formats are used to schedule employees. These are the **8/80 *work rule*** and the **40-*hour workweek rule.*** The 8/80-work rule has been used by hospitals for many years and they are the only employer allowed to use it, as defined by wage and hour regulations. Traditionally, in hospitals, employees have been scheduled to work 8-hour days. The day conveniently divides into three 8-hour periods. The 8/80-work rule covers a two-week time frame. During this time the employee works an 8-hour day and any number of days up to 10 (80 hours) within the 2 weeks. Any time worked over 8 hours in a day or 80 hours in 2 weeks is overtime and must be paid at the overtime rate. The 40-hour workweek rule means the employee is allowed to work any number of hours per shift as long as the total hours worked in a week do not exceed 40.

Both scheduling models have their advantages and disadvantages. The 8/80 rule limits the number of hours in the day that can be worked, but more days in a row are allowed. The 40-hour workweek lets an employee work longer shifts but limits the number of days in a week to a maximum of 5. This can save the organization overtime expenses when longer shifts are needed for covering the work. In today's environment, flexibility in scheduling has become an important issue to employees. Many managers are using both work rules to provide as much flexibility as possible. This does not mean the employee can use one work rule this week and the other next week, but it does give everyone more choices. Depending on organizational needs, two employees working side by side could possibly work different types of schedules. No matter which work rule is used in developing a schedule, it should be impartial and based on organizational needs.

Scheduling begins with determining how many and what type of staff are needed to perform the average workload per shift. Workload and staffing information is usually based on historical data. This should include data for shift work, weekends, and holidays because laboratories are open 24/7 and must be staffed. This type of information needs to be used regardless of the size of the laboratory. In a large laboratory the schedule is probably more departmentalized and complicated; a smaller laboratory would be simpler and include all areas, benches, and shifts.

The schedule should start out as a generic process; this would be the "ideal" schedule based on organizational needs. Once this has been developed, then individual employees and special requests can be plugged in. Schedules should also be determined far enough ahead so that everyone has advanced notice of when to work. A schedule is a dynamic process. It is continually changing based on the needs of both the organization and the employee. The schedule should be set up based on the pay period as the working unit. A pay period is usually 2 weeks no matter which work rule is used. At the end of each pay period the employee is paid for hours worked.

In any pay period fourteen 24-hour days need to be staffed. No matter which work rule is used, a full-time employee cannot work more than 10 days in the two weeks without incurring overtime. Part-time employees are hired to provide coverage when full-time employees are off work. In the case study, a generic schedule was developed for the entire laboratory using the 8/80 rule. When using this rule, the day is divided into three shifts of eight hours each. These are called the day, evening, and night shifts. Historical data were used to determine workload and levels of staffing for each shift including both weekdays and weekends.

For the average workload, Table 14–3 shows the staff required for each shift. Once the staffing levels are established, the number of employees needed to provide the staffing must be determined. An easy way to do this is to determine the number of shifts needing to be worked for each job classification. Remember, a

TABLE 14–3. Staffing for the Average Workload

	Day Shift	Evening Shift	Night Shift
Weekdays	3 technical 2 phlebotomy 1 secretary	2 technical 1 phlebotomy	1 technical
Weekends	2 technical 1 phlebotomy 1 secretary	1 technical 1 phlebotomy	1 technical

shift using the 8/80 rule is eight hours and in a 2-week period there are 14 days. A full-time employee works 10 of the 14 shifts. A part-time employee usually works the other four. Knowing this information we can now calculate the number of people needed (Table 14–4). Once this information has been determined a generic schedule can be developed (Table 14–5).

After the generic schedule is established, the names of the employees are filled in, taking into account special needs or requests such as vacations. If necessary, determine who will provide coverage for the special requests. Then add the work assignments. This can be done using numbers, colored dots, letters, or whatever works for this department (Table 14–6).

TABLE 14–4.   Staffing

Day Shift

Weekdays   3 technical staff needed for 10 shifts = 30 shifts to cover
Weekends   2 technical staff needed for 4 shifts = 8 shifts to cover
                                                    14 days   38 shifts to cover

If a full-time employee works 10 shifts, divide the 38 shifts by 10. This equals approximately four. Four full-time people are needed to provide this coverage.

Weekdays   2 phlebotomy staff needed for 10 shifts = 20 shifts to cover
Weekends   1 phlebotomy staff needed for 4 shifts = 4 shifts to cover
                                                    14 days   24 shifts to cover

Divide the 24 shifts by 10. This equals 2.4, which means 2 full-time people and 1 part-time person is needed to provide this coverage.

Weekdays/ends   1 secretary needed for 14 shifts = 14 shifts to cover

Divide 14 shifts by 10. This equals 1.4, which means 1 full-time person and 1 part-time person is needed to provide this coverage.

Evening Shift

Weekdays   2 technical staff needed for 10 shifts = 20 shifts to cover
Weekends   1 technical staff needed for 4 shifts = 4 shifts to cover
                                                    14 days   24 shifts to cover

Divide the 24 shifts by 10. This equals 2.4, which means 2 full-time people and 1 part-time person is needed to provide this coverage.

Weekdays/ends   1 phlebotomy staff needed for 14 shifts = 14 shifts to cover

Divide 14 shifts by 10. This equals 1.4, which means 1 full-time person and 1 part-time person is needed to provide this coverage.

Night Shift

Weekdays/ends   1 technical staff needed for 14 shifts = 14 shifts to cover

Divide 14 shifts by 10. This equals 1.4, which means 1 full-time person and 1 part-time person is needed to provide coverage.

TABLE 14-5. Generic Schedule

Day Shift	Sun	Mon	Tue	Wed	Thu	Fri	Sat	Sun	Mon	Tue	Wed	Thu	Fri	Sat
FT Tech	x	o	x	x	x	x	o	o	x	x	x	o	x	x
FT Tech	x	x	o	x	x	x	o	o	x	x	x	x	o	x
FT Tech	o	x	x	x	o	x	x	x	o	x	x	x	x	o
FT Tech	o	x	x	x	x	o	x	x	x	o	x	x	x	o
FT Phleb	x	o	x	x	x	x	o	o	o	x	x	x	x	x
FT Phleb	o	x	x	x	x	o	x	x	x	x	x	x	o	x
PT Phleb		x		x	x	x							x	
FT Sec.	o	o	x	x	x	o	x	x	o	x	x	x	x	o
PT Sec.	x	x	x	x	x	x	x	x	x	x	x	x	x	x

Evenings

	Sun	Mon	Tue	Wed	Thu	Fri	Sat	Sun	Mon	Tue	Wed	Thu	Fri	Sat
FT Tech	x	x	x	x	x	x	o	o	o	o	x	x	x	x
FT Tech	o	o	o	x	x	x	x	x	x	x	x	x	x	o
PT Tech		x	x				x		x	x				
FT Phleb	x	o	x	x	x	x	o	o	o	x	x	x	x	x
PT Phleb		x	x				x	x	x	x				x

Nights

	Sun	Mon	Tue	Wed	Thu	Fri	Sat	Sun	Mon	Tue	Wed	Thu	Fri	Sat
FT Tech	x	x	x	x	x	o	o	o	x	x	x	x	o	x
PT Tech		x					x	x	x					x

Key x = Working
    o = Off
    FT = Full-time
    PT = Part-time
    Tech = Technologist/Technician
    Phleb = Phlebotomist
    Sec = Secretary

TABLE 14–6. Specific Schedule

Day Shift	Sun	Mon	Tue	Wed	Thu	Fri	Sat	Sun	Mon	Tue	Wed	Thu	Fri	Sat
Bob	C	o	C	C	C	C	o	o	H	H	H	o	H	H
Sally	H	H	o	H	H	H	o	o	BB	BB	BB	BB	C	C
Susan	o	BB	BB	BB	o	BB	C	H	o	C	F	H	C	o
Joan	o	C	H	F	BB	o	H	C	C	o	C	C	BB	o
Jessica	0400	o	0400	0400	0400	0400	o	0400	0400	0400	0400	0400	0400	0400
David	o	0400	0700	0700	0700	o	0400	o	o	0700	0700	0700	o	0700
Cynthia		0700	0700			0700				0700			0700	
Linda	o	o				0700	0700	0700	o	0700	0700	0700	0700	o
Cathy	0700	0700	0700	0700	0700	0700		0700	0700	0700	0700	0700	0700	0700

Evenings	Sun	Mon	Tue	Wed	Thu	Fri	Sat	Sun	Mon	Tue	Wed	Thu	Fri	Sat
John	1430	1430	1430	1430	1430	1430	o	o	o	o	1430	1430	1430	1430
Stephanie	o	o	o	1530	1530	1530	1530	1530	1530	1530	1530	1530	1530	o
Amy	1500	1530	1530	1500	1500	1500	1430	1500	1500	1430	1500	1500	1500	1500
Dan		o					o	o	o					
Mary	1500	1500	1500	1500	1500	1500	1500	1500	1500	1500	1500	1500	1500	1500

Nights	Sun	Mon	Tue	Wed	Thu	Fri	Sat	Sun	Mon	Tue	Wed	Thu	Fri	Sat
Judy	2300	2300	2300	2300	2300	o	o	o	2300	2300	2300	2300	o	2300
Jean						2300	2300	2300					2300	

Key H = Hematology/Urinalysis(UA)/Coagulation (Coag)
C = Chemistry
BB = Blood Bank
F = Float
o = Scheduled day off
Numbers indicate shift start time in military time.

274

Return to the case study and the microbiology department. The current staffing consists of two full-time technical employees and one part-time technical employee. During weekdays two people work and on weekends one person works. There are no evening or night shifts worked in this area. The department is open from 0600 to 1700 (which is 6 AM to 5 PM expressed in military time). Since most laboratories operate 24/7, military time is often used in the scheduling process. Thus all times in this discussion are expressed in military time. One person reports at 0600 and the other at 0830 during the week and one person works 0700 to 1530 on weekends. If a stat Gram stain is needed at other times, the technical staff in the rest of the laboratory has been cross-trained to do them. Cultures received during those other hours are set up by the same staff (Table 14–7).

With the projected increase in work and with the addition of a new piece of equipment, it has been determined that nontechnical staff employees will also be added and will be needed everyday. If someone is needed every day, that means there are 14 shifts to cover in the pay period. This means one full-time person and one part-time person will have to be hired to provide the coverage (Table 14–8).

The schedule in Table 14–5 was developed using the 8/80-work rule. Some of the employees work six shifts in a row and others ten. If this schedule had been developed using the 40-hour workweek rule, the schedule could still look much the same as long as 8-hour shifts are still worked and the employee works every other weekend. When using the 40-hour workweek, the week is defined as Sunday to Saturday. It splits the weekend, which still allows employees to work six days in a row (or ten), but it must include the weekend.

In our case study the 8/80 work rule is being used for scheduling. It has worked well for the department and will not be changed. Suppose though that for some reason the workload does change in the general laboratory. The schedule will need to be adjusted to provide coverage. For this example, the workload has changed at two specific times of the day. The first time is from 2100 to 2400.The emergency room work has increased fourfold during this time and the evening shift is having trouble keeping up. To provide some relief it was decided that the night shift tech would start work two hours earlier at 2100 and work a 10-hour shift. The second time of the day that workload has significantly changed is from 1400 to 1500 because of blood arriving from off-site clinics. This occurs in the middle of the change of shift from days to evenings, and overtime is occurring because the day shift is unable to leave on time. An overlap is needed to provide coverage and reduce this expense. To reduce overtime, it was decided that one dayshift tech would start working 10-hour shifts from 0700 to 1700 (Table 14–9). Note the differences between Table 14–9 and Table 14–5.

A third option for scheduling is called *self-scheduling*. Generational studies have shown that inflexible scheduling is considered poor working conditions by the newest to the work world. An increased number of younger workers willingly forego higher wages to achieve an agreeable work-life balance. Some companies have improved retention and recruitment by introducing such programs as self-scheduling into their organizations. Successful self-scheduling takes teamwork but the rewards for letting team members have some control over their schedules is well worth the effort.

TABLE 14–7. Current Microbiology Schedule

Micro	Sun	Mon	Tue	Wed	Thu	Fri	Sat	Sun	Mon	Tue	Wed	Thu	Fri	Sat
John	0700	0600	0600	0600	0600	o	o	o	0600	0600	0600	0600	o	0700
Karen	o	o	0830	0830	0830	0600	0700	0700	o	0830	0830	0830	0600	o
Larry		0830				0830			0830				0830	

Key 0600 = Bench 1 Set Ups/Gram Stain/Specials
0830 = Bench 2 Read Plates/Set Up MICs
0700 = Employee on duty covers both benches (1 & 2)
   o = Scheduled day off

TABLE 14–8. Projected Microbiology Schedule

Micro	Sun	Mon	Tue	Wed	Thu	Fri	Sat	Sun	Mon	Tue	Wed	Thu	Fri	Sat
John	0700	0600	0600	0600	0600	o	o	o	0600	0600	0600	0600	o	0700
Karen	o	o	0830	0830	0830	0600	0700	0700	o	0830	0830	0830	0600	o
Larry		0830					0830			0830			0830	
FT New	0700	o	0700	0700	0700	0700	o	o	0700	0700	0700	0700	o	0700
PT New		0700					0700	0700					0700	0700

Note: In this projected schedule there are 2 employees working both Saturdays and Sundays. On these days, 1 employee works bench 1, the other works bench 2.

Key 0600 = Bench 1 Special Cultures
0830 = Bench 2 Read Plates/Set Up Susceptibility Tests (MICs)
0700 = Set Ups/Gram Stains/Ordering
  o = Scheduled day off
Numbers also indicate start time in military time.

TABLE 14–9. Generic Schedule 2

Day Shift	Sun	Mon	Tue	Wed	Thu	Fri	Sat
FT Tech	o	*0700	*0700	*0700	o	*0700	o
FT Tech	o	0600	0600	0600	0600	0600	o
FT Tech	o	o	0900	0700	*0700	0900	o
FT Tech	0600	0700	0600	0700	0700	0600	0600
PT Tech	0700					0700	0700
FT Phleb	o	o	x	x	x	x	x
FT Phleb	x	x	x	x	x	o	x
PT Phleb		x	x			x	
FT Sec.	x	o	x	x	x	x	o
PT Sec.	x	x				x	x
Evenings							
FT Tech	o	o	x	x	x	x	x
FT Tech	x	x	o	x	x	x	o
PT Tech			x				
FT Phleb	o	o	x	x	x	x	x
PT Phleb	x	x					
Nights							
FT Tech	*2100	*2100	*2100	*2100		o	o
PT Tech		*2100	*2100		*2100	*2100	*2100

Key FT = Part Time
     PT = Full Time
     Tech = Technologist/Technician
     X = Scheduled work day
     o = Scheduled day off
     * = 10 Hour Shifts

Numbers indicate start time in military time.

Note: The full time tech that works 2 ten hour shifts is on a 40-hour work week and works 6 hours on two other days in order not to work more than 80 hours in the pay period.

Self-scheduling guidelines will need to be designed to meet the needs of the particular department. Two important points to remember as you create these guidelines are:

I. No one is guaranteed a specific schedule.
II. The needs of the department must be covered.

The following is an example of a successful self-scheduling plan:

1. Team members are divided into 2 groups, RED and BLUE. The scheduling groups alternate signing up first on the new blank schedule. Each group has 4 days to sign up. There is a maximum and minimum number of staff needed each shift. (The minimum number is the number of staff needed to perform the average daily workload and the maximum number is the most the budget affords working in one shift – these numbers are determined by the manager). When the maximum number of staff is achieved, that date will be X'd out on the schedule. There is a week to make revisions after which the schedule is finalized and posted. Unbalanced schedules will not be finalized.
2. The second group to sign up should be the first group to make schedule changes. It is the responsibility of the second group to review the schedule at revision time and attempt to balance the schedule.
3. The manager tracks changes made to help balance the schedule. Changes to the schedule must be made in red ink to get credit for changing. (Pencil is used until revision time).
4. If the schedule is not balanced after revisions, the manager will change staff according to the following guidelines:
   a. Staff not meeting their weekend commitment
   b. Per diem staff
   c. Staff in the second group who have not made changes to balance previous schedules according to past schedules
   d. Staff in the second group who have not made changes to balance the schedule in progress
   e. Staff in first group
5. If your schedule is changed without your approval, the manager will make every effort to notify you and it will be your responsibility to either work the shift or find an even trade.
6. 4 weekend shifts per schedule are required. Dayshift and evening weekend shifts are Saturday and Sunday. Nightshift weekend shifts are Friday and Saturday.
7. During revision time, if you switch off a weekend shift, you must sign up for another weekend shift if another weekend shift is low.
8. The manager may decrease the weekend commitment of a team member if it is in the best interest of the schedule.
9. A maximum of 2 "R" (request) days per schedule will be granted. Only 2 team members may be granted PTO (paid time off) days on any one shift.
10. Vacation requests must be in the vacation request book. Only 2 team members per shift will be guaranteed vacation at the same time.

11. No vacation can be scheduled if the TM does not have the PTO time in their bank.
12. All schedule change requests after the schedule is finalized must be approved by the manager. Every attempt must be made on the part of the team member to find an even trade for their request if the request would short that shift.

Retaining

Retention of team members is well worth putting forth a good effort. As the number of people entering the workforce decreases, people have more choice in the job market. Work-life balance, as mentioned earlier, is very important to workers in their 20's and 30's. This age group is not nearly as loyal to an employer as previous generations. The cost of recruiting, hiring, and orienting a new team member is approximately the cost of that position's annual salary. Remember, you will be paying 2 people to do one job for several weeks as they orient. If the person stayed long enough to accumulate benefits, they will be taking some of those benefits (PTO) with them when they leave. You may also be paying overtime to other team members to cover the vacated shifts while you recruit.

Retention may be as simple as recognizing each of your team members every day, giving praise where due, and treating the team fairly when making assignments or counseling them. Giving employees time for continuing education opportunities will also help retention. If an employee sees promotion in their future, they will be more likely than others to stay with the organization.

SUMMARY

A process design serves as a blueprint for completing work or a task. It may be complicated or simple based on the size of the task and the setting for which it is being developed. Workflow and staffing are integral parts of process design development, providing the details of the blueprint. Further, the development of a process design is influenced by many other factors, each of which should be examined and analyzed.

As previously stated, workflow is an essential aspect of process design development. Three workflow phases must be considered: (1) preanalytical, (2) analytical, and (3) postanalytical. Of these the preanalytical phase is the most difficult to control. The development of a workflow chart that identifies the specific points within each of these phases is indicated when performing workflow analysis.

Process Management is the management strategy of continuously monitoring the performance of processes and identifying opportunities for improvement using proven problem-solving methods. Many variations and methodologies are available in the literature and on the Internet. These may be dictated by your organization or you may research and choose the best approach for your department. Successful organizations continue to strive for perfection in processes without sacrificing quality.

Staffing is critical to process design development. Four components are involved in staffing. The first is hiring, which consists of two parts: (1) the written application and (2) the oral interview. Each part of the hiring phase provides specific information about the prospective candidate so that a good hiring decision can be made. Once an employee is hired, the second component, training, comes into play. Training consists of orientating the employee to the facility, the department, and to policies and procedures associated with performing the job. The third component is scheduling. The assignment of workers to jobs can be a complex task that consumes much of a laboratory manager's time. Two work rules may be used in scheduling employees in a hospital setting: the 8/80 work rule, or the 40-hour work week rule. The development of a generic schedule will provide a basic plan from which a specific schedule may be designed and implemented. Self-scheduling is an option that offers flexibility and control to team members. Retention is the fourth stage of staffing. Once you have hired a good employee, effort should be made to retain that employee. Successful retention is cost effective and may improve outcomes as experienced employees become more proficient in their work.

The key to developing successful process designs is by approaching it carefully, one step at a time, addressing each appropriate issue. Along with the use of flowcharts, where appropriate, a successful process design may be developed.

SUGGESTED PROBLEM-BASED LEARNING ACTIVITIES
Chapter 14: Process Designs-Workflow and Staffing

Instructions:	Use Internet resources, books, articles, colleagues, etc., to present solutions to the problems listed below. There is no one correct solution to any problem.
Note to Instructor:	Students in class may be divided into groups and given the problem-based learning activity to discuss and solve. Once the group has reached consensus as to a solution, the group may present it to the other students in the class. This activity will provide all students with information regarding solutions to the problem.

Problem #1
Choose a laboratory discipline, such as hematology or chemistry, and implement new technology/instrumentation for this discipline. How would this affect your current work processes?

Problem #2
Suppose your institution just contracted with a physician group to provide laboratory services. As laboratory manager, you must design a process to acquire samples, provide testing on the second shift and produce results by the next morning.

Problem #3
Suppose your institution has merged with another institution and all redundant services will be eliminated. As laboratory manger, you must design an efficient laboratory operation to provide the necessary services at both institutions.

BIBLIOGRAPHY

Chester, Eric: *Getting Them to Give a Damn: How to Get Your Front Line to Care About Your Bottom Line*, Dearborn Trade Publishing, Chicago, 2005.

Cornacchione, K.S., Forrest, I., Harmon, C., Hicks, S., McLeay, K.L., Molas, G., et al. (2003, February). *Revised MSICU Self-Scheduling Guidelines*, Self-Scheduling Committee Meeting conducted at Morton Plant Hospital MSICU, Clearwater, Florida.

George ML: *Lean Six Sigma for Service.* McGraw-Hill. New York. 2003.

Gitlow H, Levine D: *Six Sigma for Green Belts and Champions: Foundations, DMAIC Tools, Cases, and Certification.* Pearson Prentice Hall. Upper Saddle River, NJ. 2005.

Jacobson J, Johnson M: Lean and Six Sigma: Not for Amateurs. Lab Medicine. 2006 Mar: 37(3): 140–145.

Pande P, Neuman R, Cavanagh RR: *The Six Sigma Way Team Fieldbook: An Implementation Guide for Process Improvement Teams.* McGraw-Hill. New York. 2002.

Internet Resources

American Academy of Family Physicians. (2006). How to Conduct Quality Projects. Retrieved January 8, 2006 from
http://www.aafp.org/x3858.xml

Curious Cat Management Improvement Library–Dictionary. (1996-2006). PDSA, PDCA, Deming Cycle, Shewhart Cycle. Retrieved July 8, 2005 from
http://curiouscat.com/management/pdsa.cfm

iSix Sigma. (2000-2006). Six Sigma—What is Six Sigma? Retrieved August 12, 2005 from
http://www.isixsigma.com/sixsigma/six_sigma.asp

Laboratory Design Guidelines
http://www.uky.edu/FiscalAffairs/Environmental/ohs/ labdesign.html

McNamara Ph.D., Carter. Employee Task and Job Analysis
http://www.mappnp.org

Prudent Practices in the Laboratory Handling and Disposal of Chemicals
http:// www.nap.edu/readingroom/books/prudent

Tilden, E.(1999, May 3). Re: PDSA-Proposed Operational Definition. Message posted to Deming Electronic Network Discussion List, archived at
http://deming.eng.clemson.edu/pub/den/archive/99.05/msg00001.html

Workflow Principles.
http://www.outsights.com

15

Computer-Based Laboratory Information Systems

ANN TIEHEN, MT(ASCP)SBB

Chapter Outline

Objectives

Following successful completion of this chapter, the learner will be able to:

1. Describe the hardware components of a laboratory information system.
2. List the functions of the software components of a laboratory information system.

3. Identify the components of a database.
4. Outline the process for selecting a laboratory information system.
5. Name the standard operating procedures needed to maintain a laboratory information system.
6. Describe the kinds of testing that should be performed to validate a laboratory information system.
7. Identify the training needs of laboratory and hospital staff in the use of the laboratory information system.

Key Terms

Database
Definitional Database Table
Descriptive Database Table

Hierarchical Database
Relational Database
Validation

Case Study: Computer-Based Laboratory Information Systems

You are a manager of a clinical laboratory at a medium-sized community hospital. The laboratory includes chemistry, hematology, immunology, microbiology, and transfusion service sections. In addition there is a laboratory support section that includes phlebotomy services, data entry, and customer service. A technical specialist heads each section. A computer-based laboratory information system (LIS) has been in use at your facility for 10 years and is supported by a system manager. You have just learned that your computer system vendor will no longer be supporting the version of software that is currently in use. You must now select a new system and plan the installation.

Issues and Questions to Consider

1. *How will you approach selecting a new LIS?*
2. *Which personnel should be involved in selection, training, and implementation of the new LIS?*
3. *How will you ensure that current laboratory operations will proceed during implementation of the system and training of laboratory staff?*
4. *What tasks must be performed to tailor the software to the laboratory's operations?*
5. *What revisions or additions will be needed in the written standard operating procedures of the laboratory?*
6. *What testing should be performed to validate the functionality of the new system?*
7. *How will the laboratory staff be trained to use the new system?*

INTRODUCTION

Information, in the form of test results and clinical consultations, is the primary product of the clinical laboratory. To meet the needs of the laboratory's customers, it is essential that this information be accurate, available, and timely. In some smaller laboratories it may be possible to meet these needs with a manual information system, but most of today's laboratories require a computer-based laboratory information system to handle the large volume of data that it both receives and reports out. Another product of most hospital laboratories is blood and blood components issued by the transfusion service. With the vast array of special blood product needs of many patients, it is useful to have a computer system that will help ensure that those needs are consistently met.

Selecting and installing a computer-based laboratory information system (LIS) is a lengthy and labor-intensive process. It includes many tasks and involves all members of the laboratory staff. (Table 15–1). The purpose of this chapter is to introduce the reader to these tasks and basic corresponding computer terminology.

Before beginning the process of LIS selection and installation, it is useful to have an understanding of the basic components of a computer system and how they interact with each other.

System Components

A computer system includes two basic components: **hardware** and **software.** Hardware components are the physical pieces of equipment. Software is a set of instructions written in special computer language that tells the computer how to operate and manipulate the data. Many laboratory information systems also use special **interface** hardware and software that allows the system to communicate with other computer systems and/or automated analyzers.

Hardware

Most computer systems have three kinds of hardware components. Each piece of hardware performs a specific function in the handling of information. The three main functions performed by hardware components are information processing, input/output, and storage. The input/output and information storage components are also referred to as peripheral devices.

TABLE 15–1. Tasks and Responsibilities in LIS Installation

Task	Responsibility
System selection	Medical director, laboratory manager, section supervisors, system manager, technical staff
Allocation of human resources	Laboratory manager
Building definitional tables	Technical staff, section supervisors
Revision/creation of standard operating procedures	Medical director, laboratory manager, section supervisors, system manager
System validation	Section supervisors, technical staff
Training and competency assessment	Section supervisors, technical staff, trainers
Go live	All staff

The core piece of hardware in a computer system is the **central processing unit (CPU).** It controls the interpretation and execution of instructions provided by the software. Other pieces of processing hardware include ROM and RAM. ROM stands for read only memory and contains the "start-up" instructions for the computer. RAM, random access memory, is where data are temporarily entered while being processed. When a computer is turned on the CPU, ROM and RAM interact with each other and the operating system software to prepare the computer to accept data and instructions from its users.

Input devices are tools connected to the CPU that allow the entry of commands and data in a format that the computer can understand. They include such equipment as keyboards, pointing devices, barcode readers, and testing instruments. Keyboards are used to type instructions that tell the computer what to do, or to enter data such as patient demographic information and test results. Many systems will also accept barcoded information from sources such as test tubes or blood component labels. Entry of information by a barcode reader is much more accurate than manual entry methods.

Output devices transfer data out of the computer usually in the form of text or images to a display screen or printer. The most common output device is the monitor, which displays information as it is typed on the keyboard. Together, the monitor and keyboard make up the user terminal or workstation. The monitor can also display historical information at the request of the user. Another output device essential to the laboratory computer is the printer, which provides hard copy output on paper. Printers can produce specimen labels, specimen collection lists, patient chart reports, blood component compatibility tags, and management reports. The kind of printer chosen for any of these applications depends on the quality of print desired. For example a barcode label printer requires a high resolution printing capability for accurate interpretation by the barcode reader. Patient reports should also be printed using high quality print; management reports, which are usually used internally, can be of lower quality print.

A modem is an example of a combined input and output device. Modems allow computer systems to communicate with each other over telephone lines. Laboratories can use this mechanism to connect remote facilities to the main computer system so that all sites will have access to the system's databases. This configuration is found in laboratories with several collection or testing locations or in a system of hospital affiliates. Software vendor technical support staff also use modems to investigate and solve system problems or to transfer files to the customer.

The vast amount of information processed by the LIS requires two kinds of information storage hardware: short-term and long-term. Short-term storage is for the information that is most frequently requested and therefore requires efficient retrieval such as the most recent laboratory test results. This information is usually stored on a disk made of metal coated with a magnetic film called the hard disk. It contains software applications (programs) as well as user entered data. The hard disk may be contained in the main system unit or exist as a peripheral device. The information on the disk is accessed by entering commands, usually with a keyboard connected to a display terminal. These commands are then executed by the disk drive. The storage capacity of the hard disk is finite, and at some point older information must be transferred to long-term information storage hardware to keep the computer operating at an acceptable speed. Long-term storage can be accomplished using optical disks or magnetic tape.

The hardware components and the way in which they are connected to each other are called the system configuration. In the past laboratory information systems were stand-alone systems. In a stand-alone system configuration, the CPU of the LIS is usually located in the laboratory, and all the peripheral devices, including the terminals, are directly linked to the CPU. The terminals are known as "dumb terminals" because they do not have any information processing power of their own; they consist of a monitor and a keyboard, and their only function is to allow entry and display of LIS information. Now, in many laboratories the LIS components are connected to each other and to other information systems through network connections. A network is simply a system of communication links that allows users access to multiple information systems. In the hospital this could include the LIS, the hospital information system (HIS), the pharmacy computer, the radiology information system, and the materials ordering system. In a network configuration, the dumb terminals are replaced by workstations that consist of a monitor, keyboard, and a separate CPU. At a workstation, users may access other information systems, word processing programs, and spreadsheet programs, as well as the LIS. One example of a laboratory information system configuration is illustrated in Figure 15–1.

Some information system vendors have begun offering software that connects remote laboratories and physician offices with a centralized LIS through web-based portals. This allows remote customers to enter orders and review results on their own computers. The internet is expanding the reach of the classic laboratory information system configuration.

Software

Software programs provide the computer hardware with the instructions for organizing and presenting all of the information it has received. Software can be divided into two general categories: application software and operating system software.

Application software is designed to perform specific tasks. For example personal computers (PCs) often have application programs such as word processing, spreadsheets, and databases. LIS application software allows users to perform tasks that are specific to laboratory operations. Some of these tasks might include ordering laboratory tests or blood components, entry of test results and quality control data, and issuing blood for transfusion. These are specialized laboratory tasks and would be difficult if not impossible to perform in an application not specifically designed for laboratory use. The primary function of the LIS applications is management of the *database* of patients and laboratory tests. Older laboratory information systems used *hierarchical database* management systems, and most systems currently on the market use a *relational database* management system.

The hierarchical database has an inverted tree structure that looks similar to a company organization chart. The disadvantage to this type of structure is in the

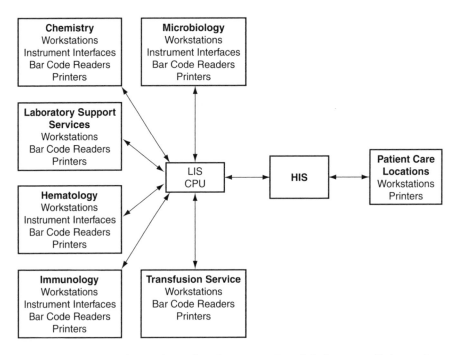

FIGURE 15–1   Configuration of a Computer-Based Laboratory Information System.

restricted way that information can be accessed. Records can be retrieved only through the top level of the structure. For example in the illustration of a hierarchical database in Figure 15–2, one could not easily get a list of all patients who have had a particular laboratory test result. Each patient record must be examined to determine which patients have had the test.

A relational database structure (Figure 15–3) shows that all of the data are linked. This kind of structure allows the user to quickly produce a list of only those patients who have had a particular laboratory test. Relational databases organize the information into sets of data called tables that are related to each other by common elements in the tables.

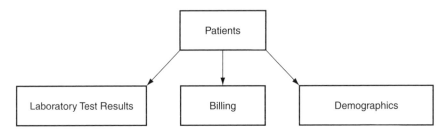

FIGURE 15–2   Hierarchical Database Structure.

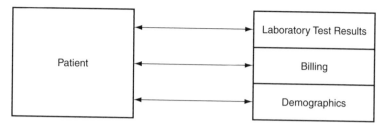

FIGURE 15-3   Relational Database Structure.

The database contains two different kinds of tables: definitional and descriptive. *Definitional tables,* often called dictionaries, remain fairly constant throughout the life of the LIS. These tables define the basic services of the laboratory and will be created during system implementation. They include test codes and definitions for each laboratory section, blood product codes, test comment codes, physician demographic data, and patient wards. Access to definitional tables is restricted to management staff, and these tables are updated only as tests or services are added or removed from the laboratory operation. *Descriptive tables* are continually updated with new information as users enter new patient and laboratory data. These tables include patient demographics, test results from each laboratory section, and blood product dispositions.

The tables are subdivided into records and each record in a table contains the same fields or data items. Figure 15–4 shows how the parts of a database relate to

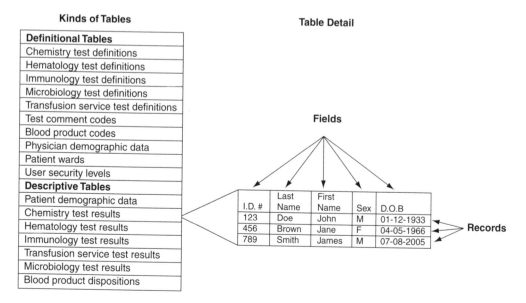

FIGURE 15-4   Database Components.

each other. Some of the fields in the database tables are designated as key fields, which serve as identifiers for the records; such key fields may include patient name, sex, and date of birth. When searching for a particular record, users will enter one or more key fields to obtain access to that record. One key field will be designated as the primary key and must be unique for each record in the database. In laboratory information systems, the primary key is the patient identification number, and the system will not allow more than one patient record to have the same identification number. When two or more tables contain the same primary field, information can be retrieved from multiple tables. For example, the table of patient demographic data and the table of hematology test results both contain the patient identification number allowing the user to obtain data elements from both tables at the same time.

Another way to think of the electronic database is to relate it to a manual filing system. The database itself can be thought of as the file cabinets that contain all the patient and laboratory test information. The file cabinets contain numerous file folders, each containing its own set of information, which are analogous to the tables in an electronic database. The folders in turn contain specific records (Table 15–2).

Many laboratory information systems will permit the creation of a second, separate database that contains the same definitional tables as the first. One database will be designated as the "production" database, and the other will be considered a "test" database. The production database is where actual patient records are stored and is the environment where day-to-day operations will be recorded. The test database will usually contain fictitious records and offers users an opportunity to practice the applications of the system (and to make mistakes) without corrupting the database containing actual patient information.

Unlike application software, operating system software works in the background of the LIS so that the tasks it performs are fairly invisible to users. It performs important functions, however, because it controls the computer's hardware, manipulates the application software, and coordinates the flow of data to and from disks and memory. For example, when data are entered into one of the application programs, the operating system software places the data on the hard disk for storage. When a user, through an application program, requests the data, the operating system retrieves it and sends it to the appropriate peripheral device such as a workstation display monitor.

TABLE 15–2. Manual Filing System versus Electronic Database Management System

Manual Filing System	Electronic Database Management System
Rules and procedures used to file patient and laboratory data	Software for management of data
Filing cabinets	Database
File folders	Tables
Patient test report	Record

Interfaces

One of the biggest advantages of a computerized laboratory information system is its potential for decreasing errors in reported information. To make full use of this potential, laboratory information systems must be allowed to share data with the hospital information system (HIS) and with the microcomputers contained in automated analyzers. Because different computers communicate in different computer languages, they need an interpreter that will allow data to flow between them in a controlled manner. The interface, which consists of specialized software and hardware connections, acts as the interpreter. An interface between the HIS and the LIS will allow patient demographic data to be transferred from the HIS to the LIS, thus reducing the potential for error in data entry of patient information in the LIS. Laboratory testing analyzers can be interfaced to the LIS to allow direct transfer of test results into the LIS, which reduces the potential for transcription error as well as eliminating a labor intensive task of typing test results into the LIS. The LIS to HIS interface also allows test result information to flow from the LIS to HIS display monitors in patient care areas.

SYSTEM SELECTION

Shopping for a LIS can quickly become confusing and overwhelming if some homework is not done in advance. There are numerous systems from which to choose, each with its own advantages and disadvantages, so it is best to take a systematic approach to system and vendor selection. Table 15–3 lists the steps that should be taken to select the best laboratory information system for the laboratory. The following section describes each of those steps in more detail.

The first task in system selection should be to analyze the information processing needs of the laboratory. This should include considerations of both software applications, hardware and interface needs. A systematic analysis of the laboratory's workflow and its customer needs will help laboratory staff define which LIS features or options the laboratory actually requires. Input should be obtained from both laboratory personnel and customers. Some of the software applications or functions that are available in laboratory information systems on the market today are listed in Table 15–4. Careful thought should be given to how

TABLE 15–3. **Steps in Selecting a Laboratory Information System**

Analyze information processing needs.
Review LIS information sources.
Request information, price quotes, and user lists from LIS vendors.
Evaluate vendor responses.
Perform reference checks.
Conduct site visits.
Choose system and vendor.
Negotiate contract.

TABLE 15–4. LIS Functionality

User security access control	Autoverification of test results
Audit trail of actions	Test reflexing
Patient identification	Requirements of individual laboratory sections
Admission, transfer and discharge	Result inquiry
Test order entry	Result reporting
Specimen collection	Report formatting
Specimen receiving	Electronic transfer
Specimen tracking	Faxing
Specimen storage and retrieval	Quality control
Result entry	Quality assurance
Manual	Laboratory management reporting
Worklist	Billing and accounts receivable
Automated instrument	Regulatory and standards compliance
Test interpretation	

each computer function can best meet the needs of all laboratory sections. Some LIS vendors will offer additional functionality that can enhance the laboratory's services. It is equally important to consider the LIS hardware needs of the laboratory. This should include the number of peripheral devices needed such as workstations, printers, barcode readers, and data storage devices. The laboratory staff should also decide which automated analyzers and other information systems should be interfaced to the LIS.

Because there are so many laboratory information systems and vendors, a review of some information sources in this area is essential before making contact with any vendors. Fortunately, good resources are available. A good place to begin is with the College of American Pathologists monthly publication, *CAP Today.* A survey of clinical laboratory information systems is published annually in November. The survey includes a useful list of characteristics of virtually all laboratory information systems and their vendors. This information can help to narrow the field of choices. For example some systems are designed primarily for reference laboratories, and others do not have transfusion service functionality. Another information source available on a regular basis is the Lab InfoTech Summit, an annual conference focusing on information technology for the clinical laboratory. This conference features presentations, as well as many LIS exhibitors. The website for this conference (*http://www.labinfotech.org*) includes PowerPoint lectures from past conferences and links to laboratory information system vendors. Other information sources are annual meetings of the American Association of Blood Banks, American Association of Clinical Chemists, Clinical Laboratory Management Association, American Society for Clinical Pathology, and College of American Pathologists. A review of current laboratory, laboratory management, and healthcare information system literature can also provide some useful information. Review of these information sources will likely limit the number of choices to about 10 or 15 systems that can meet the needs of a particular hospital laboratory.

The next step in system selection is to request information, price quotes, and user lists from those vendors identified as most likely to meet the needs of the laboratory. To obtain accurate price quotes, a document should be prepared listing all of the laboratory's identified information processing needs including software functionality, hardware peripheral devices, interfaces to analyzers and other information systems, and data storage devices. This document should also include the current test volume and a projection of that volume over the next five years. This information is important so that the vendor can adequately size the CPU and short-term data storage capacity of the system. The vendors should be asked to describe how their systems could meet the laboratory's software requirements. Some vendors may offer to schedule an on-site demonstration of their system. These can furnish a nice overview of system functionality, but the demonstration systems will not contain the laboratory database and should be viewed with this fact in mind. The vendors should also provide a price quote including both the initial purchase cost and ongoing maintenance charges. It is also extremely important to ask the vendors to supply a list of both new and long-term customers with contact names, addresses, and/or phone numbers.

After the vendor's responses have been received, the LIS selection team should evaluate the details of the responses with the goal of eliminating those vendors who are unlikely to meet the laboratory's information processing needs. Cost will most certainly be a consideration, but system functionality should be the overriding concern. Decisions based solely on cost could result in the selection of a LIS that will ultimately cost the laboratory many more dollars in lost customers or in time spent resolving problems.

Using the vendor supplied user lists the laboratory can perform telephone reference checks with laboratories that are currently using the system. The purpose of this exercise is to determine the satisfaction level of current users. The most valuable information will probably come from users whose laboratory operations are most similar in scope and size to your own. Table 15–5 lists some questions that might be asked to determine operational similarities, as well as user satisfaction. Additional questions regarding system functionality may also provide useful information.

The information received from the vendor along with that obtained from the telephone reference checks should allow the LIS selection team to narrow the choices to three to five systems. Now the team is ready to schedule site visits to see how installed systems perform in functioning laboratories. These site visits are the most valuable mechanism for selecting the LIS that will finally be installed in the laboratory. Depending on the location of the sites to be visited, some travel expenses may be incurred. However, the visiting team should include someone from each laboratory section, some bench-level technologists, managers, and pathologists. It may also be beneficial to include someone from the hospital information systems department. Visiting team members should observe how the system is used in the host laboratory. Team members should also try to discover

TABLE 15–5.   LIS Vendor Reference Checklist

What is the scope of the laboratory's services (e.g., chemistry, hematology, outreach)?
What is the volume of testing performed?
What other information systems are interfaced to the LIS?
What automated instrument analyzers are interfaced to the LIS?
When was the LIS installed?
When did the LIS go live?
How satisfactory are the following characteristics of the support staff?
    Knowledge of the system
    Timeliness of response
    Courtesy
Is there a users group?
    How often does it meet?
    Does the vendor implement user group suggestions?
What are the best features of the system?
What are the worst features of the system?
Would you recommend the system to other laboratories? Why or why not?

how flexible the system is. In other words, did the host laboratory have to change any of its operations to fit the computer? Questions similar to those listed in Table 15–5 can also be asked to determine overall satisfaction with the system.

In some hospitals or laboratory systems, a more formal process for vendor selection may be required. This usually involves submitting a request for proposal (RFP) to the vendors under consideration. An RFP is a list of questions designed to elicit information to determine if a vendor can meet the needs of the customer. The writing of an RFP and subsequent evaluation of RFP responses can be tedious and time consuming. It is difficult to write an RFP that will cover every aspect of an LIS, and it should not be used as the sole source of information for selecting a system and vendor. Often, it is the site visits that will provide the most useful information regarding a laboratory information system.

Armed with all of the gathered information, the laboratory staff should now be able to select the one LIS that will best meet the information processing needs of the laboratory. Once the vendor is identified final contract negotiations will take place, usually with the assistance of hospital materials services staff. After the contract is signed, a date for delivery of system components can be scheduled and arrangements made with the hospital information services department to install the system.

ALLOCATION OF HUMAN RESOURCES

Before the system components are delivered to the laboratory, it is advisable to begin thinking about who will be involved in implementation. One of the biggest challenges is making sure that normal laboratory operations continue while the installation is proceeding. Laboratory personnel will have to be assigned to both the computer installation project and the regular day-to-day operations of the laboratory. A system manager should be designated to coordinate the configuration of the system and the building of definitional tables (dictionaries), and to act as a liaison between the laboratory and computer system vendor. In addition someone from each laboratory section should be assigned the responsibility of building the dictionaries for his or her particular laboratory section. These staff members, sometimes referred to as "super users," do not need an extensive knowledge of computers; but they should be familiar with the test menu, workflow, and other operations of their laboratory section. In addition, they should understand any regulatory issues relating to their specialty area; this is particularly true in the transfusion service section. The super users will be busy with database building and will not be available to perform their regular duties. If the installation is to proceed expeditiously, others must be assigned to those duties. This may involve overtime pay, increasing the hours of available part-time staff members or contracting for temporary help.

BUILDING DEFINITIONAL TABLES (DICTIONARIES)

The vendor will train the system manager and super users to build the LIS definitional tables or dictionaries. Depending on the vendor this training may be held at the vendor location and or at the customer's location. If the training is held in or near the laboratory, it is essential that the trainees be freed from all operational responsibilities during the training period. Building the dictionaries involves entering data into a definitional table template that prompts for information specific to a particular laboratory. For example the physician demographics table will include prompts for physician code, name, address, telephone number, and fax machine number. Some of the more complex tables are those that define the laboratory's testing procedures and policies. Each system will have slightly different format for definitional tables, but will require input of much the same information. Figure 15–5 illustrates a simplified version of a definitional table for a laboratory test. Most systems will require much additional information for each test to be defined. One table will have to be created for every test on the laboratory's test menu.

A table of users with assigned security levels must also be defined. This table will include the identity of every user, access codes, and a list of applications that each user will be allowed to access. Some systems require a tedious and time-consuming procedure where every user must be individually assigned the applications he or she will need. Other systems allow the creation of several security classes that can then be more quickly assigned to each user.

In addition to the test definition and user tables, many other tables will have to be defined by the laboratory staff. Even in a small laboratory, this task can take many hours and should be undertaken only by those who have an intimate understanding of the laboratory's operations, policies, and procedures.

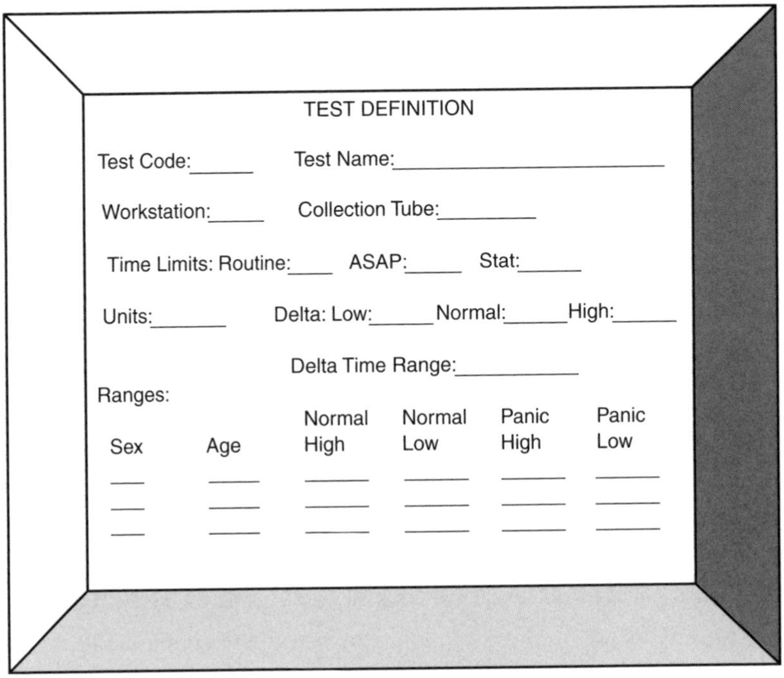

FIGURE 15–5   Sample Definitional Table (Dictionary).

Standard Operating Procedures

The introduction of a new laboratory computer system will inevitably require at least some revision to most of the existing written standard operating procedures (SOP). The computer-related tasks that are associated with technical operations can be incorporated into each technical procedure or can be written in a separate section of the procedure manual. These new procedures will be the basis for training staff in the use of the new computer system. In addition to the technical procedures, a number of LIS maintenance procedures will also be required. The subjects of these are listed in Table 15–6 and are discussed below.

Whether planned or unplanned, every computer system will temporarily cease functioning or "go down" at some time. Planned down-time may occur when the system must undergo maintenance procedures, system backup, or software and hardware upgrades. Unplanned down-time occurs when the system experiences some difficulty such as a power outage. To ensure continued laboratory operation, there must be a written procedure that addresses all tasks normally performed by, or with the assistance of, the LIS. These tasks will minimally include review of historical patient data (e.g., ABO blood group test results), recording new patient data generated during the down-time, and communication

TABLE 15–6. LIS Maintenance Procedures

Computer down-time
Hardware maintenance
Backup of software programs and data
Restoration of software programs and data
Assessment of hard disk space
Archiving data
Retrieval of archived data
Maintenance of security
Tracking and correction of errors

---

of test results. Historical data may be obtained from previously generated paper records or may be available on a personal computer where the information has been previously copied from the LIS. New data generated during down-time can be recorded on paper worksheets or forms. The procedure should also include instructions for entering such data into the LIS when the system becomes functional again.

To minimize the occurrence of unplanned down-time the LIS hardware should be properly maintained. The hardware vendor will suggest periodic cleaning, lubrication, and replacement of parts. These tasks usually require that the system be turned off for a period of time. It is best if the maintenance can be scheduled before hand so that laboratory staff can prepare for the down-time. If possible, the maintenance should be scheduled during usual periods of low activity. The SOP for this task should include the procedures that will be performed, the mechanism for notifying laboratory staff of the down-time, the frequency with which the maintenance will be performed, who will perform it, and how it will be documented.

Hardware and software failures or natural disasters such as a fire or flood can destroy all or parts of a computerized information system. With so much important patient information being stored in the laboratory computer it is essential to have a procedure for periodically copying the software programs and database to some other storage medium, such as disks or tape. This is usually referred to as a backup procedure. In the event of a catastrophe resulting in lost or corrupted software or data, the copies can be used to restore the information. The software vendor will recommend the frequency with which this backup routine should be performed based on the workload of the laboratory. The backup copies should be stored in a safe location away from the LIS so they will not be affected by a natural disaster that might befall the LIS. Another procedure for restoring the information must also be written.

The information storage capacity of the LIS is limited, and as more data are entered into the system, the hard disk will become full. This may slow down the computer response time and will have an undesirable effect on both users and other customers. Additional information storage capacity can be added to the system or old data that no longer needs to be immediately available can be transferred to long-term storage media such as magnetic tape, disks, or microfiche. A procedure for periodic assessment of hard disk space should be instituted so that data can be archived in an orderly fashion before the hard disk becomes full. Written procedures for archiving data should adhere to applicable regulatory requirements for retention of data. A procedure for retrieving the archived data must also be written so that records can be retrieved within a reasonable period to maintain patient care.

The procedure for adding users to a system, which was used in creating the user definitional table, must be written and include the basis on which security levels are assigned. For example, the list of functions or applications to which a user will have access can be created for each job description or security class. A mechanism must also be established for promptly deleting the access codes of users who leave the facility. An additional level of security can be obtained by requiring users to periodically change their passwords; many security applications can be programmed to require this at specified intervals.

Error management is required by all laboratory regulatory and accrediting agencies as part of the quality assurance program. Errors occurring in the LIS may be a result of inadequate personnel training, poor system implementation, hardware problems, or "bugs" in the software. Error management includes detection, documentation, investigation, implementation of corrective actions, and reporting to appropriate agencies. When errors are the result of poor training or system implementation, they should be corrected to prevent recurrence. When errors are caused by software problems, they must be reported to the vendor so that other users can be notified and remedies can be included in a future software revision. Error management procedures should already exist in the laboratory, but it is important to include management of computer system errors in the error management program.

SYSTEM VALIDATION

Validation is the establishment of documented evidence that provides a high degree of assurance that the system will consistently function as expected. All laboratory regulatory and accrediting bodies require some level of validation of the LIS, and laboratories that make blood products have especially stringent validation requirements imposed by the United States Food and Drug Administration (FDA). The LIS vendor is also required to validate its system, but vendors cannot simulate all the conditions under which the system will be used in every laboratory. Differences in environment, hardware, databases, standard operating procedures, and people require that each laboratory perform on-site validation testing to prove that the system will perform appropriately under those unique conditions.

The first step in validation requires the definition of a test plan. The plan should outline which computer functions will be validated and should include the testing of data entry methods, autoverification procedures, calculations on patient data, control functions, acceptance criteria, corrective action (if necessary), and final acceptance. Examples of each of these test plan components are listed in Table 15–7. The test plan will guide the next steps in validation, which are writing test scripts or cases for each function to be validated. Specific test cases are discussed in the next section. Screen printouts, written logs, or printed reports can be used to document the testing. After the testing is completed, the results should be compared with the acceptance criteria to determine acceptability. If unacceptable results are obtained, they should be investigated and corrective action implemented. When corrective action is necessary, testing should be repeated until it is found acceptable.

Validation of Software

Test cases Validation test cases should be designed to assess the system under normal situations, as well as more challenging scenarios. The goal is to ensure that the system repeatedly meets performance expectations even in the most unexpected circumstances. The test cases include step-by-step instructions to be followed by those performing the testing. The FDA and others specify five kinds of testing that should be performed. They are normal, boundary, invalid, special, and stress cases.

1. Normal testing uses typical laboratory inputs to produce routine outputs. This would include entry of test results in the normal reference ranges.
2. Boundary testing involves forcing the system to evaluate data that are slightly below or slightly above valid ranges. This kind of testing might be used to ensure that the system recognizes and appropriately flags low and high panic values for test results.

TABLE 15–7. Validation Test Plan Components

Test Plan Component	Example
Data entry methods	Keyboards, barcode readers, instrument interface, LIS or HIS interface
Autoverification procedures	Test results from interfaced instruments that can be automatically released to the patient record if they meet user defined criteria
Calculations on patient data	Test results that are generated by user defined calculations on other test results
Control functions	Decisions made by the system without human intervention (e.g., prohibiting the release of a group A red blood cell component to a group O patient)
Acceptance criteria	The expected LIS outputs that will prove the system is functioning properly
Corrective action	Actions taken when acceptance criteria are not met
Final acceptance	An approval statement indicating that acceptance criteria have been met

3. Invalid test cases assess the system's ability to recognize and reject inputs that are absurd or of the wrong data type. Invalid inputs might include entry of alpha characters when numerical values are required or entry of a blood product code that has not been defined in the definitional database table.

4. Special cases are those that make the system react to unusual inputs. A special case could be designed to ensure that the system will not allow more than one person to edit or add information to a particular patient file at the same time.

5. Stress testing involves pushing the system to its physical limits. This might be accomplished by allowing large volumes of data to be entered into the system via all available input devices.

Not every type of test case may be appropriate for each function to be tested. For example, boundary test cases will not be applicable in test result functions where the results are either simply positive or negative. Validation of the LIS is a lengthy and labor intensive process, but it provides great benefits if undertaken in a thorough manner. Extensive testing will identify potential problems in the way that the laboratory intends to use the system. Sometimes workarounds will have to be created, but when done as part of validation testing, staff can be properly trained before going live on the new system or software.

Validation testing must be performed before a new system can be implemented and whenever new software, databases, or hardware is added to the system. When validation is to be performed on an existing system, the testing should be done in the test database where it will not affect the production data.

TRAINING AND COMPETENCY ASSESSMENT

The introduction of a new laboratory computer will undoubtedly cause some anxiety in the laboratory staff. They will be confronted with many changes in the way they perform their daily operations. A well-designed and comprehensive training program can help allay these fears and reduce the number of problems that will inevitably arise when the system goes live. Training modules can be designed that will present users with the situations they will encounter in their work. They should address every function and procedure that each user will be expected to perform in both normal and unusual situations. The trainers will not be able to anticipate every exceptional situation, but staff must be able to cancel orders, correct errors, document unusual specimens, and appropriately manage atypical results. One might be able to borrow some of the test cases used in validation to present staff with many of the different operations they will have to perform in the new LIS. The training program must include documentation of competence before any staff member can be allowed to use the computer system for actual laboratory work. A convenient way to do this is to ask trainees to print the results of each operation in the training modules. Appropriate personnel can then review these documents to assess competence. Competence assessment methods can also include direct observations and written examinations.

Training of other hospital staff members should also be considered. Significant changes in the way laboratory customers will submit specimens, order tests, or receive reports or blood components should be the subject of some training activity.

GO LIVE

When all of the previously discussed implementation steps have been completed, it is finally time to start using, or go live on, the new LIS. Careful consideration should be given to the day and time that this event will occur. For example it may be wise to select a time of day when the laboratory is not normally besieged with large numbers of specimens from phlebotomy rounds. Also, if the laboratory usually experiences a high testing volume on particular days of the week, those days should be avoided when going live on the new system.

Some facilities will elect to undergo a period of parallel testing. This involves using both the old information system and the new information system at the same time. The disadvantage to this is that all work must be completed in both systems. Even so, parallel testing may offer some level of comfort to the staff who can rely on the old system if they experience problems with the new one.

It is prudent to notify all laboratory customers of the go-live date so that they may be prepared for any unanticipated problems that may arise when the new system is first placed in routine use.

SUMMARY

Selection and implementation of a computer-based laboratory information system require extensive planning and resources. When each phase of implementation is thoughtfully and thoroughly carried out, the laboratory can derive full benefit from this valuable tool for information processing.

SUGGESTED PROBLEM-BASED LEARNING ACTIVITIES

Chapter 15: Computer-Based Laboratory Information System

Instructions: Use Internet resources, books, articles, colleagues, etc., to present solutions to the problems listed below. There is no one correct solution to any problem.

Note to Instructor: Students in class may be divided into groups and given the problem-based learning activity to discuss and solve. Once the group has reached consensus as to a solution, the group may present it to the other students in the class. This activity will provide all students with information regarding solutions to the problem.

Problem #1
Suppose you are in the process of implementing a new laboratory information system (LIS). Create a plan of action and specify the tasks and individuals in your work team to provide information for the process.

Problem #2
Prepare a validation test plan for the following LIS functions: (1) Test Order Entry; (2) Specimen Collection; and (3) Specimen Receiving. Remember to include appropriate test cases for each function.

Problem #3
Research the possibilities of LIS vendors and prepare a chart itemizing the pros and cons of each. How do you make your ultimate decision?

BIBLIOGRAPHY

Aller RD, Balis UJ: Informatics, imaging, and the pathologists' workstation. In Henry JB: *Clinical diagnosis and management by laboratory methods*, ed. 20. Philadelphia, 2001, WB Saunders.

Bersch C: Laboratory information systems continue to add features that contribute to maximizing personnel and cost containment. MLO, 2003; 35(1): 36–42.

Cooper S: Laboratory information systems. In Lehmann CA: *Saunders manual of clinical laboratory science*, Philadelphia, 1998, WB Saunders.

Cowan DF (Ed.): Informatics for the clinical laboratory. New York, 2003, Springer-Verlag.

Elevitch FR: Computers in the clinical laboratory. In Burtis CA, Ashwood ER: *Tietz fundamentals of clinical chemistry*, ed 5. Philadelphia, 2001, WB Saunders.

Fowler DG: Basic concepts of a database management system. *Clin Lab Sci*, 1999; 12(3): 174–77.

NCCLS: *Laboratory instruments and data management systems: design of software user interfaces and end-use software systems validation, operation, and monitoring: approved guideline.* CLST Document GP19-A2, Wayne, PA., 2003, CLSI.

Svirbely JR et al: Computers and laboratory information systems. In Snyder JR, Wilkinson DS, *Management in Laboratory Medicine*, ed 3. Philadelphia, 1998, JB Lippincott Co.

U.S. Food and Drug Administration, Center for Devices and Radiological Health, Center for Biologics Evaluation and Research: General principles of software validation; Final guidance for industry and FDA staff. Document no. 938, January 11, 2002.

Valenstein P, Walsh M: Six-year trends in laboratory computer availability. *Arch Pathol Lab Med* 2003; 127:157–161.

Internet Resources

Aller RD: For some, newer and slicker means trouble quicker: Why labs should think twice before replacing an older but solid laboratory information system.

CAP Today. November 2004. [On-Line]. Available:
http://www.cap.org/apps/docs/cap_today/feature_stories/1104LISsystems.html

Computers and Their Applications for Medical Professionals Florida Anesthesia Computer and Engineering Team
http://www.anest.ufl.edu/computer

Friedman BA: New clinical lab products and services enabled by the web. March 2004. [On-Line]. Available:
http://www.labinfotech.org/LIS2006/Presentations2004/LIS_2004_friedman_lecture_files/frame.htm

Lab InfoTech Summit website
http://www.labinfotech.org.
Contains links to many laboratory information system vendor websites.

Rogoski R: LIS and the enterprise. Health Management Technology. February 2003. [On-Line]. Available:
http://www.healthmgttech.com.
Click on the Archives tab.

The Free On-line Dictionary of Computing Editor Dennis Howe
http://foldoc. doc.ic.ac.uk

Weiner H: System review series: Change-the biggest constant in the LIS market-place. CAP Today. November 2004. [On-Line]. Available:
http://www.cap.org/apps/docs/cap_today/surveys/1104_LISSurvey.pdf

Weiner H: The decline of the classic LIS: technical and strategic considera-tions. March 2005. [On-Line]. Available:
http://www.labinfotech.org/LIS2006/Presentations2005/Weiner_Las_Vegas_2005_files/frame.htm

Marketing Concepts

MICHAEL E. KURTZ, MS, MBA
BRIAN N. LENZ, MT(ASCP)

Chapter Outline

Objectives

Following successful completion of this chapter, the learner will be able to:

1. Define marketing and explain its role in the clinical laboratory.
2. List the elements of the marketing mix.
3. Identify and explain the elements of the marketing environment.

4. Identify steps in the marketing analysis process.
5. Analyze effective business strategies for a laboratory operation.
6. Develop and implement a marketing plan.

Key Terms

Five Forces Analysis
Market Analysis
Market Demand
Market Segmentation
Marketing
Marketing Concept

Marketing Environment
Marketing Mix
Marketing Plan
Marketing Research
Niching
SWOT Analysis

Case Study: Marketing Concepts

Laboratory Services, LLC., is a provider of specialty laboratory services to the medical, diagnostic, and pharmaceutical industry. As a result of an aggressive local marketing campaign, the laboratory has experienced double digit growth in each of the last 5 years. The rate of growth has begun to slow, and the number of potential new clients is limited. Your hospital administration expects a 15% increase in laboratory revenue during the next year. The laboratory manager and staff agree that there is excess capacity of labor and technology. The planning team decides to expand from a local laboratory operation to a national operation. As marketing manager you must develop a marketing plan to achieve the organizational goals.

Issues and Questions to Consider

1. *List possible causes of the market decline experienced by the laboratory.*
2. *What would you use to determine the root cause of the market decline?*
3. *What kind of pricing strategy would you use?*
4. *What promotional activities may assist you in reaching your goals?*

INTRODUCTION

In this age of information, consumers of healthcare have exceptionally high expectations. If we are sick we go to the doctor and expect him to fix it. If he can't, we expect him to send us to a specialist who can. And we want the full range of medical services available to us regardless of our ability to pay. Thus, the post-modern laboratory is a far different place as a result of the changes in the needs and expectations of patients and physicians.

Driven by economic necessity and technologic advances, the physician demands a higher level of accuracy from laboratory tests and better service than in the past. Patients subjected to advertising and media blitzes and who have access to the Internet are more aware of laboratory capabilities and more demanding in their expectations.

The current healthcare market environment, including the regulatory environment, the development of large integrated delivery networks, and the advent of managed care organizations, has placed additional cost pressures on laboratories. The hospital laboratory, once a significant source of revenue for the institution, is now faced with the consumer and physician demanding higher quality while the government is reimbursing laboratories less for Medicare patients. The large integrated delivery networks are increasingly demanding cost reductions, and managed care organizations are pressuring laboratories to lower fees for service.

Hospital laboratories that attempt to exist on in-patient revenues alone are doomed to a downward spiral of reducing staff and services at the same time that physicians and patients are demanding more and better services. Because laboratories have a high fixed cost structure and are capital intensive, the result is operational losses.

Faced with these pressures, laboratories have to increase revenues or face being downsized, out-sourced, or shutdown completely. In fact, many large integrated delivery networks have outsourced this function.

To lower costs, hospital administrators are shortening the length of stay. As a result, more illnesses are being treated on an outpatient basis. Thus the only source of increased testing volumes comes from outside the hospital.

Because of this new paradigm in healthcare, laboratory managers must be skilled practitioners in marketing and business planning. These skills can assist managers in increasing volume, controlling costs, and increasing profit. Managers with these skills can improve quality and add value because they know how to provide superior service and develop innovative strategies.

This chapter covers basic marketing concepts and explores ways to incorporate them into strategic business planning in the laboratory.

MARKETING CONCEPTS

Businesses today operate using different philosophies or tenets. What philosophy or tenet they choose may be directly related to their industry, market, or product.

A business philosophy held by many modern companies is called the *marketing concept.* This philosophy holds as its central tenet that the key to achieving the goals of the organization consists of being more effective than the competition in satisfying the needs, wants, and demands of the customer. Thus, the primary focus of a marketing-oriented organization is the customer. Successful companies applying the marketing concept integrate customer needs into their marketing program and increase profit by improving customer satisfaction. Every aspect of their operation has as its single purpose, value delivery to the customer. The organizational structure of this type of organization would appear as a triangle with the customer at the top (Figure 16–1). This type of organization is exemplified in the mission statement of Southwest Airlines "The mission of Southwest Airlines is dedication to the highest quality of Customer Service

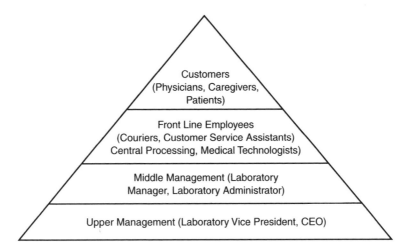

FIGURE 16–1 Organizational Structure of a Marketing Oriented Laboratory Business. In a marketing oriented laboratory, customers are represented at the top of an organizational chart represented by a triangle. All marketing decisions flow from the customer rather than the product or sales teams. Employees that directly interact with the customer are higher on the chart than upper management who may have no direct contact with the customer.

delivered with a sense of warmth, friendliness, individual pride, and Company Spirit."

This more recent business philosophy is the **production concept.** According to this concept, customers will buy goods produced in adequate volume at a low enough price. An example is the Texas Instrument Company that sells calculators.

The **sales concept** entails factory products sold by aggressive selling and promotion. These types of companies such as General Motors profit by selling high volumes of cars. They frequently use sales incentives such as rebates and premiums.

Marketing in a company employing the marketing concept can be defined as a process by which individuals and groups obtain what they want through creating, offering, and exchanging products or services of value with others. All the activities associated with providing the means by which buyers can purchase a product or service and the process of inducing them to do so are marketing activities. Even though marketing is a business function as is financing, human resources, or research and development, it does not take place within the confines of a marketing department. Rather, it entails every activity a company does, from product conception until the product wears out or is consumed.

This exchange of goods and services for something of value takes place in a **market.** A market is a web of interactions among those who have commercial relationships or the potential for such relationships with other buyers and sellers of similar commodities. All the potential customers sharing a particular need or want who might be willing and able to exchange something of value to satisfy that need or want make up a market. A market may be defined mathematically as M=qnp, where q equals the average quantity purchased, n equals the number of consumers and p equals the average price paid for a product or service. A market does not belong to the company but is external. Abundant markets exist. Californians, teenagers, homemakers, outdoorsman, women, teachers, train hobbyists, hospitals, and laboratories are all examples of markets. People over 50 years old make up one of the fastest growing markets. Markets exist for goods and services, for money and credit, for communication and technology services, and for information.

Market segmentation allows the marketing manager to break up markets into smaller more manageable pieces. This is possible because occupants of the market have similar wants, needs, and demands. They also respond similarly to market stimuli such as advertising and distribution. A plastic surgeon and a neurosurgeon are both surgeons; but the plastic surgeon's preferences may not be shared by the neurosurgeon. Teenagers and senior citizens both share a need for clothing; however, their preferences for certain styles may be quite different. Market segmentation is a legitimate business strategy used by companies to create a competitive advantage. Focusing on a specific subsection of a market is a strategy called *niching.* Saint Louis University Coagulation Consultants is a specialty laboratory that provides only testing for the diagnosis and management of patients with bleeding and thrombotic disorders. Southwest Airlines is the only short haul, low fare, high frequency, point-to-point airline. A teenager is more likely to shop at Old Navy than at Lord and Taylor's.

THE MARKETING MIX

The role of marketing in an organization is to achieve its strategic objective by deciding who will sell what, where, to whom, in what quantity, and how. The set of tools that the firm uses to pursue their marketing objectives is referred to as the *marketing mix.* This includes product, price, place, and promotion (Table 16–1).

Product

Product is what the firm offers to the public for sale. This would include the product quality, brand, packaging, features, or service options. It also includes delivery, training, warranty, repair, and other value-added product or service options, which would provide a competitive advantage to the firm. Product or service is the cornerstone of the marketing mix. Companies using the marketing concept view product as a solution to a customer's need. Different laboratories may emphasize different products. A specialty laboratory may only offer microbiology, coagulation, blood banking, or toxicology. Another may emphasize routine testing requiring a fast turn-around-time. Still others may concentrate on services that provide interpretation of laboratory results and advice on the medical management of patients that receive laboratory testing.

TABLE 16–1. The Marketing Mix

Product: *what the firm offers to the public for sale.*
Includes product quality, brand, packaging, features or service options, delivery, training, warranty, repair and other value added product or service options which would provide a competitive advantage to the firm.
Price: *the amount of money a customer pays for a product or service.*
Pricing options include selling wholesale or retail, offering discounts, sales, and credit.
Place: *how and where the product is offered to the buying public.*
Includes warehousing, distribution, and retail or wholesale outlets and the Internet.
Promotion: *the means by which a company communicates and promotes its products to its target market.*
Includes sales and marketing personnel, advertising, public relations, direct marketing, telemarketing, and on-line marketing.

Price

Critical to the marketing mix is **price.** This is the amount of money a customer pays for a product or service. Pricing options include selling wholesale or retail, offering discounts, sales, and credit. Price is part of the total marketing package offered to the customer referred to as **value.** If a customer perceives the price as higher than the value received in purchasing the service or product, the customer will either buy a substitute product from another supplier or will forego purchase of the product. Laboratories may offer discounts to client accounts because they do not incur the cost of billing the patient.

The laboratory market environment today is almost totally cost-driven and may dictate a pricing strategy based on matching the competition's price. Products or services that are purchased strictly on the basis of price are called commodities. As healthcare becomes more cost-driven, laboratory testing is increasingly viewed as a commodity, or basic material or good, instead of something of higher value, by hospital administrators who search for low-cost solutions with little consideration to the value of laboratory testing.

Pricing strategy may also be determined by the profit margin imposed on the laboratory by hospital administration. Other laboratories may determine price on a cost plus basis. They determine how much it costs to perform the test and add a percentage to cover overhead expenses and profit. Using price as a competitive weapon is risky because it could lead to a price war.

The purchase of a product or service may be value driven rather than price driven. A department store such as Nieman-Marcus may offer the same quality product of another department store, but the name and personal service provide the perception of increased value to the customer who is willing to pay a higher price.

Place

Place is how and where the product is offered to the buying public. It is difficult to walk in any building and not encounter either a Coca-Cola or a Pepsi vending machine. Most companies now offer their products via the Internet. Place also includes the use of marketing to make its product available to its customers. This also includes warehousing, distribution and retail, or wholesale outlets. Many hospital laboratories will choose to market only in their local area, whereas others may have regional, national, or even global market interests. Most large commercial laboratories have located phlebotomy stations in physician offices for the convenience of the patient, and some physician's offices have even placed laboratories in their office suites. Place includes how laboratory results are transmitted to the customers. Many laboratories have direct electronic or web-based computer links to their client's laboratory information systems (LIS) or physician office practice management systems. These links allow the electronic exchange of patient demographic information, test orders, and test results between information systems. This benefits the client by eliminating duplicate and manual data entry, decreasing transcription errors and personnel time involved with reference laboratory/client transactions. Most reference laboratories also have their test directories and other user information available on-line or on compact discs.

Promotion

The means by which a company communicates and promotes its products to its target market is called **promotion.** This includes sales and marketing personnel, advertising, public relations, direct marketing, telemarketing, and on-line marketing. Many promotional channels exist for laboratory services. Numerous national publications such as the Clinical Leadership and Management Review, Medical Laboratory Observer, CAP Today, or Advance for Laboratory Administrators are available. This kind of exposure requires an ample marketing budget. Less expensive solutions for laboratories serving only a local market include local business newspapers or publications of the local medical society. A web page provides ample market coverage, can be changed rapidly, and is relatively inexpensive. Desk top software such as Microsoft Frontpage or Macromedia Contribute, can help the novice produce an informational website for around $400.00. A professional website design company can produce a site that includes client functionality and interactivity for under $3000.000. Client communiqués such as test updates, new tests announcements, or laboratory service brochures can often be produced on the desktop inexpensively and can be direct-mailed or e-mailed to the customer. These same documents can double as a marketing tool by laboratory sales staff during client visits.

An excellent and inexpensive way to promote laboratory services is to provide customers with continuing education opportunities. Because travel and education budgets in laboratories are disappearing, a laboratory can add value to its product by solving this problem for clients. This can be in the form of local seminars, providing speakers to client hospitals or laboratories, producing an educational newsletter, or posting educational material on-line. Many professional organizations such as the Clinical Laboratory Management Association or the American Society of Clinical Pathology offer onsite continuing education teleconferences which can be offered to clientele.

Promotional approaches should be linked to what products and what approach is the most consistent with the total marketing strategy. The laboratory-marketing manager should interact with the marketing personnel from the hospital to make sure that the laboratory strategy does not conflict with the overall strategy.

To meet business objectives each element of the marketing mix must be consistent and complement the overall business strategy of the organization.

THE MARKETING ENVIRONMENT

Markets exist in a *marketing environment.* A successful company recognizes the needs and wants of its customers. It keeps a close eye on trends that may provide the company with opportunities to expand its markets. John Naisbit refers to these opportunities as megatrends or economic social, political, and environmental changes that influence the environment for a long time. Factors that influence the marketing and business planning of a company include demographics of the market occupants; the existing economic climate; political, legal, and societal structures; available technologies; and natural resources.

Demographic Environment

People make up markets. Therefore, demographic information is vital to the success of any marketing program. Population numbers stratified by age and gender, educational levels, ethnic backgrounds, and growth rates are all aspects of the **demographic environment.** The graying of American baby boomers has created healthcare market demands as well as significant opportunities. The travel and leisure industry has responded to this market demand. Choice Hotels has created its Prime Pricing program for people over 50 and offers them a 30% discount. Numerous healthcare plans such as MC (Medicare) Plus have been aimed at the Medicare eligible health consumer.

Economic Environment

The people that make up a market cannot buy products or services without purchasing power. This can be affected by elements of the **economic environment.** Savings rate, debt load, interest rates, money supply, inflation, availability of credit, and employment levels all can have tremendous impact on the amount of disposable income or money available to purchase products. If interest rates are high, sales of automobiles, boats, and houses all decrease. If interest rates are low and credit is available, sales of these items increase.

Political and Legal Environment

The **political and legal environment** can dramatically and quickly affect business. Legislation regulating business has steadily increased. Laws governing pollutants, advertising, business practices, and employer-employee relations have proliferated. Larger companies employ full-time lobbyists to favorably impact legislation in their favor. Rulings by regulatory bodies such as the Food and Drug Administration and the Federal Trade Commission can significantly impact the way companies conduct business. Recently, lawsuits against tobacco companies and gun manufacturers have produced large product liability settlements. The threat of legislation requiring small businesses to offer healthcare to all employees, along with other burdensome regulations, threatens their well-being and discourages entrepreneurs from venturing into the marketplace.

The government has not ignored the laboratory industry. The Clinical Laboratory Improvement Act of 1988 (CLIA 88), administered by the Department of Health and Human Services, mandated laboratory practice changes. Its purpose, which was to ensure quality laboratory testing, has placed demands on clinical laboratories. These regulations can be found in the Code of Federal Regulations Section 353 of Chapter 42. The Occupational Health and Safety Administration (OSHA) implemented new blood-borne pathogen standards in 1993. In 1996, the Centers for Medicare and Medicaid Services (formerly the Health Care Financing Administration) issued guidelines requiring medical necessity documentation for laboratory tests billed to Medicare. These guidelines continue to evolve and impact laboratory management functions. The Stark Ban, named after Peter Stark, chair of the Subcommittee on Health of the House Ways and Means Committee, prohibits self-referral of laboratory testing to physician owned laboratories. More recently, the Health Insurance Portability and Acceptability Act (HIPAA) will have a huge impact on healthcare providers including laboratories. Direct billing initiatives passed by some state legislatures, reflect the recent national trend to eliminate the client billing arrangement. A client bill relationship is generally described as a monthly itemized statement of account, paid in full by the client within 90 days. Direct billing legislation, if passed into law, will impact the business plans of every laboratory outreach program, especially those laboratories who's business plans center around deep discount pricing rather than enhanced service.

Technological Environment

Today's firms spend a large percentage of their revenues on research and development. The rapid pace by which technology changes has necessitated large expenditures to gain or maintain competitive advantage. Success in the **technological environment** plays a key role in the success of a firm. New markets exist in communications for cellular phones, satellite television, and global positioning devices. The advent of DNA technology has opened markets in agriculture for genetically modified seeds and in the pharmaceutical industry in the development of new drugs, and has expanded product lines in laboratories with new test development to diagnose and monitor genetic abnormalities. It is estimated that as a result of the mapping of the human genome, tens of thousands of new drugs may be marketed in the next 5 to 10 years.

Natural Environment

The **natural environment** affects companies. They need access to raw materials and available energy supplies to manufacture their products. These aspects of the natural environment can fluctuate. Oil prices increased from $2.23 a barrel in 1970 to $34.00 a barrel in 1982. The big three American automakers, with their gas guzzling big cars, lost significant market share to Japanese automakers that responded to the market with smaller more fuel-efficient autos. A shortage of wood has caused prices of new homes to rise resulting in a decrease in new home sales.

MARKETING RESEARCH

Marketing research is a crucial part of a marketing program. It is a technical and systematic approach to obtain data relevant to a specific market. It may be defined as a systematic design, collection, analysis, and reporting of data and findings relevant to a specific marketing situation. For example, a community hospital located in a metropolitan area wants to place a billboard along a highway leading into town. It hires a market research firm to investigate whether or not the cost of placing the billboard will exceed the benefits. The marketing research firm will determine what market to target, what services to advertise, where and when to place the billboard, and what the results of the advertising campaign achieved.

Sources of market research information are abundant. Syndicated research firms such as A.C. Nielson gather consumer and trade information and make this information available for a fee. Marketing research firms such as Maritz Market Research operate on a contract basis and participate in the design, collection, and reporting of data to a firm's marketing department. Market researchers can provide specialized research such as going into the field and collecting data through interviews, focus groups, and market surveys. The laboratory diagnostic equipment manufacturers conduct numerous focus groups as part of their design and build process.

A typical company may budget 1% to 2% of annual sales to market research. For smaller companies this may be much less. For a typical hospital laboratory, a budget line for market research may be nonexistent.

However, it is possible to collect useful information from a variety of alternate sources. Internal publications such as the balance sheet, income statement, customer lists, and other hospital or laboratory records are sources of marketing information. Government publications such as the US Industrial Outlook, Statistical Abstracts, and County and City Data Book are available at any public library. Other government organizations including the US Chamber of Commerce can provide useful information. Trade associations or professional organizations such as the College of American Pathologists, American Society of Clinical Chemistry, American Clinical Laboratory Association, American Hospital Association, and the Medical Group Practice Management Association conduct studies and make them available without cost to their membership. The Washington G-2 Report,

Modern Healthcare, and the Healthcare Trends Report provide updates on trends and current opportunities in healthcare.

The marketing research process begins by identifying a problem and developing the research plan and methodology. Data are then collected and analyzed. The process culminates with a final report and presentation describing the findings.

This scenario can be played out as follows. The laboratory outreach business in a hospital laboratory has declined by 25% over the last 6 months. The hospital vice president in charge of the laboratory asks the laboratory administrator to explain the variance for budgeted revenue. The laboratory administrator in turn assigns the laboratory-marketing manager to look into this situation. The laboratory-marketing manager develops a market research plan. A customer survey is constructed and mailed to all laboratory customers who have sent specimens for testing to the laboratory within the past two years. The survey reveals that a price increase at the beginning of the current fiscal year has changed the market positioning of the laboratory and revealed that they are no longer the low-cost supplier in this market. The results are presented to the laboratory administrator who decides to lower testing prices to maintain the laboratory's competitive position. Three months after prices are lowered, 5% of the lost market share has been regained.

MARKET ANALYSIS

The basic marketing concepts discussed here must be integrated into a marketing plan developed in the context of the organization's overall business strategy. This is accomplished by a continuous process of analyzing market opportunities, known as *market analysis,* developing a marketing strategy, planning and implementing the plan, and revising the plan by responding to market forces. This cycle, if successful, leads to improved products, added value to the customer, and higher sales and profits for the company (Figure 16–2).

Market Demand

An analysis of market opportunities should begin by an assessment of the *market demand.* For a laboratory, this would be the total number of laboratory tests performed in a particular market. For example, the number of physician offices plus the average number of tests performed per patient visit plus number of patient visits constitutes the market demand for laboratory testing from physician offices. Other market segments may include nursing homes, skilled nursing facilities, hospital laboratories, industrial clients, or government facilities. The total market demand would represent the sum of these individual market segments.

If sufficient demand is present, assessment must be made of how much of this total market demand the organization desires to capture. If the market demand is 1 million laboratory tests and a 30% share of the market is desired, you must have the capacity to do 300,000 laboratory tests. How much you capture may be a direct result of how many resources the organization is willing to expend and how aggressively this market opportunity is pursued.

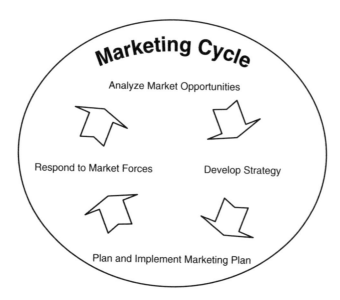

FIGURE 16–2 The Marketing Cycle. The marketing process is a continuous cycle because market forces and the market environment are changing continually. Revisions to the marketing plan are made in response to these changes.

SWOT Analysis

Decisions to pursue marketing opportunities are determined by analyzing factors internal and external to the company. Internal factors include identification of the company specific (S)trengths and (W)eaknesses and external factors include identification of industry specific (O)pportunities and (T)hreats. This process is often referred to as a *SWOT analysis.*

Five Forces Analysis

Michael Porter has expanded this model to include the personal values of the key implementers as an internal factor. For example, in a laboratory that is trying to start an outreach program, it is important to establish that hospital management, key in the implementation of a marketing program, understands the goals and objectives of the marketing plan because their buy-in is essential to the program's success.

Porter also developed the *five forces analysis* model as a framework for analyzing external opportunities and threats. These five forces are the bargaining power of suppliers, the bargaining power of buyers, the threat of new entrants, the threat of substitute products, and the rivalry among existing firms (Figure 16–3).

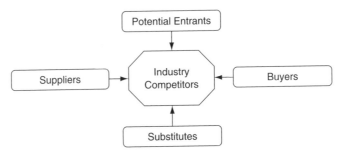

FIGURE 16–3   Porter's Five Forces Model. Michael Porter of the Harvard Business School developed this model to analyze the competitive environment that exists external to a company by considering five forces depicted above.

For example, in a particular local market there may be five community hospitals all with laboratories, two of which have outreach programs. In addition, there are three commercial laboratories doing business there. Now suppose a community hospital with no outreach program desires to share in this market.

The business or marketing manager analyzes the five forces. In this case, the threat of substitute products is a strong force because the physician's office has several choices of laboratory testing suppliers. This weakens the laboratory testing supplier's ability to raise prices. The threat of new entrants is probably low owing to the large number of suppliers already in this particular market, and the bargaining power of buyers is strong because of the number of suppliers. The business manager concludes that the ability of an outreach program to control pricing and earn profits is limited in this market and decides not to invest in an outreach program.

DEVELOPING MARKETING STRATEGIES

Porter identified three generic business strategies for dealing with the five forces: cost leadership, product differentiation, and focus. Cost leadership requires tight cost control, efficiencies of scale, and a structured organization. Product or service differentiation requires a strong research and development function, skilled marketing, and highly skilled labor. The focus strategy is a combination of both cost leadership and differentiation.

Other models of industry and competitor analysis have been developed. A well-known model is the growth share matrix developed by the Boston Consulting Group. This model describes a scenario in which an industry's growth and a firm's market share are proxies for competitive position and cash flow required for operating. The matrix is divided into stars (modest growth/positive cash flow), question marks, (high growth/negative cash flow), cash cows (low

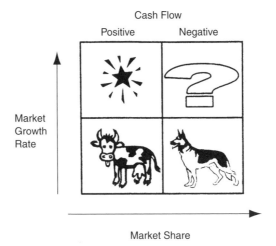

Cash Flow

Positive Negative

Market Growth Rate

Market Share

FIGURE 16–4 Boston Consulting Group Market Model. The Boston Consulting Group model was developed to assist business to analyze their competitive position in the market.

growth/large positive cash flow), and dogs (low growth/negative cash flow). This model has limitations because of many underlying assumptions and conditions imposed on the model (Figure 16–4).

Regardless of the model, a competitive strategy that fails to produce a competitive advantage is a failure. The Gap has broadly outperformed J.C. Penny on a consistent basis. What resources, capabilities, or distinct competencies does the Gap have that J.C. Penney does not? Should J.C. Penney reengineer their competitive strategy? The Gap has built a competitive advantage and created more customer value that is positively reflected in profit and growth.

Michael Porter described the process of creating customer value as a chain. This **value chain** has four levels of support activity, the horizontal links in the chain, placed on top of the primary activities of a firm represented by the vertical links of the chain. The support activities include firm infrastructure, human resource function, technology, and materials management. Primary activities include inbound and outbound logistics, operations, marketing/sales and customer service. Both vertical and horizontal links in the chain lead to increasing profit margin (Figure 16–5).

Laboratory inbound logistics apply to getting the specimen into the laboratory. The decision to contract courier service or provide that as an in-house function or even at all can have an effect on customer perceived value. Are the couriers polite? Do they provide "knock your socks off" service? Are they on time? Are they professional?

Operational activities are all the preanalytical and analytical variables intrinsic in laboratory testing. Attention to detail in your QA program, selection of

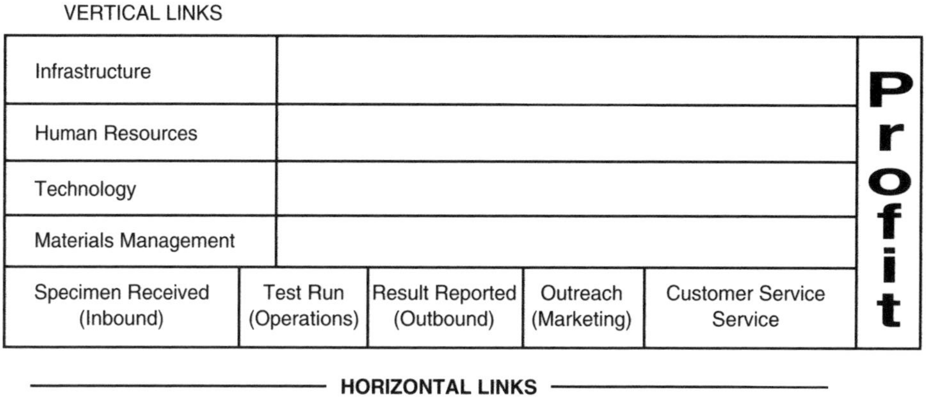

VERTICAL LINKS

		P
Infrastructure		
Human Resources		r
Technology		o
Materials Management		f
Specimen Received (Inbound)	Test Run (Operations)	Result Reported (Outbound)	Outreach (Marketing)	Customer Service Service	i t

──────── HORIZONTAL LINKS ────────

FIGURE 16–5 The Customer Value Chain. Horizontal links represent company-wide support activities. Vertical links represent primary activities of a company.

instrumentation, methodology, or suppliers can add or detract value to the product or service.

Outbound logistics or putting the results in the hands of the customer is where many laboratories fail. The processing department and medical technologist/clinical laboratory scientist can turn out a result, but it means nothing until a physician reads the result. Creating value is a team effort. Marketing/sales and customer service are vital links in the chain. Most laboratories are adept at finding new business but are not adept at providing good customer service.

Value creation can also be defined mathematically as Value-Cost (V-C). A company is profitable if the value of a product or service to a customer is greater than the cost. Companies can create greater profit by lowering costs or increasing value.

Laboratory tests account for more than 50% of the objective data used to diagnose and treat disease but represent only 3% to 5% of the average total charge for inpatient admissions (<3% for patients admitted for surgery, invasive procedures, or who are treated in the ICU). Thus, laboratory tests are the most cost-efficient source of objective medical data. The value of a laboratory test to a hospital or patient is greater than the cost to them. Results of inexpensive clinical laboratory tests are frequently used to determine the need for more expensive diagnostic procedures or to guide the selection of expensive therapeutic options. Accordingly, the costs for performing clinical laboratory tests are more than offset by the savings generated by efficient resource allocation. For example, a patient presents in the emergency department with chest pain. A cardiac troponin is ordered. The result is negative. The patient is given a consult for risk factor modification such as diet and exercise. The total cost of the consult was $200. Without the negative test result, the patient may have undergone a stress test and/or cardiac ECHO (cost $800 to $1800). The price of the troponin assay was $25. The value was above $800. The total value to the hospital of the cardiac troponin assay was $775 ($800–$25) even though this number is not accounted for in the hospital accounting system.

The basic building blocks of competitive advantage are elements that either raise value or lower costs. These are superior quality ($\uparrow$V), superior efficiency ($\downarrow$C), superior customer service ($\uparrow$V), or superior innovation ($\uparrow$V).

Healthcare consumers today consider superior quality a given. A physician with a laboratory result that does not match a clinical picture will begin to question the integrity of the laboratory result. Providing superior quality means building in quality to prevent errors beginning with specimen referral until the physician releases the patient from care. Mislabeled, lost, or damaged specimens and errors in result reporting are among common errors that separate high-quality laboratories from laboratories that provide superior quality.

Superior efficiency can lower costs and increase profit. Being able to provide batch testing while maintaining competitive turnaround time is an example of superior efficiency.

Saint Louis University Coagulation Consultants is a specialty coagulation laboratory that provides a written interpretation and recommendations for further investigation and/or patient management. In addition, consultation is available on a 24-hour basis from hematologists with special expertise and experience in the laboratory diagnosis and management of patients with bleeding disorders and thrombosis. This is provided at no additional cost to the customer and adds product value.

Expanding test menus; keeping up with the latest available technology; and finding new and innovative ways to meet the customer's needs, wants, and demands increase value. When value exceeds price the customer is induced to buy. When price exceeds value the customer will find a substitute product.

PUTTING IT ALL TOGETHER: THE MARKETING PLAN

The market analysis and strategic plan are synthesized into a written marketing plan. A *marketing plan* is an action plan or a roadmap to guide the company from one place to the next. It describes products or services and their benefits and features, target markets and its buying habits, competing products or services, and the customer problem that the product or service solves.

The plan contains the goals and objectives of the program. Goals specify the necessary levels of achievement, and objectives are the specific actions taken to achieve the goals. The marketing objectives should lead to sales. They should be distinct and measurable and have a time limit for accomplishment. If the plan has multiple objectives, the objectives should be consistent and not in conflict with each other. All parts of your marketing plan should support these objectives.

In addition to the market analysis and product or business strategy, the plan should include the marketing and sales strategy, distribution channels, and advertising and promotional plans using the concepts of the marketing mix. It should also contain a realistic budget detailing the cost of implementing the plan.

It is important to remember that market fundamentals in place when the plan was written may change. A contingency planning component based on assumptions may be important in a volatile healthcare atmosphere that exists today.

Finally, the plan should contain or reference the mission and vision of the organization. Vision describes where the business is headed and how the business gets to where it is headed is referred to as mission. Mission statements are developed to share with managers, employees, and customers and to provide a shared sense of purpose and direction.

SUMMARY

Today's healthcare environment demands a new skill set among laboratory professionals. Successful managers will need to understand basic business concepts such as marketing and finance. Knowledge and expertise in analyzing marketing opportunities and developing business strategies is essential to adding value for purchasers of laboratory services. Quantitating this value in terms of increased business, lower operating costs, increased revenue, and higher profit is essential to create buy-in from hospital administrators, managed care companies, and third-party payers whose buying power you are trying to attract.

SUGGESTED PROBLEM-BASED LEARNING ACTIVITIES
Chapter 16: Marketing Concepts

Instructions: Use Internet resources, books, articles, colleagues, etc., to present solutions to the problems listed below. There is no one correct solution to any problem.

Note to Instructor: Students in class may be divided into groups and given the problem-based learning activity to discuss and solve. Once the group has reached consensus as to a solution, the group may present it to the other students in the class. This activity will provide all students with information regarding solutions to the problem.

Problem #1
Suppose your administrator instructed you to provide him/her with alternatives for acquiring additional revenue by eliminating the excess capacity.

Problem #2
Develop a marketing plan for providing services to a long-term healthcare facility.

Problem #3
Develop a marketing plan for providing services to a government-supported dialysis center.

BIBLIOGRAPHY

Baker, M.: The Marketing Book. Butterworth-Heinemann. An imprint of Elsevier Science, Burlington, MA., 2003.

Drozdenko, RG and Drake, PD.: Optimal Database Marketing Strategy, Development, and Data Mining. Sage Publications, Inc. Thousands Oak, CA., 2002.

Evans, R. and Berman, B. marketing 9th ed. Atomic Dog Publishing, Cincinnati, OH., 2005.

Kalb, Ira S. E-Marketing: What Went Wrong and How to Do It Right. K&A Press, 2004.

Kotler, P: According to Kotler: The World's Foremost Authority on Marketing Answers Your Questions. Amacom. a division of the American Management Association, New York, NY., 2005.

Kotler P: Marketing Insights from A to Z. Concepts Every Manager Needs to Know. John Wiley and Sons, Inc. Hoboken, NJ., 2003.

Lamb, CW, McDaniel, C, Hair, JF.: Marketing With Infotrac. Thompson South-Western, Mason, OH., 2006.

Internet Resources

STATLINE Federal and State News Briefs, March 16, 2005, 2005 College of American Pathologist
<http://www.cap.org/apps/docs/statline/billing_iowa.html>

Interview with J.C. Penney Chairman, James Oesterriecher
http://www.industrywatch.com.

Saint Louis University Coagulation Consultants
http://www.slucare.edu/clinical/ pathlab/coagulation

ARUP Laboratories
<http://www.arup-lab.com/>

Clinical Laboratory Management Association
<http://www.clma.org/>

American Society of Clinical Pathology
http://www.ascp.org/

It is imperative that laboratory managers not only prepare themselves but also groom their employees for a successful career in laboratory medicine. Promoting professional development, as introduced in Section II chapter 7, developing a career plan and creating opportunities provide the basis to successful career planning resulting in career success.

Success in your career is also dependent on incorporating values of ethics and morality into the ethics of management.

Section V focuses on strategies for career success and consists of two chapters, one that focuses on ethics and one that discusses career planning. Chapter 17 discusses ethical issues in laboratory management. Laboratory managers encounter daily some of the issues related to personnel, training and education, financial, billing, following standards and regulations, and marketing. Ethical conduct plays a role in these daily activities of the laboratory manager. Chapter 18 presents strategies for career planning. Utilization of the tips provided in this chapter is designed to assist learners in their own career planning as well as to help that of others.

Section V Contents:

17

Ethical Issues in Laboratory Management

ADIL E. SHAMOO, PhD, CIP

Chapter Outline

Objectives

Following successful completion of this chapter, the learner should be able to:

1. Discuss the importance of ethical issues in laboratory management.
2. Identify the ethical principles at stake when faced with a moral dilemma.

3. Identify areas of laboratory management that may face ethical issues.
4. Recognize boundaries of ethical laboratory management and its value.
5. Delineate and discuss the ethical decision-making process for laboratory management.

Key Terms

Moral Dilemmas in Management
Ethical Theories and Principles
Autonomy, Justice, and Maleficence/
   Non-Maleficence
Confidentiality

Conflict of Interest
Ethical Decision-making Process
Risks and Benefits
Regulatory Compliance

Case Study:

A colleague and a friend of the technologist asks the technologist for the results of a pregnancy test of his girlfriend. The technologist obliged after telling his friend that he is doing him a big favor and that he should not tell anyone that he told him. The test was positive. The manager was told about it through another employee.

Issues and Questions to Consider

1. *Evaluate the information and the problem.*
2. *Identify the stakeholders.*
3. *What are the values at risk?*
4. *What are the moral responsibilities of the laboratory technologist?*
5. *What are the moral responsibilities of the laboratory manager?*
6. *How should the laboratory manager proceed?*

INTRODUCTION

In order to achieve a task (small or large) that requires a group of individuals with the same or complementary skills, management of the group or the organization is an essential component of a successful organization charged with completing a task. Even though modern management principles of an organization are relatively recent phenomena, nevertheless the management practices have been in existence for thousands of years. The Romans were great engineers with great management skills to achieve complex and large tasks such as building roads, bridges, and aqua ducts. Effective management requires: knowledge, leadership, competence, and moral authority. Managers of organizations operate in a community and the society. Therefore, our human values of ethics and morality must be incorporated into the ethics of management. This is because management ethics involves management activities that can encompass all of the good or bad of our humanity. Managers, by virtue of their job, are leaders. Therefore, the ethical or unethical behavior of the leader clearly would heavily impact the effectiveness of the leader on the outcome of the organization. Laboratory managers encounter daily some of the issues related to personnel, training and education, financial, billing, following standards and regulations, and marketing. Ethical conduct plays a role in the daily activities of the laboratory manager.

Some of these activities as they relate to ethical laboratory management may involve, in part, the following:

1. Confidentiality of the information
2. Fraud and abuse of charges
3. Fraud and misconduct of data
3. Marketing and advertising
4. Quality of services
5. Profits
6. Human resources issues: workers salaries, working conditions, drug-testing, etc.
7. Conflict of interest
8. Regulatory compliance

Dealing with all of these managerial issues intersects with our individual and societal ethical values that will have a crucial impact on all of these activities as well as on our society at large.

This chapter will explore ethical theories, ethical decision-making, potential ethical issues in some of the items listed above, and give some case examples of how to deal with it.

ETHICAL THEORIES

Most ethical theories, concepts, and principles deal with the most important three parameters: (1) Actor; (2) Act; and (3) Outcome. Of course some theories deal simultaneously with any combinations of the three parameters in order to become more generalizable. The theories that deal with the Actor and his/her character traits are called virtue ethics. Ethical conduct, therefore, is determined by the person's virtuous character such as: honesty, honor, courage, humanity, benevolence, fairness, and temperance. Aristotle was a strong proponent of virtue ethics. The virtue of integrity is the consistency of virtuous behavior such as honesty and fairness. Ethical behavior requires learning the good behavior and practicing it. This is similar to playing an instrument or learning mathematics; it requires learning and a lot of practice as Aristotle stated. Moreover, these characteristics are developed within the context of the community. The individual influences the community and certainly the community influences the individual. Ethical leadership greatly depends on virtue ethics. The leadership sets the tone for the organizational culture in terms of honesty, courage, fairness, and wisdom of decisions. Members of the organization emulate, in large part, their leaders.

The theories that deal with the Act itself by the moral agent (Actor) are within the second category of "Act". The moral agent ought to know the difference between right and wrong action. The eighteen century German Enlightenment philosopher Immanuel Kant was the proponent of this approach. Kant emphasized that the reasons for action (i.e. motives of the agent) matter a great deal. Therefore, he advocates doing the right thing for the right reason. He introduced the concept of categorical imperative (CI) of "what if everyone does it". This is basically a re-statement of the 'Golden Rule" where it requires that you treat others as you want them to treat you. In addition, proponents of the natural law also have advocated that life, health, happiness, and pleasure are naturally good. Whereas, death, suffering, disease, and pain are bad. Also, advocates of natural rights may fall into this category since they contend that certain rights are endowed to us such as life, liberty, prosperity, freedom of thought and freedom of religion without any duties or obligations to others. The seventeenth century British philosopher John Lock was the champion of natural rights.

The theories that deal with outcomes (Third category) are concerned with the consequence of the action by the "actor". The individual's motive is less important than the outcome. The eighteenth century philosophers Jeremy Bentham and nineteenth century philosopher John Stuart Mill developed the theory of utilitarianism. The basic tenet of the theory is that our actions should have the best overall consequences for the largest number of people. For example, the political system of socialism is derived from this theory. Cost/Benefit analysis is a derivative of this theory. The social contract theory also falls within the outcome domain since people living in a society have obligations to the society at large by the very nature of accepting to live in a community and society.

APPLIED ETHICAL PRINCIPLES

Let us imagine a very large circle representing the domain of ethical conduct in life. The ethical conduct governs societies in all areas of life from family, community, education, business, and government. Imagine a small concentric circle within this large circle representing the domain governed by laws and related legal structures. The laws are areas that the society has decided to make those unethical behaviors illegal and provided remedies including punishment. But, the remaining area between the two circles are the ethical norms, for whatever reason, the society expect us to abide by them (See Figure 17–1). If a society abides only by what is legal, the civil society will cease to exist. These are the norms all societies utilize to enforce social controls. Usually, societies enact laws to govern a specific area in such a manner as when a continuous and flagrant infringement on the societal expectation of ethical norms. This is not to say that all laws in every society are ethical. The best example is that slavery was legal but yet unethical. The more the society is free, the greater the likelihood that their laws are ethical. There is always a tension between increasing the legal circle and reducing it in order to lessen the regulatory compliance burden on the society. It is also important to note that when we discuss unethical behavior, one may erroneously get the impression that everyone is unethical. Most individuals are noble people and well intentioned. Discussing pathology in ethical behavior is not different

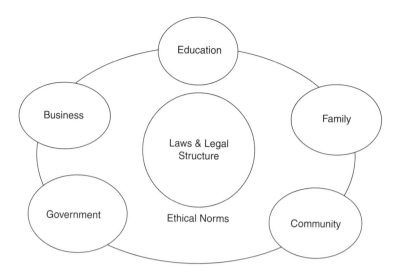

FIGURE 17–1. **Ethical Conduct in Life**

than discussing and studying pathology in medicine. Pathology in medicine affects only a very small percentage of population. Nevertheless, studying pathology helps us to learn how to prevent and treat the pathology. Moreover, we like to have the best possible treatment that will not introduce more pathology. In ethics, this is no different in that we study pathology in ethical conduct in order to prevent it and remedy it in the most ethical manner.

It is important to derive simple ethical principles. The following ethical principles can be deduced from the above brief discussion of ethical theories and from the fact that they can be considered to be prima facie principles. (See Table 17–1) These principles are not absolute rules. It is recommended to use these principles but when they come in conflict with each other, we should choose among them which ethical principle will have a higher priority than others. As a matter of fact one can find a case whereby each of these ethical principles falls apart. We

TABLE 17–1. **Categories of Ethical Principles**

Integrity of Conduct	Honesty
	Objectivity
	Openness
Respect for Persons	Fairness
	Loyalty
	Respect for subordinators/colleagues
Social Responsibility	Do good; Do no harm
	Public responsibility
	Obeying laws and regulations
	Efficiency

will list the three broad categories of ethical principles with few sub-categories. We will only discuss a limited number of the most important sub-categories.

1. *Integrity of Conduct.*   This is an area of ethical duties for managers that involve multiple specific areas such as:

a) honesty,
b) objectivity, and
c) openness.

Honesty is a crucial characteristic for managers in acquiring, recording, and manipulating the data. Trust among subordinates for honest leadership is important to promulgate good practices. Objectivity in reporting the information to patients, subordinates, or upper management is at the heart of the truthfulness of the data. Openness engenders public trust in the system. For example, if conflict of interest exists, then transparency and managing the conflict of interest become an important part of good management practices.

2. *Respect for persons.*   This is an area of ethical duties for managers that involve issues of:

a) respect and the protection of autonomy;
b) fairness;
c) loyalty; and
d) respect for subordinators and colleagues.

In the area of respect and the protection of autonomy, each individual should have free and full rights for decision-making. We should all respect the rights of each individual to exercise their rights. Assuming a rational individual, then the individual should be able to make an informed and responsible choice. Even if the choice is not a responsible one and it does not infringe on someone else's rights, we must respect it and the individual will bear its consequences. However, none of us in a position of management is left alone to make decisions. Managers have to comply with numerous oversights from upper management as well as from the inside policies and outside regulatory agencies. Therefore, autonomy can be limited because other forces of good come into play such as issues of justice and serving the public good.

In the area of fairness, Aristotle said that "equals should be treated equally and unequals unequally". In a society, we should allocate resources fairly. Also, we should distribute the risks and benefits to the largest number of population (i.e. the greatest good). This is what is called "social justice". We should not have a segment of society reaping benefits while having another segment of society take all the risks that brought the benefit. There should be justifications as to why people are treated differently.

Respect for subordinates and colleagues is an extension of respect for others and giving deference to others to make their own free choice.

In the area of loyalty, one should be loyal to their organization and to their colleagues as long as it is ethical.

3. *Social responsibility.* This is an area of ethical duties for managers that involve issues of:

a) do good and do no harm;
b) public responsibility;
c) obeying the laws and regulation; and
d) efficiency.

In the area of do good and do no harm, the two concepts are interrelated principles of doing good and preventing or not inflicting harm. "Do good" connotes a positive action whereas "do no harm" is a passive state of refraining from harm. However, preventing harm could be a positive act. This is why these two principles are so inter-related. Some argue that beneficence should be optional on the individual rather than mandatory. I think in some cases beneficence can be optional like giving financial aid to the needy but it is obligatory when you see a car accident and you are the only one who can stop and help.

It is of interest to note that the American Society for Clinical Laboratory Science (ASCLS) in 2002 issued a Code of Ethics to its members. Among the ethical principles they enunciated are: a) duty to the patient requiring competence and strict confidentiality; b) duty to colleagues and the profession with respect to all involved; and c) duty to society to adhere to laws and regulations.

ETHICAL DECISION-MAKING PROCESS

Now that we have discussed the ethical theories and principles, we can utilize them to guide us to make an ethical decision. An ethical decision is usually needed when there is a moral dilemma. In other words, there are moral choices one has to make. For example, when shopping for a car, selecting what color you should buy is not an ethical dilemma. However, if an individual has to decide to have his older brother to write his term paper for him or not is a moral dilemma? In a moral dilemma, you have two choices or more. What is the right thing to do? How do you arrive at an optimal ethical decision? What values are involved and which ones have priority and why? These are all factors involved in an ethical decision-making process. (See Table 17–2)

Let us discuss the process of ethical decision-making. As we mentioned earlier, there has to be a moral dilemma first in order to go through the process.

1. *State the Problem.* For the case study above, the problem is that the technologist revealed confidential information and the moral dilemma for the manager is what to do about it.

Let us take the case study above and analyze it. The manager clearly has a moral dilemma of what to do to the employee and other related issues within the

TABLE 17–2.   Steps of Ethical Decision-Making Process

State the Problem
Collect and Verify the Information
Identification of the Primary Stakeholders
Determine any Violation of Laws
Delineate Harm
Delineate Options
Make a Decision
Defend the Decision

laboratory. Moreover, the manager has to deal with it in a fair and just manner in order to set the moral standards and to maintain or increase the moral of the laboratory. Furthermore, resolving the issue will reflect a great deal of the manager's skills.

2. Collect and Verify the Information.   Did we verify that the technologist gave the information regarding the pregnancy test? Let us assume the answer is yes. How much information was disclosed? The employee is a valuable employee with five years of excellent working habits. Apparently, several other employees learned of the incident. Let us assume we have all of the information.

3. Identification of the Primary Stakeholders.   The stakeholders are: the friend, girlfriend, technologist, and the manager. The secondary stakeholders who will be affected by this problem are: other employees, and the organization. The tertiary stakeholders are: the profession, and the society at large.

4. Determine any Violation of Laws.   Have anyone violated the law? The answer is yes since confidential information has been revealed. There are state and federal laws prohibiting such disclosure. The manager can take action according to the law. However, legal actions are not usually prescribed to deal with the individual in such cases. In this case, the act or its outcome of revealing confidential information is unethical. You will need to go to the next step of delineating options. If the act (not like in this case) was legal, then the question ought to be: Does it violate any organizational policies? At this stage, the manager can take action.

5. Delineate Harm.   We can all agree that the primary harm from this infringement can occur to the girlfriend. Her confidential information has been revealed and thus her autonomy has been violated. The girlfriend may even suffer dignitary harm from being embarrassed that others have such private information on her and so on. She may lose her boyfriend and thus harm may occur to her by a possible loss of her boyfriend, and her job. If the information leaked, some employers under the guise of competence, may not want a sick person employed for various reasons. The harm also could be done to the technologist himself since he may be fired or reprimanded. The harm also could be done to the manager since he/she will have to deal with it and spend valuable time on it. Secondary harm also could come to other employees since they have been tainted and the manager and the upper management may become more suspicious. The tertiary harm could come to the profession by casting dark clouds on the integrity of the profession. Finally the society, at large, may be harmed since no one would like to see a society in which such behavior is the common norm.

6. Delineate Options.   In part, the following options are available:

a. Do nothing
b. Fire the technologist
c. Suspend the technologist for a short period of time with or without pay
d. Reprimand the technologist and require education and training
e. Inform the girlfriend and apologize
f. Require all laboratory personnel to undergo education and training
g. Institute a new policy for the laboratory in order to protect confidentiality

There are many more options in between the one listed. Also, we can choose to do one or more of the listed options.

The option of doing nothing is unethical since harm has been done without accountability and responsibility. Doing nothing sends the wrong message to all involved. Firing a valued technologist for a first offence may be an over-reaction and not commensurate with the infringement. Some may recommend firing the technologist. However, for every suggested resolution we need to discuss the risks and benefits. Firing the individual may inhibit others in the future from coming forward. Firing could cause a hardship to the technologist and his family way over and above the harm done to others due to infringement. So, we can all argue among the four options listed above or their combination depends on more detailed information. Honest individuals can differ into the proposed solution within the ethical boundaries. It is important to note that option (a) is unethical and option (b) may be unethical. One cannot simply make all options as ethically equivalent because they are not. More detailed information may even eliminate other options as unethical. We have in this section related and evaluated the options to different values and principles.

7. Make a Decision.   Let us assume we chose options (d), (e), (f), and (g). This is probably the most comprehensive resolution.

8. Defend the Decision.   Now we have to address the final step of whether we are comfortable if this information becomes public and we must determine if our decision can be defended. The reason for this final question is to eliminate the factor that we may be hiding something unethical. If the answer is yes in that we are comfortable with the decision if everyone knows about it, then we should act. Otherwise, we should start the evaluation all over again. However, there are unique circumstances that may render going public as inappropriate and could

cause even more harm to the individual. This is one of these cases because going public would bring greater harm to the girlfriend. The girlfriend could be subjected to more embarrassment as well as to loss of potential jobs (unlikely) since we do not know the circumstance and implications of her positive Pap smear test and may invite speculation.

ETHICAL CHALLENGES IN LABORATORY MANAGEMENT

As we have mentioned earlier, societies determine which ethical issues, if violated, will result in punishment. The area of laboratory management is a good example of how the legal circle was widened at least twice in the past twenty years in order to provide legal remedies for violators of the ethical norms. There are billions of public dollars annually spent by the federal government on government supported health care such as Medicare and Medicaid. Prior to 1988, various laboratories set their own standards for the quality of their tests (for example for cholesterol and Pap smear evaluation). Due to serious violations and concerns, in 1988 the federal government enacted into law the Clinical Laboratory Improvement Amendment (CLIA) (Public Law, 1988). CLIA established quality standards for all laboratory tests to ensure accuracy and reliability. The society no longer was willing to risk the public good on the ethical and professional standards alone of those in the field.

The second example is the passage in 1995 of the final rule for "Medicare Program; Physician Financial Relationship" (42 CFR Part 411) which addressed the issue known as self-referral. A good number of laboratories were owned by physicians or members of their families. In some cases, physicians would order tests (or unnecessary tests) for their patients to be conducted in the laboratory next door in which they or members of their family had a financial interest. There was a clearly a conflict of interest issue and a great opportunity for abuse of public money. This practice was clearly unacceptable to the public and the government. This was the reason why in this new rule, the Health Care Financing Administration (HCFA), now called the Center for Medicare and Medicaid Services (CMS), issued in 1995 the final rule forbidding self-referral "except under specified circumstances".

In the introduction, I listed eight categories of potential areas of questionable ethical conduct in laboratory management. We will not be able to discuss all of these areas. However, we would like to expound on several of them. In our case study, we discussed the importance of confidentiality of the information. One of the most important ethical areas in this field is the area of fraud of charges and fraud and misconduct of data. There are literally hundreds of millions of dollars annually lost for fraud and abuse. In part, because the federal government is paying the bill, patients do not check what they were billed for and thus makes it easy to commit fraud. The most prominent areas of fraud and abuse are: charges for services not performed; unnecessary testing (i.e. not medically necessary); waiver of co-payments and deductibles; fraudulent or inaccurate data; and unbundling of laboratory tests so that the laboratory charges are higher than if the charges were all part of one service. Another area of concern we mentioned earlier is marketing and advertising. In some fraudulent practices, the laboratory advertises for free testing for a particular disorder; however, the laboratory requires all patients fill a form which in essence is used for billing purposes.

Another example of an ethically troubling issue in a laboratory occurred in 2004 in Maryland General Hospital in Baltimore, Maryland. Apparently the allegations are that in over a year, hundreds of patients received incorrect HIV and hepatitis test results and the patients were not notified. Some patients were HIV positive and were told the test was negative and some the reverse. The laboratory personnel overrode the results from the controls. Moreover, a former laboratory worker complained to the management about the quality of tests without any results. A state official, once he learned of the laboratory practice, was quoted as saying: "I think this is unconscionable behavior; people not being told about the status of their test".

SUMMARY

Training and education in ethical issues in laboratory management is an essential component of a student's education. Students as potential laboratory managers need to be aware of potential ethical problems they will face. They need not only to deal with that particular problem but also to set the standard for ethical managerial competence to set an example for others. In order for laboratory managers to be effective, they need to understand the ethical decision-making process in order to be able to analyze the particular moral dilemma he/she is faced with. Ethical managerial leadership provides a milieu for all to work in a cooperative and successful manner as part of being a true professional.

SUGGESTED PROBLEM-BASED LEARNING ACTIVITIES
Chapter-Ethical Issues in Laboratory Management

Instructions: Use the library and internet resources, articles, textbooks, and your colleagues to solve these problems.

Note to Instructor: Group activities in order to provide division of labor as well as discussions are encouraged.

Problem #1
Develop a code of conduct for the laboratory for employees and managers.

Problem #2
Develop a case study of an ethical issue in the laboratory. List right and wrong solutions and why.

Problem #3
Develop an educational program that you may require for all employees of the laboratory in ethics.

BIBLIOGRAPHY

National Commission for the Protection of Human Subjects of Biomedical and Behavioral Research. 1979. The Belmont Report. Available at: *http://www.fda.gov/oc/ohrt/irbs/belmont.html.* Accessed: September 21, 2004.

Shamoo A and Resnik D. 2003. Responsible Conduct of Research. New York: Oxford University Press.

Internet Resources

American Society for Clinical Laboratory Science (ASCLS) Code of Ethics (2002), Accessed on 5/10/05.

DHS
http://www.state.ar.us/dhs/aging/10-LaboratoryFraudAndAbuse.pdf

DOJ
http://www.usdoj.gov/dag/pubdoc/health98.htm

HCFA: 42 CFR Part 411, HCFA
http://www.dwt.com/practc/healthcr_compliance/publications/OIG_Hosp_Compliance/docs/StarkI.pdf.

This addresses issues of: Medicare Program; Physician Financial Relationships With, and Referrals to, Health Care Entities. (i.e. Self-Referrals), 1995.

OIG
http://www.dwt.com/practc/healthcr_compliance/publications/OIG_Hosp_Compliance/docs/StarkI.pdf

Public Law 100-578, Section 353 Public Health Service Act (42 U.S.C. 263a) October 31, 1988. The title of the regulation is: Clinical Laboratory Improvement Amendments of 1988 (CLIA'88).

The Baltimore Sun
http://www.baltimoresun.com/news/health/bal-te.md.general22apr22,1,2395129.story? coll=bal-health-utility
http://www.baltimoresun.com/news/health/bal-lab0311,1,1804926.story?coll=bal-health-utility

Acknowledgment

This paper was supported in-part by a grant from: Fogarty International Center/NIH 1R25TW007090-01.

Career Planning

DENISE M. HARMENING, PhD, MT(ASCP), CLS(NCA)

Chapter Outline

Objectives
Introduction
The Successful Career Plan
Career Imperatives
Professional Development Programs
Creating Opportunities
Strategic Development Plan

Continuing Development
Summary
Self-Assessment Questions
Answers to Self-Assessment Questions
Bibliography
Internet Resources

Objectives

Following successful completion of this chapter, the learner will be able to:

1. Define the responsibilities of professional life.
2. List the elements of a successful career.
3. Describe several skills related to the planning and implementation of a professional development plan.
4. Describe a unified view of a professional career in light of the professional community, the workplace, personal needs and interests, and collaboration with colleagues.
5. Outline a customized plan for professional development and identify the main skills needed to make that plan succeed.

"The secret to success is that there is no secret to success."

Anonymous

INTRODUCTION

The necessity of career planning and management is one of the many challenges facing the laboratory scientist today. These challenges come to us from all directions: new regulations and technologies, the relocation and restructuring of the workplace, the reorganization of institutions in response to changing national perspectives and priorities, economic pressures from government and the private sector, and the need for a lifelong process of continuing education in the aftermath of the "knowledge explosion."

These issues are the product of larger concerns: the healthcare crisis, the information explosion, quantum leaps in technologic innovation, and economic shifts keenly felt inside and outside the workplace. The long-term effects are just starting to surface and be identified; the short-term effects, dictating the way we conduct our day-to-day lives, are what we must all cope with—and somehow adjust to.

This chapter explores the elements of successful career planning by describing career imperatives and professional development programs. In addition, strategies for creating opportunities and the use of a strategic development plan as well as participating in continuing development are addressed. Self-assessment questions over the material presented in this chapter are located after the summary section. Learners are encouraged to complete these questions and then review the answers provided at the end of this chapter.

THE SUCCESSFUL CAREER PLAN

The time is past when we could operate on a safe routine within a narrow specialty with set procedures, feeling confident that nothing dramatic would change from year to year. No longer can we afford to be out of touch with political, social and scientific developments, or to ignore our connection with related disciplines within the layer context of medicine. The pressure is on to determine our own destiny in our institutions, professional associations, and work environments. Vital to any successful career is a plan. Success is the outcome of the ability to create a custom-designed, multifaceted professional development program that facilitates lifelong learning. A personal commitment to professional development must be made in at least one of the following areas: expansion of the applied body of knowledge, growth through professional activities, scholarship, teaching, research, and/or community service.

A philosophy of life that focuses on attaining and maintaining high standards of practice in educational, professional, and/or research activities must be developed. Professionals are obligated to share knowledge and expertise with co-workers and colleagues at all levels of practice: local, state, and national. Each has the responsi-

TABLE 18–1   Advantages and Benefits of Networking in the Profession

* Exchange of research and teaching techniques and technologies
* Extension of professional contacts and networks for departments and staffs
* Opportunities for joint ventures and collaborative development of grants, scholarships, and other support and subsidies
* Productive matching and complementary working between and among facilities, administrative systems, and operations, leading to interaction, enrichment, and resource sharing for faculty, staff, and administrations of all participants

bility to contribute to and expand the overall body of knowledge within the profession. Exchanges through networking play a key role in professional development, providing an immeasurably valuable range of advantages and benefits.

CAREER IMPERATIVES

Learn to network and capitalize on the knowledge and expertise of colleagues. Learn to extract information from peers, encouraging and partaking in collaborative efforts. You are not alone. Cooperation and the "team approach" are the keys to any successful career whether in nonprofit, service-oriented organizations or industry. Knowledge and resources in the field are not a zero-sum issue—they expand when shared (Table 18–1).

PROFESSIONAL DEVELOPMENT PROGRAMS

Professional development can be defined as the establishment of activities and procedures to assist acquisition of the knowledge, skills, and attitudes that enable increased effectiveness in performing all functions related to professional life.

Personalized professional development programs should seek to prepare competent practitioners while developing professional attitudes, attributes, and values. Specifically, the programs should be designed to accomplish one or more of the following goals:

1. Develop personal attributes to enhance scholarship, productivity, and exchange of ideas.
2. Promote contributions to the profession and community.
3. Cultivate awareness of professional issues and responsibilities for enhancement of the scope of practice.
4. Serve as a catalyst to fulfill goals and maintain high standards of practice as set out in both our philosophy of life and professional philosophy.

Figure 18–1 outlines some of the self-directed professional development aspects that could be activated to accomplish these goals.

Three elements are critical to this basic approach:

1. Flexibility: Flexibility is a "read" capability to adapt to new, different, or changing requirements. This is the time to take new directions and opportunities as they emerge. This often means looking at crises and obstacles as an invitation to re-define, rethink, and respond with enthusiasm and energy rather than with pes-simism and anxiety. Creative problem solving will be called into play. Implicit is an open-mindedness about who we are, what we can do, where we're headed, and our growing roles and potential power as part of the healthcare team.

SELF-DIRECTED PROFESSIONAL DEVELOPMENT ACTIVITIES

Development of Expertise

PUBLISHING	EDUCATIONAL	RESEARCH
• Submit letters, editorials, book reviews, articles, chapters, monographs for publication • Collaborate with co-workers within or outside your immediate circle to write articles, proposals, grants	• Participate in educational activities at work locally, regionally or nationally • Read current journals, newsletters, etc in your field • Audit courses, enroll in a new degree program, take a continuing education course	• Participate in collaborative research or institute projects • Participate in consortium projects

Contributions to the Profession and the Community

WORK-RELATED	COMMUNITY ACTIVITIES	CULTURAL EXPERIENCES
• Network with individuals outside of your department • Cross-departmental activities • Membership in professional associations	• Volunteer work • Community activities • Fund raising • Association endeavors • Career advising	Consult • with science centers • with museum institutes Participate in • Association-sponsored study-tours abroad

Personal Development

PHYSICAL	EMOTIONAL/SPIRITUAL	COGNITIVE SKILLS
• Form a focus group for activity • Learn a new hobby or sport • Jog with a group of colleagues	• Form a focus group for activity • Meditation • Build in support mechanisms for emotional well being	• Form a study group • Explore a new language • Expand computer literacy

FIGURE 18–1   **Self-Directed Professional Development Activities.**

2. Dedication to the profession: The term reflects a profession broader and more demanding than the traditions of subspecialties alone. The new language is an invitation, a challenge to live up to the new image of ourselves based on a broader scope of practice. The concept of dedication as "self-sacrificing devotion" is timely and appropriate.

3. Positive attitude: Optimism and the vitality it generates, independent of changing circumstances, are essential for personal and professional advancement and achievement. We are being asked to think above and beyond the problems of today to create momentum to carry us into a new era of competence, pride, and influence. This is a task we must take upon ourselves; its rewards will not be conferred from the outside. Power is born from within. We ourselves must take control of our profession and determine our own destiny.

As practitioners, we are steadily becoming more assertive, creating our own opportunities rather than complacently waiting for them to be handed to us.

Professional development must become a new part of the career process for all laboratory scientists—practitioners, faculty, and students. It cannot remain an optional activity to be considered only if and when time and funds permit. The benefits are many, ranging from job security to the satisfaction of service to society to the joy of personal and professional growth—both collective and personal.

CREATING OPPORTUNITIES

We must learn to foster the growth and development of our own careers. This entails expanding our general knowledge base and cultivating skills such as quantitative reasoning, problem solving, decision making, communications, interpersonal exchange, and legal and ethical sensitivity.

Identifying strengths and weaknesses is helpful as part of the process of getting to the answer of WHO you are and who you want to become. One plan for professional development consists of capitalizing on strengths while addressing weaknesses to neutralize or make assets of them. Assessing your personality in terms of work ethic, standards and values, personal style, and preference in the work environment is a worthwhile investment to begin the process (see Keirsey Temperament Sorter and other self-assessment tools).

STRATEGIC DEVELOPMENT PLAN

We must learn to create our own opportunities, know how to capitalize on them, and formulate a strategic development plan based on answers to the following five "Who, Where, What, How and When" questions.

1. Who am I as a professional and as a person?
2. Where do I want to be in 1 year, 3 years, 5 years, 10 years and by the close of my career?
3. What are the steps to get there?

TIMETABLE FOR CREATING YOUR OWN OPPORTUNITIES				
	YEAR 1	YEAR 3	YEAR 5	YEAR 10
WHO				
WHERE				
WHAT				
HOW				
WHEN				

FIGURE 18–2   Timetable for Creating Your Own Opportunities.

4. How do I make opportunities happen?
5. When do I start?

Figure 18–2 consists of a suggested timetable for creating your own opportunities. The strategic plan must include a way to acquire the requisite knowledge, skills, and attitudes for approaching your primary goal. There must be built-in mechanisms for maintaining your effectiveness, improving your approach to fulfilling responsibilities, and making satisfying adjustments to changes in your environment and circumstances. You can expect your overall goal to bring about improvements in the overall quality of your life.

CONTINUING DEVELOPMENT

It is your responsibility to enhance your continuing development in order to meet your own needs, as well as those of your employer and others important in your life.

You must continually be prepared to meet the demands for new knowledge, skills and attitudes inherent in a changing society and workplace. This includes learning to intuit and anticipate the "pulse" of the era and to take a broad view of the world you live in.

TABLE 18–2   Key Problem-Solving and Decision-Making Skills

- Ability to analyze, store, and retrieve theoretical knowledge.
- Ability to coordinate or modify human behavior in complicated structures.
- Ability to engage in participatory decision making.
- Ability to regulate and modify individual and group behavior.
- Ability to resolve conflicts.
- Ability to respond to change creatively.

You must learn to increase your "copeabilty"—to effectively clarify your goals and values in order to relate to others and choose among competitive alternatives you have created and discovered for yourself. For this planning process, problem solving and decision making are crucial processes. Both require the development, fine-tuning, and polishing of a range of abilities. Table 18–2 lists the basic abilities pivotal to effective problem solving and decision making.

SUMMARY

A strategic development plan, using the techniques of opportunity creation, can clarify and even plot your professional goals. It will put your planning perspective in immediate visual terms. By this process, the "perfect" job can suddenly take shape as a three-dimensional reality, replacing a vague cloud of hope. Having "seen" this shining future image, you can then advance confidently, creating excellence as you go. Personally or professionally, there is no more satisfying venture.

SELF-ASSESSMENT QUESTIONS

1. Outline the responsibilities of professional life.
2. What three elements are basic to achieving the goals of professional development?
3. List three abilities essential to effective decision making and problem solving.
4. List three areas of professional development.
5. Define professional development in terms of operative skills.
6. Outline the Five-Question Strategy for Creating Your Own Opportunities.
7. Explain why professional development has become so important to laboratory science.

BIBLIOGRAPHY

Chappelow C, Leslie J: *Keeping Your Career on Track: Twenty Success Strategies.* Center for Creative Leadership. Greensboro, NC., 2005.

Drucker P: *Management Challenges for the 21st Century.* Harper Business, New York, 2001.

Keirsey D, Bates M: *Please Understand Me: Character and Temperament Types.* Prometheus Nemesis, Del Mar, CA., 1984.

Kelly A: *Decision-Making using Game Theory: An Introduction for Managers.* Cambridge University Press. Cambridge, England. 2003.

Marion P: *Career Tune Up.* Artemis Arts Library. San Francisco, CA. 2005.

McConnell C: *Umiker's Management Skills for the New Health Care Superviso,* 4th ed. Aspen Books, Denver, CO., 2005.

Pittiglio D: Harmening A Journal for a United Profession, (with K. Doig and M. Posey, 1:1) Clinical Laboratory Science: Image, Challenge and Opportunity, (1:2), Professional Development for Faculty and Students: New Opportunities and Directions (2:2), The Ultimate Advantage Writing Power, (2:6), Editorials, Clinical Laboratory Science, 1988–1989.

Powell C: *Career Planning Strategies*, 5th Ed. Kendall/Hunt Publishing Company. Dubuque, IA., 2004.

Simmers L: *Health Science Career Exploration*. Delmar Learning. Clifton Park, NY., 2004.

Tracy B, Fraser C: *TurboCoach: A Powerful System for Achieving Breakthrough Career Success*. AMACOM Div American Mgmt Assn. New York, NY., 2005.

Warner J: *Problem Solving & Decision-Making Profile Facilitator's Guide*. HRD Press, Inc. Amherst, MA., 2003.

Yeung R: *The Ultimate Career Success Workbook: Tests & Exercises to Assess Skills & Potential!* Kogan Page Limited. Sterling, VA., 2004.

Internet Resources

Career Builder
http://www.career-vision.com
E-Span Career Companion
http://www.careercompanion.com
Mapping Your Future
http://www.mapping-your-future.org/planning/
Career Planning
http://careerplanning.about.com/
Career Planning
http://www.focuscareer.com/

ANSWERS TO SELF-ASSESSMENT QUESTIONS

1. **A.** Attaining and maintaining high standards of practice; share knowledge and expertise; contribute to and expand overall body of knowledge.
2. **A.** Flexibility, dedication to the profession, and a positive attitude.
3. **A.** 1. Ability to analyze, store and retrieve theoretical knowledge.
   2. Ability to coordinate or modify human behavior in complicated structures.
   3. Ability to engage in participatory decision making.
   4. Ability to regulate and modify individual and group behavior.
   5. Ability to resolve conflicts.
   6. Ability to respond to change creativity.
4. **A.** Expansion of the body of knowledge, growth in professional activities, scholarship, teaching, community service, professional activities, research.

5. **A.** Establishing activities and procedures to assist acquisition of the knowledge, skills, and attitudes that enable increased effectiveness in performing all functions related to professional life.
6. **A.** **1.** Who am I?
   2. Where do I want to be in _____ years?
   3. What are the steps to get there?
   4. How do I make the opportunities happen?
   5. When do I start?
7. **A.** Response to challenges: new regulations and technologies, the knowledge explosion, restructuring of the workplace, reorganization of institutions to respond to changing perspectives and priorities, economic pressures, and growing need for continuing education.

GLOSSARY

This alphabetized glossary contains definitions of the bolded terms found throughout the text as well as select related terms pertaining to the principles of laboratory management.

40-hour work week: A work rule consisting of varying hours worked per shift with a maximum of 40 hours per week. Overtime is defined as any time worked over 40 hours in one week.

8/80 work rule: A work rule consisting of ten 8-hour work shifts for a total of 80 hours worked within a two-week period. Overtime is defined as any time worked over 8 hours in one day or 80 hours in two weeks.

Accountability: Acceptance for success or failure.

Affective domain: A category of learning that is focused on attitudes, feelings, and behaviors. It also includes professional development issues, in this case pertinent to laboratory work, such as ethics, initiative, interpersonal skills with others, patient confidentiality of laboratory results, and professional interaction with other members of the healthcare team.

Affirmative action: A duty imposed on certain federal contractors and subcontractors to not discriminate and take proactive measures in employment decisions on the basis of race, color, sex, and national origin.

Age Discrimination in Employment Act (ADEA): A federal law passed in 1967 that prohibits discrimination in employment against persons aged 40 years and older.

Ambulatory payment categories (APCs): A prospective payment system for hospital-based outpatient services. Services that are similar in terms of resource consumption are grouped into categories and a payment rate is calculated for each category. Patients may have more than one APC per visit.

Americans with Disabilities Act (ADA): A federal law that prohibits employers from discriminating against qualified individuals with a disability in employment decisions.

Analytical phase: The phase of workflow consisting of actual testing.

Anchoring trap: A decision-making trap in which the mind gives disproportionate weight in favor of the first information it receives.

Application: A written document that details a perspective employee's education, qualifications and work experience.

Appropriation budget: A type of budget commonly associated with government agencies and characterized by an authorized spending level for a specific period of time.

Assets: The resources owned by the organization.

At-will employment doctrine: A common law employment standard that defines the employment relationship as terminable at the will of either party, at anytime, for any reason.

Authority: The right to make decisions.

Autocratic style: A group-decision making technique in which the leader of a group makes a decision without consulting with the others in the group.

Autonomy: Allows rational individuals to make their own decisions and act on them.

Balance sheet: A financial statement that depicts the financial position of an organization at a particular point in time, usually at the end of an accounting period.

Behavioral approach: An approach to leadership that is focused on what a leader "does" rather than what a leader "is."

Benchmarking: The process of determining a standard used in measuring and/or judging quality.

Beneficence: An ethical principle that entails an obligation to protect persons from harm. The principle of beneficence can be expressed in two general rules: (1) do not harm; and (2) protect from harm by maximizing possible benefits and minimizing possible risks of harm.

Billable procedure: A laboratory test that is billed to a payer (the payer may be an individual or a private or government insurer).

Bona Fide Occupational Qualifications (BFOQ): Requirements that are required for successful performance of the job, despite the fact that they may be related to a legally protected classification such as age, sex, or religion. Race can never be a BFOQ.

Brainstorming: A method for developing creative solutions to problems by focusing on a problem, and then deliberately coming up with as many unbounded solutions as possible and then pushing for ideas as far as possible. In this phase, "the sky is the limit."

Break-even analysis: A process performed using the costing information to determine if the total of all fixed and variable costs equals the amount of revenue generated (the break-even point). One of the uses for this method is to help determine the best alternative between several possibilities (i.e., decisions about providing in-house testing versus using a reference laboratory).

Break-even point: The point at which there is no profit or loss from performing a laboratory test; the total cost of all fixed and variable costs equals the amount of revenue generated by performing the test.

Browser-server model: A computer model, fundamental to Internet interactions, from which end-users may directly access (browse) specialized information that is available on demand from powerful server computers, thus creating a user-friendly interface for navigating the network.

Budget: A financial plan for allocating funds to cover the expenditures such as supplies, salaries, and overhead involved in the operation of the laboratory.

Budget justification: A report that compares the budget to actual events (particularly actual expense). The report highlights any variances present and should propose concrete solutions for any encountered.

Budgeting: A system for formalizing in writing a quantitative financial plan supportive of the institution's financial mission, for a given period of time.

Budget – Performance Report: A document that provides forward looking financial information for a given time period based on past performance and analysis of the future. It compares budget expectations with actual performance.

Bureaucracy: A form of organization with functional specialization, clear delineation of authority, and decision making based on rules developed to pursue organizational goals consistently and efficiently.

Capital budget: A plan that identifies anticipated purchases of capital assets and the expected source of funds required to make the purchases.

Capitation: A payment methodology used to reimburse managed care plans whereby a provider is paid a set amount per member per month for contracted services regardless of the number of services used by the patient.

Carve out (carved out): A type of payment plan in which the reimbursement rate is based on the type of care being provided. For example, a hospital room rate may be at a set reimbursement rate unless the patient is in a special care unit (such as ICU). These special care unit days are "carved out" of the set reimbursement rate and may have a separate per diem rate, or they may be reimbursed on a fee-for-service basis.

Case mix: The mix of patients seen by the provider based on diagnosis, severity of illness and utilization of services.

The higher the case mix, the more costly the care.

Cash flow projection: A projection of all changes affecting cash in the categories of operations, financing, and investments.

Cash Sources and Uses Statement: A document that analyzes the sources of cash inflows and uses of cash.

Centers for Medicare and Medicaid Services (CMS): A federal agency who partnered with the Centers for Disease Control and Prevention (CDC) to develop the CLIA'88 regulations. These two groups were also charged with informing the laboratory community of their work. Formerly known as the Health Care Financing Administration (HCFA).

Central Processing Unit (CPU): The core piece of hardware in a computer system. It controls the interpretation and execution of instructions provided by the software.

Character: A suggested leadership quality that refers to a person who promotes ethical decision making and expects ethical behaviors from others.

Chargemaster: A list of all billable services, their associated billing codes, and the price that is charged to the patient or insurance carrier.

Clinical Laboratory Improvement Amendments of 1988 (CLIA'88): A set of quality standards mandated by the federal government to ensure accuracy, reliability, and timeliness of patient test results.

Cognitive domain: A category of learning that is focused on acquiring and applying knowledge.

COLA (Formerly known as the Commission of Office of Laboratory Accreditation): A voluntary organization that initially accredited only physician office laboratories. Today, COLA also accredits other test sites including those located in small hospitals.

Collaboration: The act of working together with other individuals to achieve a common end.

Collaborative management: A scenario in which individuals feel appreciated and understood; they are not forced to comply by a mandate from their supervisor. Individuals work with their supervisors to make decisions and to solve problems. The four basic principles of collaborative management are trust, understanding, independence, and solutions.

Communication: The act of disseminating and receiving information using either written or oral transmission; may be formal or informal in nature.

Competency: The knowledge, skill, ability, or characteristics associated with high performance on a job such as problem solving; definitions of a competency include motives, beliefs, and values.

Competency-based performance evaluation: An evaluation based on a limited number of specifically defined tasks that are taught and assessed by direct observation during orientation and then periodically thereafter.

Competency modeling (model): A performance evaluation design that uses core competencies (organizational capabilities or strengths—what an organization does best).

Compliance: The adherence to rules, standards, regulations, and guidelines.

Confirming-evidence trap: A decision-making trap in which there is a mental bias that leads managers to seek out information to support their existing point of view while avoiding information that contradicts it.

Congruence model: An organizational model that shows detailed elements of an open system and the dynamics involved; used to analyze environmental relationships of an organization and to assess the relationships of its constituent parts.

Consensus: General agreement of an issue/solution reached by more than one individual; individuals may not like the decision made but are willing to "live with it."

Consultative style: A group decision-making technique in which the leader obtains suggestions and ideas from group members and then makes a decision that may or may not reflect the group members' influence.

Controlling: A performance measurement of implementation whereby adjustments and corrective actions can be taken to ensure that organizational goals are achieved.

Coordination: The blending of functions so that they are intertwined and build on each other thereby minimizing the risk of duplication or redundancy.

Co-payments: A dollar amount representing a predetermined proportion of total medical costs that the insured has to pay out of pocket (that is, self-pay) each time health services are received after the deductible has been paid.

Core competency: A term that refers to organizational capabilities or strengths—what an organization does best.

Cost: The charge (in dollars) associated with providing a billable procedure; also known as an expense; assets that have been purchased such as inventories of lab supplies that have yet to be used, or equipment whose cost has not been expensed through depreciation.

Cost accounting: A system for providing analysis or forecast of information to be used in financial decision making.

Cost/benefit analysis: One approach for determining and comparing costs, benefits, and values of solution alternatives. It is designed to determine if the results are of significant benefit to justify the cost of taking the action.

Cost center: An organizational unit for which revenue and expenses are accumulated separately in the accounts.

Cost per test: The sum of the expenses required to perform one laboratory test. Also referred to as microcosting.

Courage: A suggested leadership quality that refers to the willingness to make change and accept challenges to the status quo.

Credibility: A suggested leadership quality that refers to excellent credentials, substantive knowledge, and sound practical experience that a successful leader possesses.

Criteria-based performance evaluation: An evaluation based on rating the performance of the employee on specifically defined criteria such as knowledge, judgment, attendance, and reliability.

Cultural: See culture.

Culture: Basic assumptions, values, and norms shared by members of the organization.

Current value of money: The value of money today versus its value at a point further out in time (the future).

Database: A set of data organized into tables. The rows of the tables are made up of records, and the columns of the tables are fields that contain the same kind of data elements.

Debt Ratio: A ratio used to determine the organization's ability to meet long-term debt obligations.

Decision making: The process of choosing among several alternatives.

Decision tree: A graphic diagram consisting of nodes and branches used for visualizing alternative choices facing managers in a given situation or problem.

Deductibles: Dollar amounts that insured individuals must pay first (usually annually) before benefits of an insurance plan are payable.

Definitional database table: A collection of records arranged in rows that define the procedures and terminology of a computer-based information system. In a laboratory information system (LIS), these tables contain such information as test definitions, patient ward locations, and physician demographics.

Delegation: A group decision-making technique in which a leader turns over a problem to the group and lets them generate and evaluate alternatives and attempt to reach agreement on a solution without any leader involvement.

Demographic environment: An aspect of the marketing environment that is focused on the people who make up the market; consists of population numbers stratified by age and gender, educational levels, ethnic backgrounds, and growth rates.

Department: A cost center or group of cost centers with one person given responsibility for operations.

Depreciation: A dollar amount determined by the number of years over which a piece of equipment is accounted for on the general ledger; typically the dollar amount that is "written off" is the same over the useful lifetime of the equipment.

Descriptive database table: A collection of records arranged in rows that contain the historical events that have occurred in a database. In a laboratory information system (LIS), these tables contain such information as patient demographics, test orders, and test results.

Diagnostic Related Groups (DRGs): A classification system used in the prospective payment system for inpatient care for Medicare patients. Services that are similar in terms of resource consumption are grouped into categories and a payment rate is calculated for each category.

Direct expense (cost): All of the charges (in dollars) directly related to performing a laboratory test. Examples include reagents, consumables, labor, and benefits.

Directing: The use of leadership skills to obtain unified action through issuing directives, building participation, and achieving consensus. Also known as leading.

Economic environment: An aspect of the marketing environment that focuses on the purchasing power of the people in the market; this environment may be affected by many factors including the savings rate, interest rates, money supply, and inflation.

Emotional intelligence: A suggested leadership quality that refers to the basic emotional competencies that allow leaders to manage themselves as well as their relationships with others effectively.

Empower: A suggested leadership quality that refers to the ability and willingness of a leader to share power/authority. This may be done by delegating responsibility to others whenever possible.

Environment: External forces that affect an organization's ability to achieve its objectives and goals. Environment may include suppliers, customers, competitors, and regulators and encompasses economic, political, cultural, and technological driving forces.

Equal Employment Opportunity Commission (EEOC): A federal agency with the duty of administering a variety of federal laws including Title VII of the Civil Rights Act of 1964, the Americans with Disabilities Act (ADA), the Age Discrimination in Employment Act (ADEA), and the Equal Pay Act (EPA).

Equal Pay Act (EPA): A provision of the federal Fair Labor Standards Act of 1938 that prohibits discrimination in the payment of wages based on gender.

Essential functions: Those duties and responsibilities that are critical for successful performance of the job.

Expense: The charge (in dollars) of providing a billable procedure; also known as cost.

Expenses: Outflows of assets and are recognized when incurred.

Expense budget: A document that identifies planned expenditures based on forecasted units of service.

Fair Labor Standards Act of 1938 (FLSA): A federal law that defines how and when employees shall be paid and setting standards for minimum wage, wage classification such as exempt or nonexempt status, hours of work, and overtime payments.

Family and Medical Leave Act of 1993: A federal law that provides eligible employees with up to 12 weeks of unpaid leave for the employee's own serious health condition, to care for an immediate family member who has a serious health condition, after the birth of a child, or placement of a child in the employee's home for adoption or foster care.

Fee-for-service: A payment method whereby a provider is paid a specific amount for a specific service. Fees charged will increase if the corresponding costs increase.

Feedback skills: Skills that supervisors find necessary to effectively communicate with their employees about things such as work performance. Such skills include communicating clear goals and objectives, listening, praising the positive aspects and diplomatically identifying situations in which corrections may be necessary to make before they become a problem.

Financial accounting: The process of generating financial records and forecasts and performing strategic planning for an entire entity; often produced by the department of finance in the institution.

Financial management: The process of planning, organizing, directing, controlling, and evaluating available monetary resources. The primary goal of financial management is to ensure the profitability and survival of the organization.

Financial ratios: A tool consisting of ratios that managers use to manage finances and thus maintain internal control of these finances. It is based on the premise that ratios mean nothing un-

less it can be compared to something else.

Financial Ratios and Analysis: Used to evaluate financial statements.

Fishbone diagram: A diagram that systematically analyzes cause-and-effect relationships and identifies potential root causes of a problem.

Five forces analysis: A marketing analysis model that serves as a framework for analyzing external opportunities and threats. The five forces are the bargaining power of suppliers, the bargaining power of buyers, the threat of new entrants, the threat of substitute products, and the rivalry among existing firms.

Fixed budget: A type of budget that contains estimates for a single level of activity.

Fixed costs: Expenses that do not change over a given amount of time regardless of testing volume. Examples include administrative salaries and rent.

Flexible budget: A budget that takes into account the fact that certain costs vary with the level of activity, and other costs remain fixed over a relevant range of activity. Flexible budgets are designed to anticipate the possibility of change and show planned revenues and expenses at various levels of activity.

Flowchart: A picture or diagram of a process.

For-profit entity: A company that is privately held (such as a corporation). Profits are distributed to the owners, and its primary purpose is to generate adequate revenue to be profitable. The profits generated are taxed by the government.

Framing trap: A decision-making trap that deals with how one views one's own choices or how one frames the questions around the problem. A frame may lead individuals into other decision-making traps such as anchoring.

Full-time equivalent: The equivalent of one employee working full-time; that is, 2080 hours per year.

Functional structure: An organizational model that is hierarchical and bureaucratic in nature; specialized units within the model report in an upward chain of command; responsibility and authority within the organization are clearly understood.

Functions: A management term referring to a process and strategy for dealing with issues of change.

Goals: Outcomes that one strives to achieve.

Government payers: Public sources of funding (such as Medicare and Medicaid) that pay for the care of a patient.

Hardware: The physical pieces of equipment that make up a computer system such as the central processing unit, display monitors, keyboards, and printers.

Health Care Financing Administration (HCFA): See Centers for Medicare and Medicaid Services (CMS).

Health Maintenance Organization (HMO): The most common type of managed care organization. See managed care for further details.

Hierarchical database: A structured set of data organized into tables that link records together like a company organizational chart. Records can be retrieved only through the top level of the structure.

High complexity testing: The most difficult laboratory testing determined by examining seven criteria among which are test system, troubleshooting, test interpretation, and judgment.

HIPPA: Health Insurance Portability and Accountability Act.

Hiring: Choosing the person who will be doing the work.

Historical-based budgeting: Budgeting above 100% of the previous year. To budget in this way, the total spent in the previous year is divided by 12. The number obtained plus a percentage for inflation is used to budget for the upcoming year.

Human Resource Management (HRM): The overall management of the people within an organization as resources including activities related to recruitment, selection, development, staffing, scheduling, and performance.

Humility: A suggested leadership quality that refers to the ability of a leader to realize that others may also have good ideas and accept the fact that one may be wrong.

Income forecasting: An estimation of future revenues used to set goals.

Implementing: The act of putting a plan into operation by carrying out the steps and activities designated to achieve the goal.

Income statement: A financial document indicating what has transpired financially within an organization over a period of time, usually monthly or yearly; a document that represents the financial outcome of an organization over a period.

Indirect expense (cost): All of the charges (in dollars) that are part of doing business but are not directly related to the cost of the test being evaluated; also known as overhead. Examples include marketing, licenses, and information systems requirements.

Influence approach: An approach to leadership in which leadership is an influence or social exchange process.

Inpatient: A patient receiving care while in the hospital.

Input-throughput-output mechanism: A process that takes a product and/or information (concerning the product) from the environment (input); transforms, converts, and processes it (throughput); and then exports a changed product back into the environment (output).

Insight: A suggested leadership quality that refers to the ability to determine and understand clearly the nature of things, which is often accomplished through intuition.

Instructional/educational objectives: Clearly stated directives written in measurable terms for the purposes of achieving goals related to instruction.

Integrity: A suggested leadership quality that is based on the premise that the value individuals place on themselves and others is paramount to being effective.

Interface: Specialized software and hardware connections between different information systems that allow the systems to communicate with each other, even when the systems use different programming languages.

Interview: In-person, oral process that serves as confirmation of a perspective employee's application and to fill in any gaps.

Job: An arrangement through which work is done; products or services are delivered in the mutual interest of a worker and an employer.

Job analysis: The analysis and documentation of the tasks, conditions, requirements, and authority arrangements of a working situation.

Job application: A written document requesting work.

Job description: A written document describing the tasks, expectations, reporting relationships and other information relative to the employment of an individual; also referred to as a position description.

Joint Commission on Accreditation of Healthcare Organizations (JCAHO): A voluntary organization that accredits more than 80% of the US healthcare organizations.

Joint decision: A group decision-making technique, also known as democratic style, in which the leader shares the problem with the relevant team members as a group. Together alternatives are generated and evaluated. The group strives to reach a consensus that determines the decision made.

Just cause: A standard by which adverse employment actions may be assessed to determine whether they were appropriately taken and generally includes at least five factors: forewarning, proper investigation, evidence, lack of discrimination, and penalty meets the offense.

Justice: An ethical principle requiring fairness in distribution of burdens and benefits; often expressed in terms of treating persons of similar circumstances or characteristics similarly.

Keirsey four types sorter: A method of identifying and assessing personality temperament types. Individuals complete a self-assessment consisting of 16 questions that may be self-scored. The questionnaire is designed to identify 16 combinations of four temperament types.

Laboratory Accrediation Program of the College of American Pathologists (LAP-CAP): A voluntary organization that accredits only lab testing sites and not the entire healthcare organization.

Leaders: Individuals who influence the opinions and attitudes of others to accomplish a mutually agreed on task while maintaining integrity and moral purpose of all involved. Leaders are central individuals who guide others in achieving a goal.

Leadership: A quality exhibited by individuals; occurs when one individual attempts to influence the behavior of others (a group) to accomplish goals (either personal or organizational).

Leading: See directing.

Learning outcome: A desired result achieved by a learner after completing an instructional experience.

Lease: Typically the lease option is used when lump sum capital dollars are not available to outright purchase. In a lease arrangement, monthly payments are determined and spread over a specified period of time and are based on the purchase price plus interest, taxes, insurance, and maintenance.

Liabilities: The obligations that an organization has to its creditors.

Liquidity Ratio: A ratio used to determine the organization's ability to meet short-term debt obligations.

Managed care: A means of providing health care services within a network of providers with the goal of ensuring high quality and cost effective care to the patients belonging to a managed care plan.

Management: Achieving organizational goals in an effective and efficient manner by working with and through people.

Management accounting: The analysis of cost and revenue data that provides information on operations and budgeting for managers.

Managers: Individuals, usually administrators, who are able to influence decisions and actions.

Market: A web of interactions among those who have commercial relationships or the potential for such relationships with other buyers and sellers of similar commodities.

Market analysis: A continuous cyclical process of analyzing marketing opportunities, developing a marketing strategy, planning and implementing the plan, and revising the plan by responding to market forces.

Market demand: The determination of how many current customers in a particular market purchase a product or service.

Market segmentation: The breaking up of markets into smaller, more manageable pieces.

Marketing: A process by which individuals and groups obtain what they want through creating, offering, and exchanging products or services of value with others.

Marketing concept: A business philosophy whose central tenet is that the key to achieving the goals of the organization consists of being more effective than the competition in satisfying the needs, wants, and demands of the customer.

Marketing environment: The surroundings that influence the marketing and business planning of a company including demographics, economic climate, political, legal and societal structures, available technologies, and natural resources.

Marketing mix: The set of tools that a firm uses to pursue their marketing objectives. These tools include product, price, place, and promotion.

Marketing plan: An action plan or a roadmap to guide the company from one place to the next. Aspects of the plan include descriptions of the products or services, as well as their benefits and features, target markets and corresponding buying habits, competing products or services, and the customer problem that the product or service is designed to eliminate.

Marketing research: A technical and systematic approach to obtain data relevant to a specific market. It is the systematic design, collection, analysis, and reporting of data and findings relevant to a specific marketing situation.

Matrix organizations: Organizations that take advantage of the skills or functions present; this structure works best when the demands of the environment are changing and uncertainty is the norm; skill diversification, also known as cross-training, is encouraged.

Mechanistic structure: An organizational model that consists of a highly structured environment with communication from the top down and reliance on authority-obedience relationships; appropriate in environments of slow change and relative stability.

Microcosting: The process of determining the actual cost of performing a billable procedure (cost per test).

Mission statement: A document that states the purpose, attitude, and core competencies of a group, department, or an institution.

Moderate complexity testing: The middle level of laboratory testing determined by the examination of knowledge, training and experience, and calibration, quality control, and proficiency testing materials plus four other criteria.

Myers-Briggs type indicator: A method of identifying actions and attitudes associated with 16 predefined personality types. Individuals take a self-assessment and the pattern of their answers correlates with these personality types.

Natural environment: An aspect of the marketing environment that deals with raw materials and available energy to manufacture a company's products.

Net income: The amount of net revenue minus operating expenses for a given period. Net income is presented as the bottom line of the income statement.

Net Present Value: A calculation used to indicate the current value of income generated in the future discounted at an estimated percentage equal to the inflation rate over the years of income generation. This demonstrates the concept that the value of a dollar today is more than the value of a dollar in the future. The Initial Outlay - the present value of the cash inflows.

Network Structures: Structures consisting of specialized units, either internal or external to the organization, that are linked together by informal or formal agreements.

Niching: A marketing strategy consisting of a company focusing on a specific subsection of a market.

Non-billable procedure: A laboratory procedure that contributes to the generation of a billable test result, but that is not directly reimburseable; examples include standards, quality control specimens, and repeat testing of samples.

Nonmaleficence: Do not inflict unjustified harm to ourselves or other people.

Nonwaived testing: For quality control and quality assessment CLIA requirements, moderate and high complexity are grouped and referred to as nonwaived testing.

Not-for-profit entity: An organization (such as a community-based hospital) in which the profits made are held by the organization to further its cause. Such organizations exist to provide a service such as healthcare and are not taxed.

Objectives: Directives developed to accomplish established goals.

Occupational Safety and Health Administration (OSHA): A federal organization that is responsible for regulations relating to the general workplace safety and protecting the health of US workers.

Open system: A system that is in active exchange with its environment.

Operating budget: An overall plan that identifies the expected resources and expenditures of an entity for a given future period of time, usually one year.

Operating margin: Refers to the profits that are generated from the excess of revenues received for providing a service.

Organic structure: An organizational model consisting of an environment that features decentralized decision making and encourages adaptability and flexibility; appropriate in environments of change.

Organizational structure: The way in which an organization divides its tasks

and coordinates them for overall goal achievement. Commonly represented visually as an organization chart.

Organizing: The process of determining the steps needed to implement a successful plan.

OSHA's Standard Precautions: Standards set by the Occupational Safety and Health Administration (OSHA) for the handling of biological specimens, formerly known as Universal Precautions. These standards mandate that all blood, body fluids, tissue, and other potentially infectious materials be treated as equally hazardous.

Outcomes assessment: The final quantitative and qualitative evaluation of the effectiveness of the plan used to obtain an organizational goal.

Outpatient: An ambulatory patient who visits the hospital for services but is not admitted to the hospital.

Overconfidence trap: A decision-making trap in which the manager believes that they are better at making forecasts or estimates than they actually are; such individuals are overly confident about their ability to predict leading to a narrow range of possibilities.

Overhead: See indirect expense (cost).

Owner's Equity: The book-value of the organization.

Pareto chart: A graphic technique designed to help identify major factors and distinguish between the "vital few" causes and the potentially less significant ones of a given problem. It is based on the Pareto principle, which states that approximately 80% of the problems can be attributed to 20% of the causes (also known as the 80/20 rule).

Passion: A suggested leadership quality that refers to the excitement and enthusiasm a leader possesses about the leadership role and all of its components as well as about the field, in this case, of laboratory medicine.

Patient test management: The aspect of laboratory testing concerned with maintaining sample integrity and positive patient identification throughout the testing process. Defined polices and procedures must be in place to ensure proper patient preparation, sample integrity, and identification from sample collection through test result reporting.

Payback analysis: A calculation that identifies the length of time it will take to recover the initial expenditure for a project or providing a service. The calculation used is P/I where P = the purchase or investment cost and I = the annual income or revenue generated by the service.

Payback period: The time it will take to generate the incoming revenue that compensates for the money paid out for an item such as a piece of equipment; a ratio that identifies the time it will take for revenue or other positive cash flows to cover the initial outlay related to an investment project.

Payer: The individual, government agency, or insurance group that pays for the care of a patient.

Per case: A type of reimbursement payment methodology whereby a provider and insurer agree on a per case reimbursement rate. This rate is based on the premise that certain diagnoses and procedures have a relatively similar treatment protocol.

Per diem: A type of payment methodology whereby a set amount of reimbursement is agreed upon based on a per day rate that a patient is in the hospital.

Performance development: An actively ongoing two-way process between employee and supervisor for communicating about the employee's job performance designed to help them achieve excellence in their position and create job satisfaction. Processes involved include goal setting, feedback, guidance, motivation, evaluation, and development planning.

Performance evaluation: The periodic comparison of measured actual performance to the requirements stated in the job description.

Performance objectives: Specific directives developed for the accomplishing of established goals that deal with job performance.

Personnel budget: The portion of the expense budget that includes all expenses related to personnel such as salaries, fringe benefits, vacation, holidays, and shift differentials.

Personnel development: A function of management that refers to encouraging and providing opportunities to staff employees to gain additional knowledge for personal and professional growth. In-services and continuing education lectures are examples of such opportunities.

Place: A marketing mix tool that refers to the "how and where" a product is offered to the buying public.

Planning: The management function that clarifies the process of attaining organizational goals. It includes activities such as data gathering, assessment, risk calculation, and determination of strategy.

Plus/minus/interesting: A tool developed to evaluate the pros and cons of decision-making options. It consists of a table with space for writing in the information that matches these three columns: plus (positive points of taking the action), minus (negative points of taking the action), and interesting (extended implications of taking the action, both positive and negative in nature).

Political and legal environment: An aspect of the marketing environment that consists of pertinent political and legal issues related to federal government agencies, legislation, and lawsuits.

Position description: A listing of all of the essential and nonessential functions of a job, including requirements related to education and experience; also referred to as a job description.

Positive self-esteem: A suggested leadership quality that refers to the ability of leaders to believe in themselves by working selflessly to support others working toward the common good of the organization.

Postanalytical: The phase of workflow that consists of finalizing and reporting test results.

Preanalytical: The phase of workflow that consists of the steps taken before actual testing.

Premiums: The dollar amount charged by the insurer to individuals to insure against specific risks.

Price: A marketing mix tool that refers to the amount of money a customer pays for a product or service.

Private accounting: The activities performed by an entity for its own managerial activities.

Private payers: Refers to commercial insurers (such as Blue Cross) that pay for the care of a patient.

Problem solving: The process of identifying and defining a problem, determining what happened to cause it, and what steps or possible solutions will be necessary to solve it.

Process design: A broad overall plan for completing work or a task.

Product: A marketing mix tool that refers to what a firm offers to the public for sale.

Production concept: A business philosophy that suggests that customers will buy goods in adequate volume at a low enough price.

Proficiency testing: A mechanism to assess the internal quality for CLIA-regulated analytes in testing sites performing moderate and/or high complexity testing. Laboratories enroll in a program whereby they periodically receive "unknown" specimens and are required to test them just like the patient samples. Results are sent to the program administrator for grading. Corrective actions are in place for laboratories that do not meet the criteria established by the administrator.

Profitability Ratio: A ratio that demonstrates the organization's efficiency of operations.

Program budget: A type of budget created based on a specific program matrix that includes all proposed services and the resources required.

Promotion: A marketing mix tool that refers to the means by which a company communicates and promotes its products to its target market.

Prospective payment system (PPS): A payment system in which hospitals receive a set amount of reimbursement per patient discharge. This system incorporates the diagnostic related group

(DRG)-based reimbursement system for all Medicare inpatients.

Provider: A hospital, physician, or group that provides care to a patient.

Provider-Performed Microscopy [PPM] certificate: A CLIA certificate issued to a laboratory for physicians, midlevel practitioners or dentists to perform a predetermined list of tests (such as a microscopic urine examination) as well as tests on specimens collected during a physical examination. Laboratories with this category CLIA certificate may also perform waived testing.

Prudence trap: A decision-making trap that managers fall into when faced with a high-stakes decision. These individuals tend to adjust their estimates or forecasts "just to be on the safe side."

Psychomotor domain: A category of learning that involves the actual performing of identified tasks, such as performing laboratory tests, or skills.

Public accounting: The making available of financial activities to regulatory, government, and private accounting firms for both informational purposes and to meet regulatory requirements.

Quality assurance: Ensuring the overall quality of the testing process accomplished by the development of a written plan that includes a mechanism to evaluate the effectiveness of the laboratory's policies and procedures, identify and correct problems, ensure reliable and prompt reporting of results, and testing performed by competent individuals.

Quality control (QC): The testing and documenting of known samples in conjunction with testing the unknown patient samples. In addition, quality control includes having written proce-dures in place for the monitoring of and evaluating the quality of the analytic testing of each test performed to ensure accuracy and reliability of patient results and reports.

Rate of return: The ratio of the annual revenue to the price of the project calculated as follows: I/P where I = the annual income or revenue generated and P = the cost of providing the service or original investment in the project.

Ratio analysis: The use of ratios to compare an aspect of one organization to that of another; a specific example is comparing laboratory operations of one institution to those of another.

Reagent rental: An agreement that usually commits the laboratory to a minimum volume of reagent purchased over a specified period at a set price. The cost of the instrument is included in the reagent cost.

Reasonable accommodation: A duty incumbent on employers under the Americans with Disabilities Act (ADA) to provide qualified employees and candidates with remedial measures or devices, absent an undue burden on the organization.

Recallability trap: A decision-making trap associated with bias in terms of "it worked before." Managers in this trap get caught in using past experiences to forecast the future and are thus overly influenced by those past events that left a strong impression on them.

Reciprocal approach: An approach to leadership in which a shared process includes a strong emphasis on follow-ership.

Registration certificate: A CLIA cer-tificate issued to enable laboratories to conduct waived, moderate and/or high complexity laboratory testing.

Relational database: A structured set of data organized into tables that link records together through common data elements in the tables. Records are retrieved from multiple tables by matching the common data elements in those tables.

Resource allocation: The distribution of resources.

Resource based relative value scale (RBRVS): The payment system used for reimbursing physicians for services rendered. A payment rate is calculated based on geographic region, service performed, malpractice costs, and practice overhead.

Resource management: The justification and accountability of resources.

Respect for Persons: A principle stating that (1) individuals should be treated as autonomous agents, and (2) persons with diminished autonomy are entitled to protection.

Responsibility: Assignment for accomplishing a goal.

Return on investment: A dollar amount that is used when evaluating the cost versus rent or lease option; calculated by taking the profit margin and multiplying it by asset turnover. The goal is to at least break even on the return.

Revenue budget: A document that identifies each of the different types of revenue to be earned, according to the period in which it will be earned.

Revenues: Monies that the laboratory receives or is entitled to receive (i.e., income) for the services and testing it has provided.

Rolling budget: A continuous budget that is updated periodically in preparation for the next budget cycle; a rolling budget for a 12-month period is typically reviewed and revised every quarter.

Sales concept: A business philosophy that promotes factory products sold by aggressive selling.

Scatter diagram: A plot of one variable versus another to see if there is any relationship between the two variables.

Scheduling: Assigning a worker to a specific task or work area.

Self-contained unit structure: An organizational model that centers around a common basis such as a discipline, location, customer group, or technology; in this model, the components that make up the common basis function using their own expertise and supervision, hence the term self-contained.

Self-esteem: A suggested leadership quality that includes selflessly supporting people toward the common good of the organization.

Self payers: Those individuals who do not have any other type of insurance and must pay for their own healthcare.

Semivariable costs: Expenses incurred in the laboratory that will vary but only incrementally based on workload volume change. An example of such a cost is technologist salary.

Sense of humor: A suggested leadership quality that refers to the ability of leaders to incorporate laughter (humor) at appropriate times, especially during highly stressful instances.

Shewhart cycle: A problem-solving approach that incorporates scientific principles of analysis. It is a continuous circular process that includes four steps: Plan, Do, Check, and Act (PDCA).

Situational contingency approach: An approach to leadership that centers around explaining leader effectiveness as it relates to the context of a particular situation.

Software: A set of instructions written in a computer programming language that tells the computer how to organize and present information.

Staffing: Personnel required to complete the work.

Statement of cash flows: A financial document analyzing the source of cash (revenues) and cash outflow (expenses).

Status-quo trap: A decision-making trap in which individuals protect their egos from damage by avoiding to change the status quo. Individuals prefer to instinctively stay with the familiar (i.e., stay with what they know).

Sunk-cost trap: A decision-making trap, also known as "the justify-past-actions trap" in which individuals, because of past decisions, believe that they must continue in that direction, although the reason is no longer valid.

Surcharge/cost plus method: A calculation that involves first determining the actual cost of a laboratory test using microcosting and then multiplying the number obtained by a factor (such as 1.5 times the cost) or adding a dollar amount to the cost (surcharge) to arrive at the final price of the test.

Supervisory: The adjective form of supervise that means to direct or oversee work as well as workers.

SWOT analysis: A process that consists of examining and analyzing factors internal and external to the company known as SWOT. The internal factors are strengths and weak-nesses and the external factors are opportunities and threats.

System: A collection of interdependent, interconnected elements that constitute an identifiable whole.

Task/production management: Individual activities based on the manager's needs and that of the organization, not on the individual. This creates a submissive, passive, and dependent feeling in the individual. Individual frustration, resentment, and underproduction often result.

Tasks: The routine duties for which a laboratory manager is held responsible and accountable.

Taxonomy levels: Levels/categories of learning designed to aid an instructor in defining appropriate learning outcomes.

Technological environment: An aspect of the market environment that deals with advancements in technology such as the advent of cellular phones, satellite television, DNA technology, and numerous new medications.

Theory X-Theory Y: A model designed for managers to operate by that is based on the premise that two sets of expectations (known as X and Y) about employees' attitudes and abilities ultimately influence their work performance. The Theory X manager is likely to compensate for the shortcomings of the workers and tends to be dictatorial and autocratic. The Theory Y manager possesses a more optimistic set of expectations, suggesting that workers are highly motivated, self-disciplined, and creative problem-solvers, thus capitalizing on worker strengths.

Theory Z: A management model recently proposed that is based on the premise that changing societal goals must be included in the workplace. Productivity and rewards are not the only objectives of the workers. Other issues such as quality of life also have a significant impact on worker performance.

Title VII of the Civil Rights Act of 1964: A federal law that prohibits discrimination based on race, color, creed, religion, national origin, and sex.

Trait approach: An historical approach to leadership that resulted in the generation of lists of personal traits that supposedly guaranteed successful leadership to those individuals possessing them; such traits include height, charisma, and intelligence.

Training: Teaching a worker the department policies and procedures.

Trend analysis: A management tool that examines an organization's performance over a given period of time.

Unlawful harassment: Occurs as the result of an individual exhibiting inappropriate behaviors based on sex (whether or not of a sexual nature), color, race, national origin, religion, protected activity, disability, or age.

Validation: Documented evidence that provides a high degree of assurance that a system or process will function consistently as expected; the managed process of determining that something accomplishes what it is intended to accomplish.

Value: The worth of a product or service in money or goods.

Variable costs: Expenses that vary based on workload volume and change in direct relationship to that volume. Examples include reagents and supplies.

Variance analysis: The process of analyzing and evaluating differences between actual and budgeted performance.

Vision: A suggested leadership quality that refers to the ability to "see the big picture" to determine strategic/future directions of a department and/or organization. It also refers to the ability to effectively communicate such directions to others.

Waived tests: Laboratory tests considered to be simple and foolproof (such as glucose monitoring via devices cleared by the FDA for home use). Tests in this category are determined by examining seven specific criteria including reagents and materials preparation and characteristics of the operation steps.

Waiver certificate: A CLIA certificate that permits a site to perform only those test methods identified as waived.

Workflow: The process of work through a work station or department from the beginning to the final product.

Work group: A group of employees working together in various capacities with the goal of accomplishing work-related tasks.

Zero-based budget: A budgeting method by which the appropriate manager must annually reevaluate all activities to decide whether they should be eliminated or funded; projects are approved based on funds availability and funding levels are determined by priorities. Each year every department manager is required to justify the entire unit budget as though it were totally new.

Index